DATE DUE

GAYLORD   #3523PI   Printed in USA

D1378130

Computers in Health Care

Kathryn J. Hannah   Marion J. Ball
Series Editors

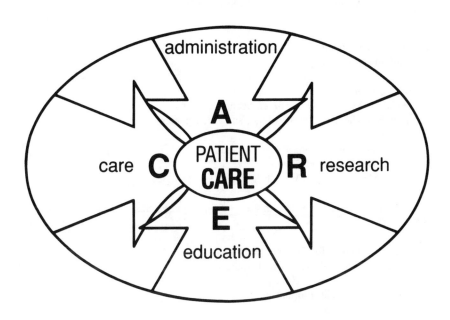

Springer

New York
Berlin
Heidelberg
Barcelona
Budapest
Hong Kong
London
Milan
Paris
Santa Clara
Singapore
Tokyo

Computers in Health Care

Series Editors:
Kathryn J. Hannah   Marion J. Ball

Patricia Flatley Brennan   Sid J. Schneider
Elizabeth Tornquist
Editors

Information Networks for Community Health

With 36 Illustrations

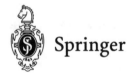 Springer

Patricia Flatley Brennan, Ph.D., R.N.
Moehlman-Bascom Professor
University of Wisconsin-Madison
Madison, WI 53706, USA

Sid J. Schneider, Ph.D.
Henry M. Jackson Foundation
P.O. Box 207
Bethesda, MD 20889, USA

Elizabeth Tornquist, M.A.
University of North Carolina
 at Chapel Hill
1700 Duke University Road
Durham, NC 22701, USA

Library of Congress Cataloging-in-Publication Data

Brennan, Patricia Flatley.
  Information networks for community health / Patricia Flatley Brennan,
Sid J. Schneider, Elizabeth Tornquist.
      p. cm. — (Computer and health care)
  Includes bibliographical references and index.
  ISBN 0-387-94697-7 (hardcover : alk. paper)
    1. Public health — Computer networks — United States. 2. Community
health services — Computer networks — United States. I. Schneider,
Sid J. II. Tornquist, Elizabeth M., 1933–   . III. Title.
  IV. Series.
RA423.2.B74   1997
362.1′2′028546 — dc20   96-21900
                                                         CIP

Printed on acid-free paper.

Production coordinated by Chernow Editorial Services, Inc., and managed by Natalie Johnson; manufacturing supervised by Jeffrey Taub.
Typeset by TechType, Inc., Ramsey, NJ.
Printed and bound by Braun-Brumfield, Inc., Ann Arbor, MI.
Printed in the United States of America.

9 8 7 6 5 4 3 2 1

ISBN 0-387-94697-7 Springer-Verlag New York Berlin Heidelberg   SPIN 10524666

Series Preface

This series is intended for students and practitioners of the health professions who are seeking to expand their knowledge of computers in health care. Our editors and authors, experts in their fields, offer their insights into innovations and trends. Each book is practical and easy to use.

Since the series began, in 1988, we have seen increasing acceptance of the term "informatics" and of the innovations it brings to health care. Today more than ever we are committed to making this series contribute to the field of healthcare informatics, the discipline "where caring and technology meet."

KATHRYN J. HANNAH
MARION J. BALL

v

Preface

Computer technology has transformed health care not only by improving the accuracy and quantity of information available to clinicians, but also by improving the flow of information among the people who provide, arrange for, and pay for health services. This book is about the new computer networks that electronically link people and organizations in the health care field. Its purpose is to explore the impact of new computer networks upon the different organizations in the field, their services to patients, and the way in which organizations collaborate and compete, share information, and guard confidential material. The book explores computer networks primarily from the perspective of public health, discussing the impact that networks have upon communities as well as individuals. In particular, the book explores new computer networks that are designed to be used by patients, altering the manner in which patients interact with, and are influenced by, health care providers.

The technology to transfer information from one computer to another has evolved extremely rapidly. The technology now exists to link physicians and other health care providers, hospitals, health maintenance organizations, preferred provider organizations, employers, health educators, nursing care facilities, pharmacies, health insurers, researchers, patients, and the public. Many communities are establishing electronic linkages among these groups, creating Community Health Information Networks, or CHINs. Several chapters in this book address the effect that CHINs are having upon health care delivery in the geographical areas in which they are established. The chapters cover the issues crucial to creating and operating a CHIN, such as who will own, control, and have access to it, what its principal functions will be, and how confidential information will be guarded.

However, most network applications in healthcare are not CHINs. Most networks are smaller and have a more limited goal to link only certain kinds of providers, such as drug abuse treatment centers. Some serve a particular purpose, such as allowing psychiatrists at urban hospitals to provide consultations for patients in distant rural communities. Because this book devotes many chapters to these kinds of networks, we could not title the book *Community Health Information Networks. Information Networks for Community Health* better conveys the breadth of the book.

We have tried to emphasize the impact of networks upon health care delivery. We asked authors not to devote much space to the technical aspects of networks, such as the hardware and software involved in networking. They do, however, share some of their experiences in transforming existing stand-alone systems into networks—a process that involves not only finding the appropriate hardware and software and resolving incompatibilities among systems, but also eliciting cooperation among many different organizations, even ones that do not usually coordinate their efforts. Authors also share their decisions about the capabilities of their networks, beyond merely providing connectivity among organizations.

A number of chapters explore the future of health information networks, when patients will have access to them. Patients may soon use information networks routinely to communicate with their providers and insurers. Increasing numbers of people have computers in their homes and work sites, which could give them access to health information networks. Also, new technologies such as computer-based interactive telephone systems can provide patients with access. It is likely that in the future, computer networks will become not merely avenues for communication, but also sources of information and health care for patients. For example, computer networks have the potential of reaching very large numbers of people with health-promotion interventions at relatively little cost. We have included in this book several examples of current network-based health promotion applications. The chapter authors discuss the issues that must be resolved so that patients can effectively use networks to obtain information, support, and help in making decisions about their medical treatment.

This book is divided into four sections. The first section, Core Concepts, explains the term "community-based" health care and describes the computer technologies that presently exist to support community-based health care. Kristine M. Gebbie, formerly the National AIDS Policy Coordinator, shares her perspective on the features of a community and the approaches to health care that emphasize the needs of a community. Alan F. Dowling explains the current state of the art of CHINs. Michael G. Kahn shows how networks are best designed to link health care organizations, and how community health care is affected by these linkages among organizations. Warner V. Slack, one of the pioneers in developing applications in which patients interact directly with computers, puts into historical perspective the new developments in patient-computer interaction described later in the book.

The second section of the book, Linking Organizations, contains four chapters describing a few of the recent computer linkages established among health care organizations. Kim R. Pemble describes the design and operation of the Wisconsin Health Information Network, a well-known

CHIN that is serving as a model for developers of newer CHINs. Richard D. Rubin and Megan C. Aukema's chapter is about the Community Health Management Information System (CHMIS) developed under the auspices of the Hartford Foundation. CHMIS is well known for its ground-breaking establishment of some of the first community-wide networks and its emphasis on research and evaluation. J. Nell Brownstein of the Centers for Disease Control and Prevention, and her colleagues, have written a chapter that outlines how networks enhance the flow of information among public health organizations. The chapter by D. Paul Moberg and his colleagues presents the Target Cities project, which is dramatically changing drug abuse treatment by linking the treatment programs in a community with a central intake unit that coordinates patient care. The Target Cities project is an example of a new approach to health care that is possible only because of computer network technology.

The third section of the book, Information Networks and the Delivery of Care, presents examples of how networks can themselves deliver preventive care. Eric W. Boberg and his colleagues discuss Community Health Evaluation and Social Support, a network-mediated system for providing information, support, and advice to a variety of persons with medical and psychological problems. Kathleen A. Smyth describes a network that provides support for caregivers of Alzheimer's disease patients. Paul Taenzer and his colleagues describe "Cancer, Me??" a network-based health risk assessment concerning cancer prevention. The system assesses each user's cancer risk behaviors and provides personalized feedback. Thomas L. Patterson, William S. Shaw, and Daniel R. Masys survey the self-help programs that are presently available on the Internet. Farrokh Alemi's chapter is about a system that uses a computerized interactive telephone system to reach crack-abusing pregnant women and new mothers to offer them information, advice, and support. The goal of this section of the book is to suggest how information networks may eventually become an important medium for health care delivery.

The final section of the book is called Logistical Issues and Information Networks. Dena S. Puskin and her colleagues describe the activity of her agency, the Office of Rural Health Policy in the Department of Health and Human Services, in the field of telemedicine. Shirley M. Moore outlines how the dynamics of patient-provider interaction change when the interaction occurs via a network. They explain what telemedicine is, how it fits in with other network approaches, and how it can reduce some of the difficulties caused by the paucity of some kinds of practitioners in rural areas. Randolph C. Barrows, Jr. and Paul D. Clayton offer solutions to the potential data security problems associated with networks. Neilson S. Buchanan and his colleagues have written the final chapter, which discusses the relationship between employers and CHINs, and how that relationship will affect the future development of CHINs.

We wish to thank all of the people who helped to make this book possible. However, we have room here for just a partial list: Ellen Nannis, Lawrence Peterson, John Lowe, Capt. Fredric Daniell, MC, USN, Lt. Col. Kenneth Hoffman, MC, USA, Jeannette Overholt, Marion Ball, Kathryn Hannah, and Patti Brennan's doctoral students, whose insights and discussions over the past few years helped stimulate the design and direction of this book.

Editing this book has brought us into contact with some of the most interesting and dedicated people—and some of the most challenging issues—that we have encountered in our professional lives. We hope that readers get much pleasure and insight from the book. Enjoy!

Patricia Flatley Brennan, Ph.D., R.N.
Sid J. Schneider, Ph.D.
Elizabeth Tornquist, M.A.

Contents

SECTION III: INFORMATION NETWORKS AND THE DELIVERY OF CARE

SECTION IV: LOGISTICAL ISSUES AND INFORMATION NETWORKS

Contributors

Farrokh Alemi, Ph.D.
Health Administration Program, Cleveland State University, Cleveland, OH 44115, USA

Melissa Alperin, M.P.H., C.H.E.S.
Behavioral Sciences and Health Education, Rollins School of Public Health, Emory University, Atlanta, GA 30322, USA

Megan C. Aukema
Communications Manager, Foundation for Health Care Quality, 83 South King Street, Seattle, WA 98104, USA

Randolph C. Barrows, Jr., Ph.D.
Department of Medical Informatics, Columbia Presbyterian Medical Center, New York, NY 10032-3784, USA

Judy M. Birdsell, B.Sc.N., M.SC.
Faculty of Management, University of Calgary, Calgary, Alberta T2N 1N4, Canada

Eric W. Boberg, Ph.D.
Center for Health Systems Research and Analysis, University of Wisconsin—Madison, Madison, WI 53705, USA

Renee Botta, M.S.
Center for Health Systems Research and Analysis, University of Wisconsin—Madison, Madison, WI 53705, USA

Earl Bricker, B.A.
Center for Health Systems Research and Analysis, University of Wisconsin—Madison, Madison, WI 53705, USA

J. Nell Brownstein, Ph.D.
Health Education Specialist, Centers for Disease Control and Prevention, Atlanta, GA 30341-3724, USA

Neilson S. Buchanan
President, U.S. Health Strategies, 555 Bryant Street, Palo Alto, CA 94301, USA

Paul D. Clayton, Ph.D.
Department of Medical Informatics, Columbia Presbyterian Medical Center, New York, NY 10032-3784, USA

Alan F. Dowling, Ph.D.
Principal, Ernst and Young National Office, 1660 West Second Street, Cleveland, OH 44113, USA

Steven J. Feinstein, B.S.
Department of Psychology, Kent State University, Kent, OH 44242-0001, USA

John Fleming
President, Fleming Associates Ltd., 6443 SW Beaverton-Hillsdale Highway, Portland, OR 97221, USA

Simon Freiwald, M.Sc., E.E.
Bell Northern Research Ltd., 16 Place du Commerce, Île des Souers, Verdun, Quebec H3E 1H6, Canada

Dorine D. Fuller
Bureau of Management and Information Services, New York State Office of Alcoholism and Substance Abuse Services, Albany, NY 12203, USA

Kristine M. Gebbie, RN, Dr PH, FAAN
Columbia University School of Nursing, New York, NY 10032, USA

J. Phillip Gossage, M.A.
Center on Alcoholism, Substance Abuse, and Addictions (CASAA), University of New Mexico, Albuquerque, NM 87106, USA

David H. Gustafson, Ph.D.
Center for Health Systems Research and Analysis, University of Wisconsin—Madison, Madison, WI 53705, USA

Robert P. Hawkins, Ph.D.
Center for Health Systems Research and Analysis, University of Wisconsin—Madison, Madison, WI 53705, USA

Elizabeth H. Howze, Sc.D.
Chief, Health Interventions and Translations Branch, Centers for Disease
Control and Prevention, Atlanta, GA 30341-3724, USA

Michael G. Kahn, M.D., Ph.D.
Section of Medical Informatics, Washington University School of Medicine, St. Louis, MO 63110, USA

Susan Kacerek, M.S.S.A.
Case Western Reserve University, School of Medicine, Alzheimer's Center,
University Hospitals of Cleveland, Fairhill Institute for the Elderly, Cleve-
land, OH 44120, USA

Patricia S. Littman, Ph.D.
Center for Health Policy and Program Evaluation, University of Wisconsin – Madison, Madison, WI 53703-2703, USA

Daniel R. Masys, M.D.
Director, Biomedical Informatics, School of Medicine, University of California, San Diego, La Jolla, CA 92093-0602, USA

S. Elizabeth McGregor, M.Sc.
Department of Epidemiology, Prevention and Screening, Alberta Cancer
Board, 1331 29th Street NW, Calgary, Alberta T2N 4N2, Canada

Fiona McTavish, B.A.
Center for Health Systems Research and Analysis, University of Wisconsin – Madison, Madison, WI 53705, USA

Kathleen R. Miner, Ph.D., M.P.H., C.H.E.S.
Behavioral Sciences and Health Education, Rollins School of Public
Health, Emory University, Atlanta, GA 30322, USA

Carole L. Mintzer, M.P.A.
Director, Rural Telemedicine Grant Program, Federal Office of Rural
Health Policy, Health Resources and Services Administration, U.S. Depart-
ment of Health and Human Services, Rockville, MD 20857, USA

D. Paul Moberg, Ph.D.
Center for Health Policy and Program Evaluation, University of Wisconsin – Madison, Madison, WI 53705, USA

Shirley M. Moore, R.N., Ph.D.
Assistant Professor of Nursing, Case Western Reserve University, Cleveland, OH 44106-4904, USA

Kevin P. Mulvey, Ph.D.
Department of Health and Hospitals, Institute for Urban Health, Policy, and Research, Boston, MA 02146, USA

Mark W. Oberle, M.D., M.P.H.
Public Health Practice Program Office, Centers of Disease Control and Prevention, Atlanta, GA 30341-3724, USA

Betta Owens, M.S.
Center for Health Systems Research and Analysis, University of Wisconsin—Madison, Madison, WI 53705, USA

Kevin Patrick, M.D., M.S.
Communiation Technology Policy, Office of Disease Prevention and Health Promotion, Health and Human Services, Washington, DC 20201, USA

Thomas L. Patterson, Ph.D.
Department of Psychiatry, University of California, San Diego, School of Medicine, La Jolla, CA 92093-0602, USA

Kim R. Pemble, M.S.
Vice President, Operations and Development, Wisconsin Health Information Network, Brookfield, WI 53005, USA

Alan Peres
Benefits Manager, Ameritech, Chicago, IL, USA

Suzanne Pingree, Ph.D.
Center for Health Systems Research and Analysis, University of Wisconsin—Madison, Madison, WI 53705, USA

Dena S. Puskin, Sc.D.
Deputy Director, Federal Office of Rural Health Policy, Health Resources and Services Administration, U.S. Department of Health and Human Services, Rockville, MD 20857, USA

Richard D. Rubin
President, Foundation for Health Care Quality, 83 South King Street, Seattle, WA 98104, USA

Sid J. Schneider, Ph D.
Henry M. Jackson Foundation, P.O. Box 207, Bethesda, MD 20889, USA

William S. Shaw, B.S.
Department of Psychiatry, University of California, San Diego, School of Medicine, La Jolla, CA 92093-0602, USA

Michael Shwartz, Ph.D.
School of Management, Boston University, Boston, MA 02146, USA

Warner V. Slack, M.D.
Harvard Medical School, Center for Clinical Computing, Boston, MA 02115, USA

Kathleen A. Smyth, Ph.D.
Case Western Reserve University, School of Medicine, Alzheimer's Center, University Hospitals of Cleveland, Fairhill Institute for the Elderly, Cleveland, OH 44120, USA

Richard C. Stephens, Ph.D.
Department of Sociology, University of Akron, Akron, OH 44325-1905, USA

Paul Taenzer, Ph.D.
Department of Psychology, Foothills Hospital, Calgary, Alberta T2N 2T9, Canada

John E. Vetter, M.A.
Center on Alcoholism, Substance Abuse, and Addictions (CASAA), University of New Mexico, Alberquerque, NM 87106, USA

Cathy J. Wasem, R.N., M.N.
Director, Information Services and Policy Development, Federal Office of Rural Health Policy, Health Resources and Services Administration, U.S. Department of Health and Human Services, Rockville, MD 20857, USA

Meg Wise, M.S.
Center for Health Systems Research and Analysis, University of Wisconsin—Madison, Madison, WI 53705, USA

Ivan H. Zendel, Ph.D.
Paradigm Solutions, 420 910 Seventh Avenue SE, Calgary, Alberta T2P 3N8, Canada

Section I

Core Concepts

Community health information networks (CHINs) represent an approach to the information infrastructure that reflects the way citizens of the late 20th century live, acquire health care, and manage clinical conditions. Taken individually, each word in this phrase contributes to the definition. "Communities" may be enduring or illusive, and may consist of geographically clustered groups of people or geographically isolated individuals brought together by a shared need. "Health," of individuals, families, or communities, encompasses both self-actualization and optimal function as well as illness care and management. "Information" comes in many forms: descriptors of health states, formal clinical knowledge, charges for clinical procedures, and the advice and interventions offered by nurses and physicians. "Network" evokes the image of linkages, formed by telecommunications pathways as well as organizational alliances.

Section I of this volume grounds the exploration of CHINs in the concept of community. As advanced by Kristine M. Gebbie, a community represents a "unified body" in which members have joint ownership in common resources. Health of communities is in part a function of the health of the members of the community. Effective information infrastructures rest on first understanding the nature of the community and its goals, and results from appropriate resolution of three dichotomies: health care versus medical care, individual versus population patterns, and preventive versus reactive approaches to health. High-functioning communities focus on health care, the population as well as the individual, and incorporate reactive approaches to treatment within a comprehensive prevention focus. The challenges of community-based care are subsumed under the general challenge of community health.

Alan F. Dowling provides an overview of the health care industry perspective on CHINs. Dowling rests CHIN development on partnerships, and he enumerates several important partnerships: federal, state, and local governments, public and private partnerships, and partnerships between the health care and technology industries. In an attempt to provide clarity, Dowling distinguishes CHINs from enterprise health information networks by the focus on community goals. Using a system life-style framework, Dowling appraises the present state of CHINs as being in the experimentation stages.

Michael G. Kahn details the technical and industrial alliances needed to develop a CHIN organized around 26 health care organizations. He advances pragmatic, operational questions and provides vignettes illustrating how they were handled. Integration of data across diverse sites represents the key challenge to CHIN development, according to Kahn. He identifies static integration as that implemented through a common, shared data repository, and dynamic integration as that provided on an as-needed basis, and justifies the dynamic integration solution as both efficient and effective.

Warner V. Slack advocates a consumerist perspective as a grounding to the treatment of CHINs. Defining patients as competent, but under-used, collaborators in care, Slack argues for computer technologies that enhance patients' participation in the health care process. CHINS should emerge from partnerships between patients, communities, the health care industry, and technology. Slack provides a history of over 30 years of evidence that patients can be effective partners in CHINs.

Section I provides an overview of Slack's four partners of CHINs: patients, communities, the health care industry, and technology. Content is presented through the unique voices of those espousing each component. Together these four chapters provide the foundation for an exploration and enumeration of this most recent innovation in health care.

1

Community-Based Health Care: An Introduction

KRISTINE M. GEBBIE

This chapter is intended to set the stage for the discussion of information systems that follows. Rather than plunging into the world of information, it describes the world within which information systems supportive of community health and community-based care must function. All of us who have tried to build an information system have learned that if you do not understand the world within which the information system must operate, understand the overall mission and goals of the broader system, and provide information that others in the system want, the information is useless. Thus, it is never a waste of time to explore context, though admittedly such exploration can be carried to pointless extremes.

The context of community health information systems in the 21st century is already evident in the rapidly changing health and illness care world of today. Fundamental to understanding community-based health care is the concept of "community"—which is the foundation for the care. The term is used with great frequency in current literature, possibly to show that the authors are not hidden in old institutions but out in the world and ready to be flexible and responsive. There is one problem, however: the term has been used so carelessly that it has begun to lose all meaning. Community is sometimes a place, sometimes an attitude, sometimes a rigid geopolitical boundary, and sometimes a fluid margin loosely denoting some commonality.

The dictionary is always a good place to start. Merriam–Webster gives three major definitions of community[1]:

1. a unified body of individuals as a) state, commonwealth; b) the people with common interests living in a particular area; c) an interacting population of various kinds of individuals in a common location; d) a group of people with a common characteristic or interest living together within a larger society; e) a group linked by a common policy; f) a body of persons or nations having common history or common social, economic, and political interests; g) a body of persons of common and esp. professional interests scattered through a larger society (the academic community)

2. society at large

3. a) joint ownership or participation; b) common character; social activity, d) a social state or condition.

The second meaning, society at large, is so general as to be useless for this discussion. Each of the other approaches, however, is useful for seeing health as something more than the absence of disease in a series of individual humans, and for understanding that health affects and is affected by the body of persons who share "community." Proper use of the term will thus enhance our capacity to effectively engage in community health practice at all levels of intervention.

There are two critical points to be made here: first, misuse of the concept of "community" is not simply careless, it is also potentially damaging to those involved; and second, a sound understanding of community is essential if we are to effectively protect and promote the health of the public. To describe a program as a "community" program when the goals or management serve only a narrow economic, political, or professional end is to exploit community, contrary to the principles of public health. Achieving full mental and physical health is only possible when people are authentically engaged as partners in a community enterprise.

The terms community center, community spirit, community involvement, community of interest, community board, community concern, community activism, community orientation (the list could be much longer) all imply that individuals concerned about an issue or a neighborhood are finding common ground and participating together in one or another activity. While staunch defenders of the status quo may blanch, those interested in working to improve any situation generally are positively impressed when the community is involved.

However, it is all too easy to take these terms at face value: a "community center" may be merely a building in a neighborhood to which no one from the neighborhood goes voluntarily; "community involvement" may mean that three people from an intended market segment were invited to taste test a new product; "community board" may be a list of people with readily recognizable names who have never met since an initial social hour, but are prominently displayed on a letterhead or sign board; "community orientation" may mean that the door has a glass panel, and there are no stairs to slow down entry.

Each of these terms has been misused as a marketing device, lulling potential critics into believing that the enterprise in question has merit because a community has expressed an interest, been consulted, or is sharing in a goal-directed activity. Anyone coming new to a community of any sort should begin with healthy skepticism about references to "community" until personal exposure to real involvement becomes convincing.

This attention to whether or not "community" is real in any one instance is not just an exercise in observation. We are a nation in continual transition, in which communities are constantly changing. We are easily distracted from community when talking about health and illness, because the dominant paradigm for discussion of health services and health status is that of medical care or clinical services rendered to individuals one by one in response to an illness or injury. Investment is measured in dollars spent on hospitals, physicians, and drugs, and outcome is measured, if at all, in discharges or 5-year survival rates. Yet our health should be measured by years of symptom-free living or by length of healthy life, and by rates of morbidity and mortality, the desired outcome being prevention of illness with an associated reduction in the need for illness treatment.

Public health, as it is generally understood, takes as its base not individuals, but communities or population groups. Thus its perspective is broader. Thinking about and responding to individuals one after another does not allow one to see how actions at the community level might reduce or eliminate risk of disease; improving the health of an entire population group takes a community that supports law, policy, and programs, many of which limit or alter the choices that may be made by individuals.[2]

The Meaning of Community

Arriving at a better understanding of community is essential, if we are to make more rational decisions about investment in health and the development of healthy communities. In the definitions of community given above, the most common feature is the sense of community as relationship. One definition is geographic, defined by lines on a map. This is the community of the village, town, city, county, or state. While we tend to associate this definition with smaller entities, in fact every state in our nation is at some level a community. This is especially true of those whose size or population is small. People who live near each other do have relationships, and thus must make some decisions as a community: Where will there be streets, and where building lots? Where will the waste be discarded? Shall we collect taxes for a police force, a health department, a recreation center? The geographical definition of community is often arbitrary, in that there is no natural barrier such as a river or cliff to mark its into beginning or end. Move across an imaginary line, and you are one of us; move the other way, and you have left the community. For many aspects of health, this definition is useful. Population density brings with it an increase in many threats to health. The way waste or drinking water is handled affects many. Traffic laws are essential to controlling injuries. If there is no effective means of community action, threats may become all too real and ill-health results. Proximity also makes possible economies of scale in sharing resources to respond to difficulties: clinics and hospitals can be built and staffed, education and public information can be quickly shared. Common frames of reference make it possible to more effectively communicate with all individuals.

In today's world, however, few people are members of only a single community defined by a geopolitical boundary. Even if we use the narrower definition of community as neighborhood, few individuals relate only to those people nearby. Community can also be defined by the place where one works or where one's children go to school, a religious group, a professional association, or a network of like-minded individuals connected via the information superhighway. This definition suggests that community is a sometimes voluntary connection that is tied to one aspect of life but may not touch other facets at all.

For some health-related purposes, we may be bound by actuarial analysis and premium payment to thousands of individuals we will never meet. Within managed care organizations—the currently favored approach to payment and delivery of care—it is expected that health education and health promotion will be pursued more actively and will therefore have a greater impact on health status than in the past. Yet we do not know if the individuals who enroll in a given plan will be influenced to change behavior in the direction of improved health more than individuals who do not participate. There is strong evidence that peer influence plays a role in health-related behavior choices[3]; can a group of coincidental fellow enrollees be considered peers? If not, how do plan executives and health workers find the networks that do work to support health? Or how does a health department, tied to a geographic boundary, work with the myriad of communities within and overlapping with its assigned population, to have the most positive impact?

Community Health

There are three dichotomies or axes that any student of community health systems should be aware of. These are the dichotomies between health care (or services) and medical care (or services); between a population focus and an individual focus; and between prevention and reaction.

The term "health care" as used in public discourse in the United States today is generally a misnomer. In the health care reform debate of 1994, it was used primarily to refer to personal medical (and related) services and to the financing of those services, rather than their organization and delivery. "Health insurance" is generally "illness care insurance," though people have begun demanding that costs of certain early detection and prevention services be covered. With proper use of clinical preventive services,[4] which include immunizations and techniques for early diagnosis of such treatable conditions as hypertension or breast and cervical cancer, medical care is expanded beyond the treatment of disease, but it remains focused on response to individuals who present themselves (sometimes only if reminded) at the office, clinic, or hospital, where an individual practitioner (physician, nurse, physician's assistant, dentist) takes action. In its most expanded form, this should be labeled personal health care to distinguish it from strictly treatment-oriented medical care. It is still not public health practice, though it contributes significantly to the public's health.

Public health is distinguished from medical care and personal health care by attention to populations or groups. A pediatric nurse practitioner is concerned that every one of his patients is properly immunized. A public health official is concerned that vaccine-preventable disease outbreaks are averted by assuring that over 90% of the children in her community are immunized. While the administration of the vaccine requires contact with individual children in either case, the measure of success and the methods of monitoring progress might be quite different for the nurse practitioner and the public health official. With a public health approach, mass clinics are effective, though they contribute little to the establishment of relationships between children and care givers. The practitioner-based system, which integrates vaccines into a regular program of well and sick child care, may have long-term benefits for individual children, but it is labor intensive and may not be possible where there is a shortage of providers or an urgent need to increase the immunization level quickly. Recent outbreaks of food- and water-borne infections (for example, in Seattle and in Milwaukee) illustrate the relationship between these perspectives: good medical care is essential for accurate diagnosis and treatment of each individual who becomes ill because of exposure to a pathogenic organism. However, public health practitioners, who look at patterns of illness in the community, are needed to trace the exposure to a system which, if not fixed, will threaten even greater numbers.

The line between individual prevention services and public health is fuzzy. A community's policies in regard to access to tobacco by minors, or laws requiring the use of bicycle helmets, or services for disposal of hazardous household chemicals are clearly public health interventions. Treating a person for tuberculosis or a sexually transmissible disease is both a public health measure and a medical measure. And ongoing management of diabetes is personal health care, although assuring the quality and availability of that care is a public health responsibility.

A community has real access to health services only if it has adequate access to both quality personal care (prevention and treatment) for every individual and a public health system that attends to removing threats to health and promoting healthy behavior throughout the community. The whole system is community-based when the community is a meaningful partner in setting goals, selecting methods for achieving them, and evaluating the results.

A complete community-based personal care system must include all levels of care, from primary through tertiary, and such services as hospice care. At its best, the focus is to provide services as early as possible, if not to prevent problems altogether, then to diagnose and treat them before prolonged, expensive institutional care is needed. For these systems to work well, information must be available to the client or patient concerning, for example, what to do to support one's own health; where, when, and how to access specific services; and how to participate effectively in a treatment regimen. The systems also need timely information—both on patients, as they move among providers or levels of care, and on the overall experiences of clients, for purposes of quality assurance and system planning or evaluation. Some of this information is collated as "report cards" on health plans and provided to participants on the assumption that they can thus make better choices among plans over time.

A community also needs a public health system that attends to the health status of all residents (and visitors!) in its jurisdiction, by monitoring trends, identifying risks, and matching needs to resources. The accumulation of information about the many disparate health-related events in the community is a major public health task. At least as important, but often not as well developed, is the responsibility for returning that information to the community in a usable form. The public health agency should publish (through some mechanism) annual reports on births, deaths, communicable diseases investigated or treated, and inspections of restaurants, water systems, or hospitals. But it should also try to link information in ways that are attention-grabbing, so that voluntary agencies, service groups, other government entities and health providers are encouraged to become partners in action to promote health.

It is important to remember that merely moving individual health and illness services out of a high-technology hospital to a storefront, clinic, or van does not transform those services into comprehensive personal and public health services. As community-based providers with strong ties to some part of the target community, their services are much more acceptable, "user-friendly," and effective than if offered only within professionally dominated facilities. For example, community health centers supported by the U.S. Public Health Service Migrant and Community Health Centers Program have been marked by close ties to an identified community of interest. This has kept enrolled patients coming back for regular care, helped reduce preventable hospitalizations, and tied health-related services more closely to other services reaching the same population. However, these clinics are not comprehensive; they are not able to assure their enrollees safe workplaces, health education in the schools, or sanitary restaurants. Other health entities carry those responsibilities.

Keeping a Focus on Prevention

The third dichotomy is that between reaction to identified illnesses and prevention of disease or risk. There is no way, even using the most optimistic forecasts about advances in our knowledge of the human organism, that we can prevent all illness. If that were achieved, the only cause of death would be collapse of the system from exhaustion at a very advanced age after an active, disease-free life. As long as illnesses occur, there must be a care system prepared to respond. But a substantial portion of the illnesses now needing treatment are preventable, either by individual action or by community health action.[5]

The dramatic and often successful responses our care system makes to some illnesses and injuries have made for good media coverage and have drawn attention to the need for sophisticated systems of care. We are also beginning to identify how to perform many of these interventions in the community—in clinics or even in patients' homes. We have been less taken, however, by equally dramatic successes on the public health front, such as the reduction in environmental lead and the subsequent drop in children's blood lead levels. Media attention to public health services more often focuses on weaknesses or potential failures, such as the emergence of infections (for example, Ebola fever) and adverse effects from a drug that already has regulatory approval.

Anyone wanting to be a successful community health practitioner must be attentive to both the need for care and the need for public health. In fact, one of the most widely agreed on statements on the role of public health (see Figure 1.1) notes that it is an essential service of public health to see that all members of the community have access to care. If that care is not otherwise available, it is to be provided by the public health entity. As a side note, some public health agencies have become so overwhelmed by the provision of clinical services to otherwise unserved individuals that their community-wide prevention mission is almost invisible to decision-makers and opinion leaders, or even to their own staff.

Despite the failure of Congress to provide a national framework for reshaping care services and financing, a massive shift is underway. The change is dominated by the view that the way to assure the most cost-effective care system is for insurers to prepay systems of care for a standard package of benefits. The assumption is that the provider of care, given a fixed payment known in advance, will make sensible decisions about what services to offer and will provide preventive and early diagnostic services rather than merely respond to advanced illness that requires more expensive treatment. It is also assumed that the services will be offered "in the community" rather than in hospitals. Some providers of public health services believe that this approach will bring new partners for supporting systemic, health-promoting changes at the community-wide level. Others fear that the incentives for prevention are not clear and the rhetoric about community services is merely a marketing ploy.

State Medicaid agencies have joined the movement, taking aggressive steps to enroll their recipients in managed care plans. While many laud the effort to assure each Medicaid client an identified care provider, they also note that many providers now seeking Medicaid enrollments are not familiar with the communities they will have to serve. Traditional care-

PUBLIC HEALTH IN AMERICA

Vision:

Healthy People in Healthy Communities

Mission:

Promote Physical and Mental Health and
Prevent Disease, Injury, and Disability

Public Health

- ❖ Prevents epidemics and the spread of disease
- ❖ Protects against environmental hazards
- ❖ Prevents injuries
- ❖ Promotes and encourages healthy behaviors
- ❖ Responds to disasters and assists communities in recovery
- ❖ Assures the quality and accessibility of health services

Essential Public Health Services

- ❖ Monitor health status to identify community health problems
- ❖ Diagnose and investigate health problems and health hazards in the community
- ❖ Inform, educate, and empower people about health issues
- ❖ Mobilize community partnerships to identify and solve health problems
- ❖ Develop policies and plans that support individual and community health efforts
- ❖ Enforce laws and regulations that protect health and ensure safety
- ❖ Link people to needed personal health services and assure the provision of health care when otherwise unavailable
- ❖ Assure a competent public health and personal health care workforce
- ❖ Evaluate effectiveness, accessibility, and quality of personal and population-based health services
- ❖ Research for new insights and innovative solutions to health problems

Adopted: Fall 1994
Source: Public Health Functions Steering Committee
Members (July 1995):
    American Public Health Association
    Association of Schools of Public Health
    Association of State and Territorial Health Officials
    Environmental Council of the States
    National Association of County and City Health Officials
    National Association of State Alcohol and Drug Abuse Directors
    National Association of State Mental Health Program Directors
    Public Health Foundation
    U.S. Public Health Service
        Agency for Health Care Policy and Research
        Centers for Disease Control and Prevention
        Food and Drug Administration
        Health Resources and Services Administration
        Indian Health Service
        National Institutes of Health
        Office of the Assistant Secretary for Health
        Substance Abuse and Mental Health Services Administration

FIGURE 1.1. Public health in America.

givers, including community health centers and health department clinics, are aware that many Medicaid clients are from traditionally disenfranchised and difficult-to-serve populations, and some do not speak English as a first language. If the new approaches are to succeed, the enrolling managed care organizations will have to become part of the communities they seek to serve.

Community-Based Health Care

As the next century draws closer, the push to provide health-related services with a community focus is becoming stronger. This is in part an economic thrust—it is less expensive to provide care in places other than hospitals, and we are prepared to label anything outside the hospital door as "community." However, moving a high-technology, professionally dominated illness treatment system to some other location does not make it a "community-based" program.

Public health programs, for example, are not always community based, especially if public health professionals are imposing programs on a population that is not involved in decision-making or the setting of priorities.[6] Some would argue that actions to rewrite public health and other regulations undertaken by state and national officials elected in the conservative sweep of the mid-1990s are anticommunity; they appear to be responsive primarily to the concerns and goals of the economic elite and regulated business community, without attention to other perspectives.

Services become community based when they become a living part of the relationships by which the community is defined. Several funding and organizational initiatives[7] have pushed this approach, noting that if clinical services are to be effectively related to the community, they must be developed using the techniques of public health, including epidemiology, health education, and system development.

A Model Approach

Features of strong community-based health systems include:

* An identified community of interest, whether defined by geography, ethnicity, language, or other ties.
* Involvement of that community in decision-making and priority setting.
* Commitment to improving the health of the community over time, while responding to immediate needs for care.
* An understanding that the determinants of health include economics, education, and other domains.

* An understanding that rarely will any one system do all of the personal and population-based health for a community.
* A commitment by each component of the community to accept some responsibility and work with others to see that the full spectrum of services is provided.

A successful community-based health service of any kind has a clear appreciation of its limitations and is prepared to become a partner with many other groups to provide the full range of services needed by a community. This may entail sharing of information, space, personnel, or other resources. Such an approach, however, runs counter to the competitive spirit long dominant in the illness care world[8] and touted as part of what will make managed care systems work.

If the focus is on "market share" and "profit margins" to the exclusion of the long-term health outcomes of the population being served, it will be possible to become a very healthy organization and do little or nothing for community health. If a managed care clinic measures annual bottom line as the critical outcome and rates of vaccine-preventable diseases are low in the locality, assuring full age-appropriate immunization might not be a priority. To take another example, many plan enrollees change plans from year to year, so that committing plan resources to finance automobile and bicycle safety programs (including subsidy of helmet purchases) might not appear sensible. The larger community must come together to identify preferred health outcomes and establish the time frames for their accomplishment, with the expectation (which might become a requirement) that all health-related organizations operating in the community will contribute.

Information Systems

In a small, homogeneous community, information about health status, threats to health, illness events, and treatment for illnesses may circulate readily and be available for use by decision-makers. Data sets may be small enough to be correlated by hand, rather than requiring large computer resources. It is almost impossible to imagine such a community today, however.

The sources of data needed to understand the components of any community from a health perspective are generated in a variety of places. Demographic and geographic data come from nonhealth sources. Environmental risk data come from state or national sources. State and local health agencies collect material on reportable conditions, but not necessarily on the clinical treatment offered those reported. Providers of care record data on symptoms, treatment, and outcome, which may or may not be correlated with the costs and charges associated with the care. Making the linkages needed can be complicated. For example, examining a community's experience with injury and trauma requires connections among systems recording traffic patterns, emergency transport systems, emergency rooms, hospitals, rehabilitation centers, and the system recording death certificates. The protections in place for assuring confidentiality of individual identifiers must be honored, while trying to examine an individual's experience across these systems.

Given the potential of modern information systems, it is possible to imagine a time when families would receive a signal on a home electronic message system that it is time to update children's immunizations. Parents would be able to schedule appointments for the service and review current information about risks and benefits of various vaccines. Through such a system, parents might then query their provider for more personalized risk/benefit assessments and arrive for the immunization visit fully informed and ready for children to be protected. It is also possible that the information recorded by the pediatrician when the vaccine is administered (or if an adverse effect were later reported) is simultaneously transmitted to the public health system for use in monitoring the level of immunity in the community and the quality of vaccines.[9]

Linkage of information systems would also allow such improvements as automatic mapping of reported diseases or environmental contaminants in order to assist epidemiologic analysis, community notification, or planning for prevention services. The combination of telemedicine and fiberoptic capacity might expand from remote transmission of clinical data about an endoscopic examination to the transmission of pictures of the interior of a contaminated well to an engineering specialist in another locale. Subsequent use of an integrated data system could then identify wells of similar construction that might need corrective attention.

Summary

A sound concept of community is essential if we are to effectively protect and promote the health of the public; full mental and physical health is possible only when people are authentically engaged as partners in the enterprise of supporting their own health. Each of us exists within multiple communities: some of voluntary association, such as our national professional community; others of legal assignment, such as the geopolitical jurisdictions within which we live.

The health care of the community encompasses the provision of personal medical and other health-related services, and the promotion of health in the total population through application of systemic public health services. At the same time that personal care is moving out of physically defined institutions and being organized with some attention to public health principles, public health services are also being redefined. These services are now being developed around the new community capacity that is available because of organized systems of care. For example, developing a community-wide education program on child safety can be very different in a community in which the vast majority of families with children are enrolled in community-oriented managed care systems than in a community continuing to rely on traditional solo and small group fee for service care.

In moving into the next century, information and information systems become critical building blocks for health systems. With good use of information, we can have systems with a clear understanding of a community of interest, involve the community in decision-making, attend to both long- and short-term health goals, link readily with systems involved with other determinants of health, and build collaboratively rather than independently.

For a community to understand health and begin participating in community-based care and in public health programs, information needs to be locally specific, accurate, accessible, understandable, and interrelated. The technical capacity to develop such systems exists; people must apply the technology appropriately. Community-based care, both personal and public health, should be the goal for all health professionals. Well-designed, effective information systems are an essential building block in efforts to reach this goal.

References

1. *Merriam-Webster's Collegiate Dictionary.* 10th ed. Ma: Merriam-Webster, Inc.; 1993.
2. Beauchamp DE. *The Health of the Republic.* Philadelphia: Temple University Press; 1988.
3. For example, see Meier KS, Smoking truths: The impact of role models on children's attitudes toward smoking. *Health Education Quarterly* 1991;18: 173–182.
4. Griffith HM, DiGuiseppi, C. Guidelines for clinical preventive services. *Nurse Practitioner.* 1994;19:25–35.
5. McGinnis JM, Foege, WH. Actual causes of death in the United States. *JAMA.* 1993;270:2207–2212.
6. Gebbie K. You, me, or us: Prevention and health promotion. *Am J Preventive Med.* 1993;9(5):321–323.
7. These include Community-Oriented Primary Care, the Health of the Public Grants supported by the Rockefeller, Pew, and Robert Wood Johnson Foundations, and the Community-Based Public Health Initiative of the Kellogg Foundation.
8. Starr P. *The Social Transformation of American Medicine.* New York: Basic Books; 1982.
9. *Forging a Powerful Connection.* Washington DC: U.S. Public Health Service National Library of Medicine; 1995.

2

CHINs — The Current State

Alan F. Dowling

Although conceived well over 20 years ago, Community Health Information Networks (CHINs) are only now emerging as a potentially important technology for health care. Their emergence is the result of the confluence of the forces of industry and technology, many which are evolutionary, some artificial. In time, the core concepts inherent in CHINs will undoubtedly become part of the infrastructure of health care in the United States. But in the near term, the formation and success of many CHIN "experiments" will remain tenuous. Darwinian natural selection would seem to apply also to CHIN efforts.

This chapter discusses the current state of CHINs in the United States and factors that lead to their emergence. Using several models and typologies to bring clarity to the different attributes of CHINs, the chapter discusses issues that currently affect CHIN formation and development, and the values and barriers that are associated with their ultimate success or failure.

CHIN Definition and Variance

Characterizing CHINs has proven difficult and, at times, divisive. Some health care professionals ignore their existence, while others argue passionately about their definition, role, and appropriateness. Some see them as a nonprofit service, others as a potentially profitable line of business. Some view them as an end in themselves, others as a natural extension of the use of other information technologies in health care. Nevertheless, the confusion and divisiveness about their roles are indicators of the interest and potential importance that they have in our society and the promise they hold for the delivery of care in the United States and in other countries.

The Hartford Foundation was one of the early agencies to fund CHIN-applied research. The Foundation promulgated the following definition:

A Community Health Management Information System collects and disseminates health care related data and analyses to meet a wide range of needs, building information resources throughout the community.[1]

The Hartford Foundation chose this definition in part to reflect that the role they envisioned for CHINs was one of advancing societal value; hence the choice of the word "community." A common dictionary definition of community stresses the concepts of *group* and *commonality of locality, interest*, and *government*. This definition legitimizes the various views of what the scope of a CHIN is. For example, a recent alternative definition was developed from the first national CHIN Users Group (CHUG) meeting:

> any electronic communication of patient/subscriber information between two or more unaffiliated organizations.[2]

However, the CHUG definition limits the scope or nature of the information and stresses the concept *unaffiliated* organization, which is defined as: "not associated with another or others . . .; independent."[3]

The juxtaposition of these definitions reveals the potential conflict in the scope of the CHIN's information and the members of the CHIN—are they independent of each other or are they a group with common interests? Practitioners of CHIN development have not let definitions stand in the way of action. A recent definition of CHIN enunciated by consultants attempts to deal with practical realities:

> A community health information network is an innovative combination of services, products, and technology that enables organizations to exchange clinical, financial, and administrative information electronically with other designated organizations. The role of a CHIN is to enhance the efficiency and delivery of health care by allowing the electronic exchange of information among health care entities.[4]

This definition implies that organizations can simply be senders and receivers, with or without business, social, or mission affiliation. The CHUG definition stresses the unaffiliated nature of participant organizations. And the Hartford definition stresses the community link. While there is logic behind each of the definitions, they are still reflective of divergence of views about the role of CHINs. This divergence reflects an openness of thinking about CHINs that has encouraged communities that represent technology providers through university researchers to look into the organism known as a CHIN and see different facets and values in it. As is the case during the development and adoption of most technologies, CHINs both suffer and benefit from the multiple perspectives about their role in society.

CHINs are in the early innovation stage of their lifecycle (Fig. 2.1). In this stage, technologies such as CHINs often incur developmental costs at the organizational or societal level that exceed their benefits. Investments in them are made because of the prospect of a net positive value stream over time. In nonmonopolistic situations, such as with the development of the automobile, multiple developers often "experiment" with different facets or

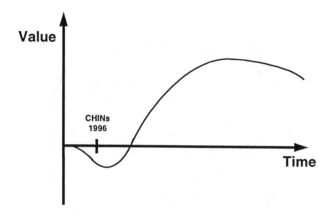

FIGURE 2.1. Value/cost ratio of technology adoption. (© Alan F. Dowling, 1985, 1995.)

aspects of the technology in the innovation stage. Hence, there appears to be, and often is, hectic, globally disorganized (although possibly locally organized) developmental activity in search of the "right answer."

Points of Agreement

While we are far from the end of the innovation stage, virtually all CHIN experimenters agree that CHINs have these minimum elements:

- Computer-based information systems and networks form the base technologies of CHINs;
- CHINs enable the transfer of data and information between organizations;
- The major domain of the data transferred is health and the provision of health services;
- Patient information is included in the information set; and
- An objective of CHINs is to improve the efficiency and effectiveness of health care delivery.

Beyond these basic elements, what else is a CHIN today? To better understand the status of CHINs in the United States, it useful to recognize that CHINs, like all computer-based information systems, are macroergonomic systems.[5] Macroergonomic systems have four key components that define their scope: mission; process or functions; humans or participants; and technology.

The mission of the organization adopting the system provides a purpose and context for the processes that define the system's interactions, or its functions, the people who initiate it, use it, or are affected by it, and the

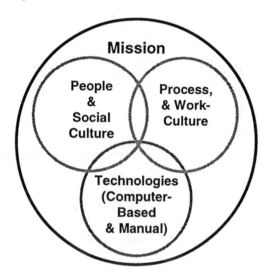

FIGURE 2.2. Macroergonomic systems. (© Alan F. Dowling, 1985, 1995.)

technologies it employs to serve the mission-based process. All of these elements interact in virtually all complex systems and the dynamics of their interactions dictate the level of success that a system will achieve. Macroergonomics gives us a framework, then, with which to decompose the CHIN environment to better understand the forces and dynamics affecting CHIN emergence and diversity. It also helps to understand CHINs' evolution through their technology adoption curves. The initial implication of CHIN macroergonomics is that the mission-related needs of potential participants are a major, perhaps *the* major, determinant of a CHIN's ability to develop and survive (Fig. 2.2).

Forces Enabling and Justifying CHINs

As with most technological innovations, the root concepts in the formation of CHINs have a long history. Sharing information in health care, an information-rich and intensive industry, has been organized for centuries through the encoding of a patient's medical information in some form of medical record. A 1974 proposal for a CHIN-like system developed by the Air Force Medical Center at Wright-Patterson Air Force Base in Dayton, Ohio, called for computer-based, interactive storage and transfer of patient information throughout the Department of Defense to improve the quality and efficiency of care of its members. Other industries, for example banking and finance, have formed "communities" around information exchange that have included the clients and providers of information-related services. So why has the concept of a CHIN gelled only recently in the health care industry? The basic forces causing change in the health care industry are the primary reasons. These forces are not unique to developing CHINs; they are motivating much wider improvements in the use of health care information technology and information management techniques in health care that enable, and are symbiotic with, CHINs. Hence, they are altering and improving the value chains associated with CHINs. They have affected health care industry participants and their missions and include:

- Clinically Oriented Information Systems Development — The earliest use of information technology in health care was for clinical purposes. However, adoption difficulties and economic incentives caused the major commercial applications to support financial, rather than clinical, processing. Later, the shift to prospective from retrospective government payment systems initiated by the Tax Equity and Fiscal Responsibility Act of 1982 (TEFRA) incented cost reduction and health resource utilization control to a degree that had not previously occurred. The resultant need to reengineer health care provider organizations (HCOs) to provide good service and survive in the new economic environment led to a realization that information systems' support of the core clinical production processes was insufficient. HCOs realized the intelligent management of information in the diagnostic, therapeutic, and management aspects of health care required improved information systems support. Therefore, to improve their care delivery processes, many HCOs significantly increased their emphasis on clinical information systems, even though the state of software for clinical informatics was still in flux. Without this increase in investment and improving clinical informatics support, CHINs could not be formed.
- Economic Risk Shift — TEFRA represented a fundamental shift in economic risk from the government to providers and, indirectly, to other payers. Employer adoption of DRGs, employer contracting for services, and the growth of capitation in payment systems have continued this shift of economic risk. In fact, the shift of risk was a major element in the Clinton health reform proposal of 1993. HCOs facing increased economic pressures and bearing increased risk found that they needed better information about the health risk attributes of their patients if they were to set economically viable prices for the services that they would undertake.
- Managed Care Expansion — Through the 1980s and 1990s, governmental, employer, and consortium purchasers of care have increasingly demanded structured and affordable care packages for those they represent. They have also increasingly intervened in clinical decisions so that now it is highly unusual to find a health plan not requiring precertification for outpatient surgery or inpatient care. It is equally unlikely to find plans that do not have some form of utilization review, at least retrospectively.

This increase in control of care led HCOs to form alliances ranging from Preferred Provider Organizations (PPOs) through Integrated Delivery and Financing Systems (IDFSs), in an effort to form economically viable health care delivery units that can provide the demanded range of services demanded across the required geographical area. As these organizations formed, they realized that increased information sharing was necessary to understand production requirements, clinical demand, resource allocation, liability, and other utilization control and coordination functions.

- Health Care Enterprise Formation—The corollary to employer or other purchaser demands for a geographically distributed set of consistent care services to their populations has been the formation of complex health care delivery organizations such as IDFSs and Integrated Delivery Networks (IDNs). Ultimately, successful health care enterprises will have made the care delivered by their geographically and functionally diverse production units efficient and consistent in care delivery coordination, quality, and contract compliance. This requires the sharing of information ranging from individual patient data through entitlement and enterprise production information in real time. As a result, sophisticated health care enterprises have recognized the need to invest in improved clinical systems, enterprise management systems, data repositories, and communication. They are, as a result, creating health information networks on an enterprise scale.

- Health Care Purchaser/Payor Involvement—The employers and other purchasers of care who have increasingly demanded consistency and coherence in the care rendered to their employees or customers have also demanded that improved information be provided to them from the health care deliverers. These demands which, from the enterprise's view, appear as external demands, often require information that the health care enterprise had not previously collected or processed in the required ways. However, health care enterprises have found that satisfying these demands is not a luxury, but a necessity. Hence, the use of information technology to provide payors and other external business agents with this information has become a cost of doing business. This push from purchasers has further increased the emphasis on building stronger information systems and information management at the health care enterprise level.

- Government Involvement—Governments are functionally schizophrenic in their health care roles; they take on, at a minimum, personalities of: provider, purchaser, and regulator/legislator. As providers of care, the federal Department of Defense Medical Services, the Department of Veterans' Affairs, and the Indian Health Service are beginning to operate more like private sector health care enterprises. As a result, these agencies will have information and information-sharing requirements like those of private sector enterprises.

The government in its role as a buyer of care has interests and requirements somewhat similar to other payers such as large corporations. Increasingly both federal and state governments are moving toward managed care and Health Maintenance Organization (HMO) options for their patient/member populations and they have analogous information needs.

- The remaining government personality, that is, the regulator/legislator, is unique. Federal agencies ranging from the Department of Health & Human Services (HHS) through the Food and Drug Administration (FDA) and the Center for Disease Control (CDC) all have roles which go beyond those of provider or payer. These obviously include basic medical research, health care research, epidemiological surveillance, quality assurance and other functions. Some quality assurance functions are delegated to authorized private sector agencies, such as the Joint Commission on Accreditation of Healthcare Organizations (JCAHO). But whether the service is produced by a governmentally franchised organization or a government agency itself, the primary roles are still those of societal advancement and protection. The resulting activities, ranging from epidemic intervention through health policy analysis, require information of a nature, consistency, quality, and specificity that are only going to increase in the future. These agencies, as a result, have dabbled with creating a health information network-like environment for years. In fact, the Clinton health care reform proposal of 1993 required the construction of a national health information network.

The technological infrastructure is to include a distributed network of regional processing centers that will 'collect, compile, and transmit information.'[5]

Further, many governmental agencies have addressed issues of relevance to the construction of CHINs. They have encouraged the development of information and technology standards, created standard medical and care delivery code structures, and created national minimum data sets and other essential elements. Proposed legislation in Congress and policy deliberations in HHS are addressing other relevant issues such as unique patient identifiers, confidentiality, privacy, and security.

- Interest of Information Technology Enterprises—Information movement and management (IMM) and information technology corporations (ITCs) have also begun to recognize that the technology infrastructure they created for other industries might be applicable to the health industry. The publicity associated with Clinton's health care reform program did much to spur their recognition of health care as an information-intensive industry. As a result, the last 3 years have seen unprecedented interest in health care information by IMMs and ITCs that had previously ignored health care. Unfortunately, many companies started health information ventures only to defund or de-emphasize them later. However, interest by a number of major vendors of information services has continued. Also, the environment has given entrepreneurial organizations many niches in which to grow and serve health informatics. As a result, many IMMs and ITCs now have an interest in furthering the development of CHIN-like information-sharing environments within health care as part of their corporate marketing direction.

- *Public/Health Services' Demands*—In addition to providers, payers, regulators, and information technology organizations, a host of community entities have a growing interest in the informatics of health care. They range from the amorphous "public-at-large" to organizations with specific missions such as advocacy groups and research institutions.

  - Institutions and think-tanks that conduct clinical, health policy, outcomes, and health informatics research have been forever hungry for improved information sources. As focus and funding shifts to more intervention- and outcome-oriented research, acquiring real behavioral and performance data from operating institutions becomes critical. Many of these organizations see CHINs as data pathways for their work. And for research into the design and adoption of information systems in health care, the CHIN, as part of the informatics armamentarium, can become the actual subject of analysis.
  - Health care performance evaluation groups, such as the National Committee on Quality Assurance (NCQA), the JCAHO, or the Cleveland Health Quality Choice (CHQC) program, which act in a quasisocietal or quasigovernmental capacity, are interested in information networks to enable their missions to proceed. For example, part of the evolving mission of the JCAHO is to be a national provider of health and quality information. Infrastructure is needed to collect clinical information remotely and enable their triennial health care delivery agency audits to become an ongoing process of continuous improvement. NCQA and CHQC similarly need access to health care delivery information through a reliable infrastructure. Timelines and accuracy of the information are important so that the health care quality evaluations they develop are fair and correct. A CHIN-based infrastructure could serve as a significant part of the infrastructure required by these organizations.
  - As consumerism and the demand for choice have become established among the consumers of health care, new demands and new services to satisfy them have developed. Health education, self-help, and triage information has appeared in media ranging from paper to interactive computer-based programs. Even the entertainment industry is working on mechanisms to provide health information services to the public. The growth in Internet activity and Web sites for consumer health, and the intention to use cable modems and cable channels to provide health information services in the home attest to the utility that CHINs could provide in the society. Health information services will depend on personal health information to "mass-tailor" services to member/patient-

specific requirements and this information could be provided via CHINs.

- The use of information technology to improve alternate site care delivery, including home care and self-care, and the increasing demand for health information for the analysis of care protocols through health policy research, are increasing the demand for the information and connectivity that CHINs could provide.

As a result of these forces, the successful fulfillment of many an organization's mission is, or will soon be, dependent upon the existence and successful operation of health information networks. Many of these organizations do not have health information networks as a primary mission component; and, therefore, they are cooperatively encouraging other agencies to create such networks — as long as they can use the networks to get the information they need to conduct their own missions.

CHIN Emergence

These forces of change affecting the providers, purchasers, regulators and others involved in healthcare delivery and management have also created a critical mass of information need, laying the groundwork to establish a high *potential* value for CHINs.

Individual health care delivery organizations have begun to adopt more robust *organizational* information communications and applications systems (Fig. 2.3) that allow them to operate more effectively and efficiently. Broadly defined, they need the information and information processes to deliver patient care, orchestrate patient management, and manage the delivery organization itself. This includes all forms of information related to health care production, resource management, payment, verification, quality, and so forth. It also includes four of the six major types of information systems shown in Fig. 2.4: task support; management control; decision support, and competition support; including composite systems such as computer-based patient records (CPRs) and executive information systems (EISs). In the near future, process control and information technology-based products systems will also be included.

Organizational-level information systems should be the easiest to justify, because the benefits they produce are self-directed. But they are not. HCOs have had ongoing difficulty justifying any systems not producing measurable cost savings. As a result, only recently have more complex, and potentially more valuable, systems (e.g., clinical pathway/protocol systems) begun to be acquired. Although their value is still difficult to measure directly, they are now being seen as a cost of doing business in a managed care environment. Nevertheless, significant problems remain at the organizational information systems level. These include cost, legacy systems, vendor supply of acceptable systems, and so forth.

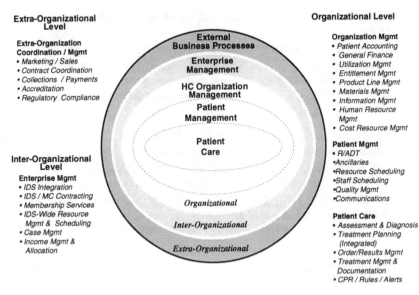

FIGURE 2.3. Three levels of HIN. (© Alan F. Dowling, 1996.)

But in a competitive health care market, newly forming health care enterprises cannot wait for organizational systems' problems to be resolved. They have realized that they need an *interorganizational*, or enterprise-wide, information system to serve as a central nervous system or they cannot coordinate and control their operations. Some individual HCOs have attempted to extend their internal technical architectures to other care delivery organizations that they acquired or with whom they partnered so as to create a common production environment. Other enterprises intended to

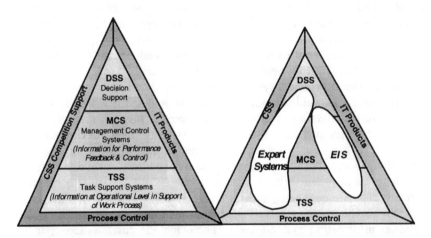

FIGURE 2.4. Information system types. (© Alan F. Dowling, 1985, 1995.)

scrap the preexisting technical environments of their constituent member HCOs, but most could not afford to do so. A partial solution to the problem is to extend the HCO's networking applications with interface engines. Thus was born the enterprise health information network (E-HIN). The value that the enterprise derives from its E-HIN is more easily identified, but still difficult to measure. These enterprise HINs enable their host enterprise to provide more effective care in a cost-efficient way throughout the geographical area required to win a managed care contract.

However, extra-organizational systems dealing with health information needs beyond and between enterprise boundaries had not yet coalesced. Agencies that focus on larger, societal health care issues, such as the Hartford Foundation, the Agency for Health Care Policy and Research, and the National Institutes of Science and Technology, began to recognize the exogenous value to be derived from health information networks and information sharing. A classic analogy is the introduction of the telephone. The existence of one telephone provides very little value to the owner — there is no one else to talk to. However, as others adopt the technology, the initial owner gains value from an increased ability to communicate, value that has not cost anything beyond the original investment. These national agencies recognized that they could take on the role of exogenous catalyst and provide the additional value push to cause enterprises to come together to create environments in which information sharing would be possible and valued. As a result, within the last half dozen years the community side of CHINs has been advanced by funding agencies, providing the economics that have enabled applied research and experimentation in CHIN formation to become viable. Other external but collateral activities have also served as catalysts. For example, in Iowa, the creation of a state-wide, fiber-based information network primarily oriented toward government agencies and educational institutions was rapidly recognized to be useful for health care delivery communities within the state. Thus, what was not started as a CHIN took on the intent, trappings, and characteristics of a CHIN as the technology was extended to Iowa's health care enterprises and organizations. Yet another force came from delivery agencies that were seeking to exploit information technology's capabilities in new ways. An example of this is telemedicine. Although telemedicine was practiced well over 20 years ago in Boston, the last half dozen years have seen a number of organizations, such as the Medical College of Georgia Telemedicine Network, attempt to create remote health care delivery capabilities that extend their care processes to other communities. Although many of these telemedicine and telehealth efforts were not initially designed as CHINs, some have gelled into forms of CHINs.

Extending an emerging technology for purposes beyond its original intent is common. That is precisely what we have seen in CHINs over the last 6 years. Figure 2.5 is a typical technology adoption curve and can be used to illustrate CHIN emergence. As noted earlier, we are now in an experimen-

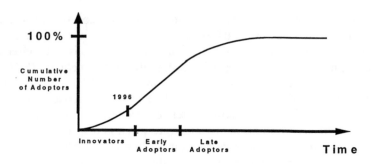

FIGURE 2.5. Technology adoption curve. (© Alan F. Dowling, 1985, 1995.)

tation or innovation stage. Numerous contemporaneous, uncoordinated "experiments" are occurring. They are characterized by macroergonomic variation: they are CHINs being formed to satisfy different missions of different participants, using or supporting different processes, used by and affecting different populations, and employing various technologies.

While most CHINs are in the innovation stage, some CHINs have begun to move into the early adoption stage. Furthering this shift are interested commercial organizations, including IMMs, ITCs, and venture capital groups, who recognize the business value of providing the technical and information services of CHINs. These typically are organizations that have rich experience in translating an innovation into a product, and have the intent and resources to help some CHINs transition productively.

Current State of CHINs

Currently, there are a large number of health information networks (HINs) in some state of formation or operation. The Community Medical Network Society (ComNet) has identified 510 HINs with "significant activity in the community arena."[6,7] Their dispersion is shown in Fig. 2.6, reflecting the fact that CHIN formation is greatest in areas of high population density *and* managed care penetration.

ComNet's research reframes one of the definitional issues discussed earlier. That is, are inter- and extraorganizational HINs really CHINs? The answer lies in one's definition of a CHIN. Based on the common tenets discussed above, the answer would be *no* and macroergonomics provides a CHIN litmus test for this conclusion (Table 2.1). ComNet also grappled with this issue and concluded that E-HINs could be viewed as embryonic CHINs that, in time, may develop true community functions.

The current state of these CHINs varies greatly. As some CHINs are being initiated, others are becoming productive, undergoing change, becoming dysfunctional, or "experiencing mortality." As with any experimen-

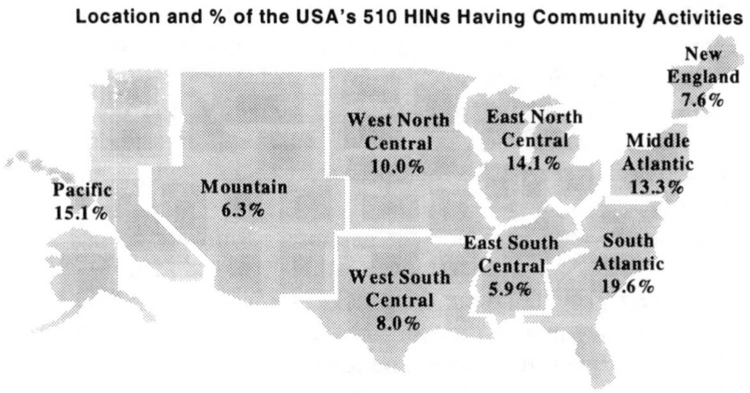

Location and % of the USA's 510 HINs Having Community Activities

FIGURE 2.6. Health networks with significant community activity. (© Alan F. Dowling, 1996. Data from market research study: *CHINs-In-Progress: Evolving to the Next Level,* © ComNet Society, 1995.)

tation in technology, risk is inherent and some CHINs will succeed while others will, quite naturally, fail.

Within the CHIN subset of HINs, we may use macroergonomics to differentiate current CHIN activities:

• Mission differences — Most CHINs have multiple mission objectives, often reflective of their participants. These have tended to be categorized as follows:

TABLE 2.1. CHIN vs. E-HIN Differentiation.

Macroergonomic component	Characteristics of an enterprise HIN	Characteristics of a community HIN
Mission	The HIN's purpose is to further the mission of a single enterprise.	The HIN's purpose is to further the common mission components of interests of two or more entities.
Processes	The aim is to support the internal production processes of a single, host enterprise even if performed by other entities.	The aim is to support the common processes of two or more entities that relate to a shared interest or mission component.
Participants	The enterprise plus any external entities that are performing functions that accrue benefit to the enterprise are participants.	Any number of common or diverse entities participate, as long as each entity has a shared function or interest with at least one other entity; and that function is supported by the HIN.
Technologies	Any information technologies that are part of a single enterprise's architecture are included.	Any information technologies that are part of a common architecture of two or more entities, or are part of an architecture that joins the diverse architectures of two or more entities are included.

1. Competitive advantage—Organizations participating in the CHIN may feel that participation gives them a competitive advantage in the market place. For example, an integrated delivery system some may see the CHIN as a mechanism of access to the community, of providing member services, or of linking providers and provider institutions to serve the geographical area required by a managed care contract.
2. Community service—Some participating organizations may recognize that participating in a CHIN can enable them to identify community needs and provide community services such as arranging for social service agency interventions or in managing an indigent case.
3. Research—Institutions with a research mission may wish access to raw demographic, epidemiological, and care information to support on-going or emerging research projects, or to research health informatics ethnographically.
4. Policy—Organizations responsible for health care policy or social service policy in an area might see participation much as researchers would. A CHIN could provide them information about the dynamics of their catchment area that would allow them to better assess community health needs and plan appropriately.
5. Care delivery—Organizations providing care could be interested in a CHIN to support care delivery, patient management, and organizational functions. In care delivery, a CHIN would allow them to share case information to better manage the care of patients, provide member services that would keep members healthy rather than converting to patients, serve members at alternate delivery sites, share best practices and outcome information, and enable better concurrent quality and utilization review. CHIN support for business processes includes health plan performance reporting, entitlement, and utilization management and business services such as coordination of benefits, billing, and collection.
6. Information or business services—Some organizations may be in the business of providing information sharing, analysis, or movement services. These organizations are interested in CHINs to open a new market or serve as a distribution channel for the organization's goods and services.

- Process differences—The processes provided by the CHIN are another way of differentiating CHINs. All CHINs support or conduct multiple processes. Among the most typical processes are the following:

1. System connectivity and integration—These processes provide the technical integration services that enable enterprises or agencies with different information technologies to communicate. These processes could address each of the Open Systems Foundation's OSI 7-Level model,[8] plus the extensions that will one day allow interoperability

(Fig. 2.7). Of current importance are the services that include physical connectivity, network protocols and services, routing, and data conversion.

2. Storage and transfer of patient information—This process involves the acquisition and centralized warehousing of patient-specific information for the purpose of providing it to other member organizations so that they may conduct valid functions using the patient data. These functions include coordination of care, coordination and adjudication of payments, and research. The warehouse need only be logically centralized. In reality, it may be a decentralized set of repositories with a central master member/patient index and pointer system.

3. Member/patient information services—This process enables members or patients in health plans to more fully participate in health education, triage, scheduling, and other such functions on their own behalf. Their participation represents a service enhancement that makes the plan providing the service more attractive and also would provide real value to the patient or member. Numerous patient education, triaging, and self-help programs can be made available though a CHIN to a member upon request. Some plans for cable modems allow the CHIN to use existing cable TV networks to reach into members'/patients' homes.

4. Application services—Many CHINs provide clinical, business, and/or financial applications to support the work processes of participating organizations. Other application services deal with enterprise or external activities, including managed care processes required to enable care delivery to move forward, such as precertification and

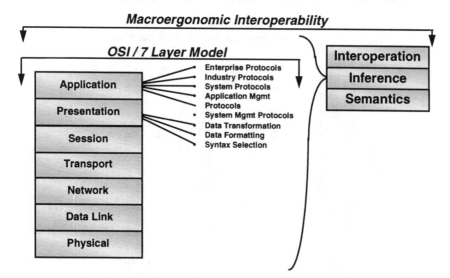

FIGURE 2.7. System interoperability requirements. (© Alan F. Dowling, 1996.)

transfer of the information necessary for utilization review and adjudication. Other services support the resale of receivables or the prefinancing of collectibles and processing the financial reimbursement associated with the rendering of care. Figure 2.8 shows the results of ComNet research into the current and planned applications of CHINs.[6,7] Clearly, applications supporting administrative (e.g., e-mail) and financial functions are most widespread. However, significant growth is planned for clinical and data repository applications.

- People differences—At the human level, the major participants in a CHIN are the controllers, the systems service providers, and the users. Those who control the CHIN may change during its life cycle. However, the issue of control via "ownership" is proving so important that it will be discussed separately below. The systems service providers are those who operate the CHIN. The users are those who execute the functions of the system or use the information that it provides. Nearly all CHINs have these groups:

1. CHIN Service Provider—Information and systems providers vary greatly in their approach, based on their corporation's business fit with the objectives of the CHIN. Some providers are members of a health care delivery organization and have great empathy with users. Others come from IMMs or ITCs and may be less familiar with health care provision. Instead they may be working to extend their corporation's core business services into health care by providing an information "utility." Their corporate perspective bears greatly on their intent and behavior. Major telecommunications companies have been primarily

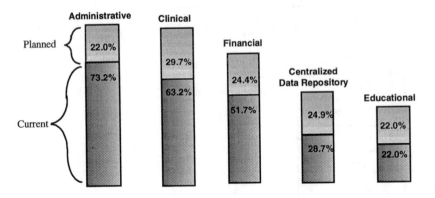

% of CHINs Having These Applications

FIGURE 2.8. Current and planned CHIN applications. (© Alan F. Dowling, 1996. Data from market research study: *CHINs-In-Progress: Evolving to the Next Level,* © ComNet Society, 1995.)

interested in CHINs that crossed regional boundaries so they could increase their inter-LATA (Local Access and Transport Area) business. Local telephone companies, on the other hand, have been more interested in intra-LATA CHINs. Some data base companies were interested in extending the repository and data management functions to a CHIN environment. Hardware and software vendors have been interested in CHINs that will make their wares the standards for a large group of customers. Many vendors have, and will, serve CHINs well. They bring a concrete value expectation, relevant experience, and a history of investing in research and development engineering—three things necessary for a CHIN to thrive.

2. CHIN Users—One major set of users is the community of health care providers, researchers, educators, and policy analysts who are aware of, or are participating in, CHINs. This group uses the CHIN for the benefit of others. They view CHIN services as tools with which to conduct their work. The second major set of users consists of health plan members, patients, and the public in general. A minority of this group are aware of CHINs and view them as a mechanism for improving the health-related services they consume. They are likely to be a more active group in the future, as in-home or in-workplace health education, self-triage, and self-care services become more widely available. They may also use the CHIN's services to order or procure health services remotely via scheduling, purchase of expendable supplies, rental, or ordering of durable medical equipment, emergency alerting, and similar services.

• Technology differences—Technology differentiation depends on the architecture for which the CHIN opts. Virtually no CHIN would be expected to have the same technology as another. However, this will change as the current CHIN experiments yield useful information about what technology designs and architectures work well. Technology will also begin to converge as for-profit CHIN service providers propagate their own technology. Currently the major areas of technology choice include:

1. Central or decentralized repositories—The object and data structures of the CHIN could support either centralized warehousing of information or distributed repositories. Ownership and the control of information often affect this technical decision.

2. Integration services—A CHIN can serve a systems integration function, but to varying degrees. Some CHINs opt for integration only at the data level; others enable data to be routed and formatted while some enable application integration. The future could bring support for participants' application interoperations.

3. Computational resources—The computational resources of a CHIN range from participants providing their own computing environment

to the CHIN providing outsourcing services for information management and systems. Many CHINs mix these modes. For example, some enterprises are responsible for their own processing while the CHIN is responsible for central network and common database processing.

In addition to these factors, the control of CHINs is central to their formation, mission, and evolution. Ownership tends to be a major differentiator. It is often associated with the prioritization of mission elements to be accomplished by the CHIN. In other words, "he who owns, dictates."
Forms of ownership include the following:

- A health care enterprise — a common form of health information network is one created by a health care delivery enterprise and later extended to a limited degree into the community. A variant is the ownership stake of physicians through their group practices, Independent Practice Associations (IPAs), PPOs, or clinic foundations. If the enterprise retains full control and provides only those services through the CHIN that it provides as a health care delivery organization, the CHIN is really an extension of an enterprise health information network. Although numerous such examples exist, the main reason for this form of ownership is to enable the health care delivery enterprise to maintain control of its market.
- An association of health care entities — In this form of CHIN, agencies that have health care delivery and/or public service commitments join to provide services to the participants for the community's business and social welfare.
- Information service providers (vendors) — These organizations initiate an ownership stake in a CHIN primarily to provide their core business services through a CHIN to an existing or new set of clients. Actors include information systems vendors, telecommunications organizations, and information services businesses.
- Payors and purchasers — Payors and purchasers have become interested in CHINs as a way to influence information availability and process consistency with respect to utilization, benefit coordination, performance, and payment services. Some also advocate CHINs' efforts to enhance their members' health-related services and education.
- Government — Government "ownership" in CHINs has come about primarily because of the need to integrate governmental business and service functions and to improve the infrastructure of the catchment area. Governments also assume an ownership stake when they believe the value to be accrued to private sector organizations for the creation of a CHIN is insufficient to enable a CHIN's services to be created and distributed. This is an example of exogenous value and is typical in the decision process as to when a government takes a role. Economists suggest that a government role is appropriate when the value to be accrued by CHIN formation is primarily at the societal level, but insufficient to motivate the market forces necessary to create the service. For example, government

support of the National Information Infrastructure (NII) and its associated Health Information Infrastructure (HII) is deemed necessary because such information infrastructure is of intrinsic value to the nation. The government's role as catalyst includes creating an economic environment that will warrant private sector investment. This role varies by jurisdiction, country, and governmental philosophy. Other governments' attempts to support CHIN creation have evolved from different belief systems. Efforts in Australia, for example, are based on the belief that the public and private sectors can both gain value from a national information infrastructure and that once such an infrastructure is created, both governmental and private sector applications would be developed to run on the infrastructure. In some European countries, health care is seen as a right of the population and governments' movement into CHINs is seen as an extension of the their role of providing services to society.

The primary forms of ownership are by an individual enterprise of some type or by an association, coalition or consortium. Enterprise-owned CHINs are likely to reflect the enterprise's mission, and coalition-owned CHINs are likely to reflect committee agreements that may or may not have business viability in the long run. Figure 2.9 shows the percentage of CHINs in which the entities shown have an ownership interest.

Ownership is one dimension of control. Control is also exercised through funding and participation. These Dimensions were also estimated in the ComNet research. Their data are shown in Figs. 2.10 and 2.11. Figure 2.10 is the percentage of CHINs in which the entities shown have provided funding for its formation and/or initial operation. Figure 2.11 is the percentage of CHINs in which the entities shown are a participant in the CHINs' operation.

Based on the variables discussed above, ranging from ownership and mission through process, actors, and technology, establishment of a broad variety of CHINs could be expected. That is precisely what has been and is

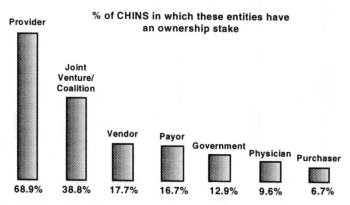

FIGURE 2.9. HIN ownership. (© Alan F. Dowling, 1996. Data from market research study: *CHINs-In-Progress: Evolving to the Next Level,* © ComNet Society, 1995.)

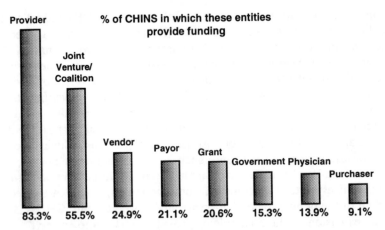

Figure 2.10. HIN funding. (© Alan F. Dowling, 1996. Data from market research study: *CHINs-In-Progress: Evolving to the Next Level,* © ComNet Society, 1995.)

happening. In spite of the differences, however, we can fit most CHINs into a summary classification that includes:

• Community-of-concern CHINs—Community-of-concern networks have a primary function, or at least an important function, of serving or supporting some element of society on a not-for-profit or not-for-business basis. These include patient member and customer services,

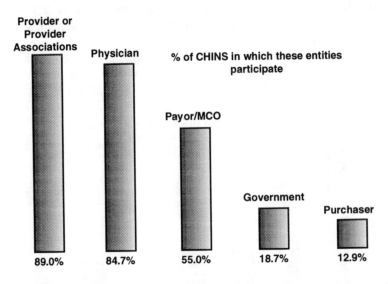

Figure 2.11. HIN participation. (© Alan F. Dowling, 1996. Data from market research study: *CHINs-In-Progress: Evolving to the Next Level,* © ComNet Society, 1995.)

functions to support policy, epidemiological and research support, health status monitoring, and other societal initiatives.

- Community-of-business CHINs – Community-of-business networks' primary functions involve tying together organizations that form a community of business interests. They include providers, payers, employers, medical service organizations (MSOs), third-party administrators, adjudicators, pharmaceutical, durable medical equipment (DME), and expendable supply distributors. The purpose is to make business transactions more effective.
- Utility CHINs – Utility networks are generally business ventures in which one or more organizations with ownership stakes create a network to provide subscription and/or transaction-based services to the health industry. The main purpose is to provide services and interconnectivity of sufficient value to warrant subscription and transaction charges. In addition, these networks provide business services ranging from adjudication to receivable financing.
- Enterprise health information networks – The final set of information network deals with the enterprise level network that could evolve into a CHIN. Theoretically this health information network forms the basis of the community of interest at the enterprise level. However, it does not meet the ComNet definition of a CHIN, which requires that the entities involved have some affinity through ownership, partnering, or outsourcing that draws them together in the provision of services to a client community.

Prognosis for CHINs – Overcoming Barriers and Establishing Value

Business, funding, and technology trends in health care are creating an environment that will bring computer-based, lifelong personal health records into existence. These records will be shared in a secure and confidential way with health care agents who have a legitimate need for the information: clinicians using patient-identified information for the patient, and researchers and policy analysts using nonascribed patient information for the development of clinical, educational, and policy interventions. Businesses insuring and coordinating care will still exist and they will use certain patient, process, and performance information generated as a byproduct of caring for the wellness and illness of patient/members. The information infrastructure that will enable this on a day-to-day basis will be electronic, photonic, and potentially biologic and will be transparent to health workers. It will be a reliable utility that they can use without having to understand its physics.

Stating this prognosis is far easier than engineering its fulfillment.

Engineering the technological base is complex but doable. Engineering its adoption in light of mission, process, and human barriers is not.

Perhaps the greatest factor in CHIN success is the ability to create value. CHINs, like any other technology or amalgamation of technology, have life cycles. A CHIN's typical life cycle (Fig. 2.1) has an initial period of negative-value creation. During this phase, resources are expended in the formation of a CHIN that are not positively offset by equal value creation for the owners or community of interest. Those CHINs that survive this infancy move to a stage in which positive value is created over a period of time. Typically this value is enhanced by exogenous variables, as noted above. Initial investment in CHIN development often assumes that the value of a CHIN will be rapidly realized by other members or users to warrant their ongoing participation. As with telephones, their involvement expands the community of users and increases the value for each preexisting user or member of the CHIN. A CHIN may not survive long enough to transition out of its early negative-value stage if its initial business proposition is faulty or insufficient value is created to sustain the CHIN to a point where exogenous value is realized. This is often the case when the origin of the CHIN is based on soft funding, rather than intrinsic business value. When the soft funding dissipates, as inevitably it must, insufficient value may be obtained to offset the ongoing costs that must now be shouldered by CHIN participants. In this situation, unless other potential members that are capable of funding and deriving offsetting value from the CHIN can be added rapidly, the CHIN will collapse. If, however, a CHIN is of sufficient utility to warrant investment in its initiation and growth, then it may survive to the point of exogenous value creation. Thus, one predictor of CHIN survivability is the initial business premise for the formation of the CHIN and the rapidity with which value can be created. Another is the willingness of a governmental agency to underwrite the funding of the CHIN until the time comes when sufficient indigenous or exogenous value is created that the CHIN can be privatized or repay taxpayers' investments.

If we extend the life cycle concept further, we can envision a point at which the value of a CHIN transitions to one of basic utility for the community. Ongoing value creation occurs at the application level by CHIN members to the degree to which innovation and evolution occurs at the application level. Although technology transfer models show an eventual decline in the utility of the CHIN, that decline is likely to be far in the future. The main reason is that we do foresee application innovation expanding in CHINs, thus rejuvenating their life cycles. Hence, we can perceive a need for ongoing CHIN infrastructure because we envision a need for evolving applications in cooperative, multiorganizational health care support and management.

In addition to difficulties and opportunities attendant on their creation of value, CHINs face ongoing management issues, the resolution of which is critical for success.

- Service innovation — Although the life cycle of products and technology includes eventual decline, a CHIN need not suffer this fate. A CHIN has the opportunity to piggy-back multiple information services on its infrastructure. If it does so innovatively, as the need — and value — of one service line declines, the CHIN can introduce other services. Hence, ongoing CHIN success is tied to its ability to innovate and provide services.

- Mission and control — Unless mission, ownership and control are based on the rational, nonconflicting business requirements of its founders, the CHIN-in-formation will probably fail. Or, it may be so conflicted that the value it could create is dissipated by instability. Competitive conflict among the CHIN's members is a major threat. Because competitive alliances ebb and flow, the premise for a CHIN should address basic needs that participants will have whether or not an alliance survives. So, too, the CHIN should not be formed to pursue markets that will soon terminate, or be significantly restructured. Forming a CHIN solely as a mechanism for a research organization to obtain soft research funds is not an enduring strategy. When the soft funding ends, the CHIN is not likely to endure.

- Distributed versus CHIN information control — This is a technological issue affected by issues such as ownership and control. It is entirely possible that the CHIN will be a set of pointers to individual information repositories that are neither owned nor controlled by the CHIN itself. The information would be "owned" by the participating organization, which would maintain its own access controls. In this kind of structure the CHIN would maintain master indices and retrieval utilities. Alternatively, if ownership and control are not an issue, information or at least relevant subsets of the information of participating organizations could be drawn into data repositories of the CHIN itself. Under these circumstances the CHIN has a higher probability of being able to generate data analysis services in addition to retrieval and connectivity services, increasing its value.

- Service reliability — As CHIN services become more routinized, they will become part of the operating fabric of participating organizations. CHINs must provide the mechanisms to assure the security and continuity of services, and recovery from damage should failure occur.

- Information validity and accuracy — A continuing barrier to CHIN services is the fear of receiving and acting on inaccurate information. There is no certain way of knowing whether clinical — or other mission-critical — information received through a CHIN is valid or accurate. As a result, receiving organizations generally choose not to completely trust it and redo diagnostic tests or incur other costs attempting to validate the information. Such actions reduce the potential value of CHINs. Unfortunately, even if the CHIN transfers information accurately, the original accuracy of the information it received is still unknown. This is a general problem with the health information infrastructure and information management practices of the society.

- Client/patient information confidentiality and privacy — Although computer-based systems have not created any new form of crime or breach of confidentiality, they can certainly be manipulated to exacerbate these problems. As consumer advocates and the public focus on this issue, CHINs will face major challenges in defining and executing information privacy and confidentiality policies. Federal legislation and regulation has been proposed to spur attention to these issues and to protect individual rights. Variously, they propose information privacy standards, mechanisms, requirements, and penalties for compliance failure. This issue alone has the potential to retard CHIN efforts, as it did in Australia.

Conclusion

As we have seen, there are a wide variety of CHINs in existence today. It is virtually certain that many of today's CHINs will, within a period of months or years, cease to exist. It is equally certain that some of today's CHINs will evolve into highly successful enterprises generating value that far exceeds cost. We may use the concepts of macroergonomics to suggest the characteristics of CHINs that will likely survive.

CHINs likely to survive will first and foremost be based on demonstrable value. Their mission, organizational structure, funding, and operation will be based on rapid return on investment consistent with the investment time line of participants or, they will have government funding to sustain the CHIN through its initial period of negative value creation until exogenous value can create a positive value flow. A number of CHINs will be successful by providing utility services ranging from interconnectivity to information analysis for marketing purposes. Other CHINs will be successful at the community level where value is derived by a larger set of participants.

Issues of ownership, control, and purpose are also vital to a CHIN's success. Wrestling over ownership and control, and over the rights to information assets, may well cause the failure of some CHINs. Other CHINs face the loss of participants when the community recognizes that the fundamental reason for the CHIN's existence may have been to further the market position of one of its members. Such CHINs may well be viable as an enterprise network. However, if they are to expand into a community network, the value they create will have to be shared among a wide variety of participants.

Functionality will also be a determinant of success. CHINs acting as simple data transport mechanisms can be supplanted easily by members of the information movement and management industry, and perhaps should be. The CHIN's value-added applications and services will distinguish it from a transport network. The functionality required will depend upon the needs and priorities of the participants. With reference to ComNet's "ideal CHIN" of the future, we envision a day in which the information network of networks in the United States will be far more robust, providing individual enterprises, governments, patients, members, employers, and other actors sufficient value to warrant their inclusion in a fairly broad-based national internetwork. Although it is operationally challenging, it is not intellectually challenging to engineer CHINs that are secure, provide patient confidentiality for patient-identifiable information, yet provide aggregation of information across patients to support policy and epidemiological analyses. It is virtually certain that such health information networks will come about.

The issue for these formative times is how to best enable these future CHINs to occur, where to be involved, and when to help change happen. Today's CHINs have not yet achieved a sustaining critical mass. But, they are social structures that can be influenced by human involvement. Thus, strong CHINs can be significantly aided in achieving critical mass by the actions that our enterprises and our government undertake. This is one reason that in a number of organizations, such as the federal government, the Koop Institute, and the Council of Competitiveness are all urging the cooperation of potential actors to create an information environment that maximizes the value to be derived from information technology, including CHINs.

References

1. The Hartford Foundation, 1994.
2. CHUG, 1995, notes, meeting held at CHIN Summit '95.
3. *American Heritage Dictionary*, Boston, New York: Houghton Mifflin Company, 1992.
4. Nutkis D, Golob R. Community Health Information Networks. *Pulse.* 1995; Ernst & Young LLP; Spring;11-15.
5. Dowling AF. Notes on the concept of macroergonomics from health care information systems course notes. Cleveland, Oh: Case Western Reserve University; 1981.
6. Furukawa MF, Peake T. Profiling America's health information networks. *COMNET's Journal of the Community Medical Network Society.* 1995;3: 25-36.
7. Furukawa MF. CHINs in progress: Evolving to the next level. *CHIN 100 Market Directory.* ComNet Society; 1996.
8. Meijer A, Peeters P. *Computer Network Architectures.* Rockville, Maryland: Computer Science Press; 1982.

Glossary of Common Acronyms

CDC   Centers For Disease Control
CHIN   Community Health Information Network

CHQC	Cleveland Health Quality Choice
CHUG	CHIN Users Group
ComNet	Community Medical Network Society
CPR	Computer-Based Patient Record
DME	Durable Medical Equipment
DRG	Diagnostic Related Group
E-HIN	Enterprise Health Information Network
EIS	Executive Information Systems
FDA	Federal Drug Administration
HCO	Health Care Organization
HHS	Health And Human Services
HII	Health Information Infrastructure
HIN	Healthcare Information Systems
HMO	Health Maintenance Organization
IDFS	Integrated Delivery and Finance System
IDN	Integrated Delivery Network
IDS	Integrated Delivery System
IMM	Information Movement and Management
IPA	Independent Practice Association
ITC	Information Technology Corporations
JCAHO	Joint Commission for Accreditation of Healthcare Organizations
LATA	Local Access and Transport Area
MSO	Medical Service Organization
NCQA	National Committee on Quality Assurance
NII	National Information Infrastructure
OSI	Open Systems Integration
PPO	Preferred Provider Organization
TEFRA	Tax Equity and Fiscal Responsibility Act

3

Enterprise-Wide Clinical Data Integration

MICHAEL G. KAHN

The basic function of a community health information network (CHIN) is to share health-care-related data among independent organizations. Because of the differences in participating organizations and in their information systems, CHINs require contributing organizations to integrate and share data among markedly diverse systems. Like CHINs, integrated health care systems need to integrate and share clinical and administrative data among entities that may have widely differing information systems. However, while similar in spirit to CHINs, health care systems need to integrate a much larger portion of their internal information to realize strategic clinical and business advantages in a competitive marketplace.

In this chapter, we describe Project Spectrum, a collaborative project designed to construct an information system infrastructure for the integration of clinical data from disparate health care entities within a newly formed integrated health care system. The focus of the chapter is on the organizational and technical challenges faced by organizations seeking to construct an integrated information-systems infrastructure. We include the description of Project Spectrum because independent organizations seeking to share clinical and administrative data within a CHIN face some of the same organizational and technical issues that newly formed integrated health care systems face.

Project Spectrum

The BJC Health System, formed in 1993 through the merger of Barnes-Jewish Inc. and Christian Health Services, consists of 18 acute-care facilities, 7 long-term care facilities, and 22 affiliate hospitals in urban, suburban, and rural communities throughout Missouri and southern Illinois. At the time of the merger, BJC had 5133 licensed beds, 22,395 full-time or part-time employees, 6013 medical staff members and $1.4 billion in net revenues.

Like many large organizations, BJC created a mission statement that set forth the key unifying goal for the newly formed organization:

Our mission is to improve the health of the people and communities we serve.

Close examination of the implications contained within this mission statement reveals three significant challenges:

1. BJC must acquire the capacity to *measure* the current health of the people and communities it serves;
2. BJC must acquire the capacity to *measure changes* in the health of the people and communities it serves; and
3. BJC must acquire the capacity to *relate these changes* to BJC interventions.

The shift in focus from single-hospital acute medical care to multifacility integrated health care significantly changes the role of information systems. Disjointed records of clinical encounters at individual facilities must be replaced by a comprehensive picture of a person's health care need and utilization, irrespective of where that care was delivered. No traditional hospital-based information systems are designed to support this change in clinical and business focus. Early recognition of the limitations of the current information-processing environment at BJC resulted in a strategic initiative to address this critical enterprise-wide need. The resulting project, called Project Spectrum, was begun in June 1994.

Project Spectrum is a joint technology development project whose major partners are BJC Health System, Washington University School of Medicine, IBM/Integrated Systems Solution Corporation, Kodak Health Imaging Systems, and Southwestern Bell. Associate partners, such as Century Analysis Incorporated, provide niche products and expertise. Project Spectrum consists of three initiatives: clinical information systems, imaging and multimedia systems, and telecommunications systems for data, image, voice, multimedia, teleradiology and telecollaboration.[1] This chapter focuses on the clinical information system (CIS) initiative.

A central goal of Project Spectrum is to create an enterprise-wide comprehensive integrated clinical information system. The term *enterprise-wide* means that the system will include data from all locations within BJC, *comprehensive* means that it will incorporate detailed data from all electronic data sources, *integrated* means it will unify patient data from independent data sources, and *clinical* means that the data will have direct utility to clinical care.

Like the BJC organization, the newly-formed Project Spectrum CIS initiative group developed a mission statement to express their goals:

We will provide comprehensive enterprise-wide clinical information to providers and administrators so that they may improve the health of our patients and the efficiency of our care.

As with the BJC mission statement, close examination of the CIS mission statement reveals two significant implications:

1. The CIS mission statement recognizes both clinical and administrative users and uses of enterprise-wide clinical information.
2. The CIS mission statement acknowledges that the systems we create will be used to improve not only the health of specific patients but also the efficiency of the healthcare system.

The mission statement and its implications explicitly acknowledge that there will be multiple users and uses of the clinical information system. The Institute of Medicine, in its seminal monograph on the computer-based patient record, listed 39 users and 37 uses of electronic patient data.[2] Users included both individuals and organizations; uses included both patient-specific decision-making and population-based analyses. Although the data contained in the Spectrum clinical information system will be more limited than a computer-based patient record, as defined by the Institute of Medicine, recognition of multiple "constituencies" with different needs for the information system is an essential feature of the CIS project. For the clinician who requires information about the care of an individual patient, Project Spectrum will integrate clinical data from all electronic sources into one database so that patient data can be presented at in a consistent workstation. For the health services researcher who requires information for clinical outcomes research, quality assessment, and process re-engineering, Project Spectrum will construct a population-focused database from patient information gathered across all practice environments within the BJC Health System. A database designed for "patient-focused" queries can be used to answer questions such as "What were the clinical laboratory results for Mrs. Smith?" while a database designed for "population-focused" queries can be used to answer questions such as "What was the average length of stay by admitting facility for all female diabetic patients admitted during the last quarter?"

The two core features of the Spectrum CIS are a single point of access to all electronic clinical data irrespective of the origin of the data or the location of the reviewer, and a long-term repository of current and historical clinical information where key data elements with lasting clinical and administrative value are stored. We have termed the first feature "one-stop shopping." This feature will necessarily be ever-expanding as areas of clinical practice currently without electronic data-capture capabilities acquire such technology. The data repository is required to provide both patient-specific historical information and enterprise-wide historical trends for epidemiological studies and process reengineering activities.

Project Spectrum was initiated on July 1, 1994 with an anticipated development lifetime of 3–5 years. Full deployment of physician workstations to the more than 3500 BJC-affiliated clinicians is likely to take a decade. The project has been divided into five phases; it currently is at the

TABLE 3.1. Clinical data locations and classes for Project Spectrum Phase One.

Data locations	Data classes
Barnes Hospital	Master patient demographics
Jewish Hospital	Clinical laboratory results
Barnes West County Hospital	Clinical pathology results
Christian Hospital Northeast	Radiology results
Christian Hospital Northwest	Cardiology results
Alton Memorial Hospital	12-lead EKG graphics
	Vital signs
	Intake/Output
	Pharmacy orders
	Transcribed histories and physicals
	Transcribed discharge summaries
	Transcribed operative reports
	Transcribed emergency dept. notes

midpoint of the 18-month first phase. For the CIS initiative, Phase One focuses on integrating 13 sources of clinical data from 6 metropolitan St. Louis hospitals (Table 3.1). Although some of the Phase One facilities share applications and not all facilities have all 13 clinical data sources, a total of 39 interfaces into existing facility-based information systems are required to meet the Phase One objective. Two facilities are large academic medical centers, three facilities are large community medical centers, and one facility is a small community hospital. Also during Phase One, the Spectrum imaging initiative will develop image-annotated computed tomography and magnetic resonance reports (limited studies with selected films). The networking initiative will establish a self-healing ring-based asynchronous transfer mode (ATM) network between all facilities, and will provide integrated services digital network (ISDN) connectivity in the homes and offices of 10 pilot internists and surgeons.

In later phases of the project, we plan to incorporate more data sources from the current six facilities; also, more BJC facilities will contribute data to the data repository, and more emphasis will be placed on cutting-edge initiatives in graphics, imaging, video, telecollaboration, telemedicine, and clinical decision support. We will restrict the remainder of our discussion to the Phase One activities because these concern the "basic" clinical data likely to be shared in a CHIN environment and because Phase One already has generated significant organizational and technical issues likely to be seen in any large-scale CHIN initiative.

The Integration of Clinical Data

Data integration involves attempting to take a collection of independent information systems and turning them into a single, unified, consistent database. Most health care organizations store patient data in more than one information system. Acute-care facilities may have a centralized hospital information system as a core or hub system, but most have specialized departmental systems that serve unique information needs. Even small organizations (such as ambulatory care centers) have separate systems for clinical, administrative, billing, scheduling, and ancillary services.

When multiple facilities merge to form a healthcare organization, the number of information systems grows with each new facility. The left column of Table 3.2 lists the type of services usually considered to be part of "clinical information systems" in acute-care facilities. Table 3.2 also shows the types of hardware and software used to supply these CIS applications in 3 of the 18 acute-care facilities at BJC. It is especially ironic to note that the three facilities listed in Table 3.2 are physically across the street from each other, yet each has chosen a different strategy for providing clinical information services.

The Organizational Challenges of Data Integration

Although health care institutions have been characterized as "islands of information," the current fragmentation of information services might be better characterized as "fiefdoms of information owners."[3] There are many information fiefdoms: departments, inpatients, outpatients, physicians, and hospitals. Departmental information system managers are better positioned than managers of large centralized systems to understand the special needs of their target users and to create systems to meet these needs. The use of unique, highly tailored information systems for specialized needs has been called *best-of-breed*. The organizational "catch-22" with the best-of-breed approach is that end-users are best served by allowing them to select information systems that meet their needs, yet an integrated health-care system requires a unified, singular view of patient-care data. The best-of-breed approach favors the needs of end-users over the desires of a central authority, but as illustrated in Table 3.2, the best-of-breed approach also results in the fragmentation of patient data. Organizations can attempt to reduce the fragmentation of patient data across specialized information systems in at least two ways:

1. "Legislate" a single system so that all patient data are in one place.
2. "Legislate" a means for exchanging data among disparate systems so that all relevant data are available to all systems.

Option One is plausible for health care organizations that have no installed information services or that have the authority to replace existing services with an "approved" system. Option Two is plausible for health care organizations that have a substantial investment in the current information services infrastructure or which are unwilling to impose a single system on

TABLE 3.2. Clinical Information Systems at three of eighteen BJC acute-care facilities. Blank table cells mean no system exists for that function. Table used by permission of the author.

Clinical Function	Barnes Hospital	Jewish Hospital	Childrens Hospital
ADT Registration	IBM 9000/820 Self Developed	IBM 9000/820 TDS HC7000	IBM 4381–92E DataCare— to be replaced
Blood Bank	IBM 9000/820 Self Developed		
Cardiology System	Macintosh Self Developed	Trinity Marquette	
Clinical Scheduling		IBM 9000/820 TDS HC7000	
Decision Support	DEC/VAX 4500 HBO Trendstar	DEC/VAX 4500 HBO Trendstar	SUN Sparc 20/ Oracle Self Developed
Dietary	IBM 9000/820 Self Developed	IBM PC CBoard/Mcounts	HP 9000/T500 Clinicom
Home Care	IBM RS/6000 INFOMED	IBM AS/400 HCIS	HAMS
Labor & Delivery	IBM 9000/820 Self Developed	HP3000	
Laboratory	IBM 9000/820 Self Developed	DEC 6220 Cerner	DEC VAX Cluster Cerner
Medical Records	IBM 9000/820 Self Developed	Meta ATC	IBM AIX RS6000 Chartflow 2000
Medication Distribution	PYXIS	SUREMED	Clinicom
Nurse Staffing	IBM PC Medicus	IBM Token Ring AtWork/ANSO	IBM Novell AtWork
OR Scheduling	Novell Enterprise Systems	IBM Token Ring ATWork/ORSUS	IBM RS6000 SurgiWare
OB/GYN	IBM 9000/820 Self Developed	IBM 9000/820 Self Developed	
Order Communications	IBM 9000/820 Self Developed	IBM 9000/820 TDS HC7000	Clinicom
POCS/ Documentation	SUN Microsystems EMTEK	IBM 9000/820 TDS HC7000	Clinicom
Pathology	DEC 3600 CoMed	DEC 3600 CoMed	
Patient Care	IBM 9000/820 Self Developed	IBM 9000/820 TDS HC7000	Clinicom
Pharmacy	IBM 9000/820 Productive Data Mgt	IBM 9000/820 TDS HC7000	IBM RS6000 HBOC
Radiology	DEC Self Developed	DEC 4000 IDX/DECRAD	DEC Self Developed
Respiratory Care	IBM Token Ring Puritan Bennet		Clinicom
Trauma	IBM 9000/820 Self Developed		Intel HTR

all end-users. Option Two is analogous to the CHIN setting because a CHIN organization is not likely to have the authority or the ability to impose the replacement of information systems. Option Two also is the approach we have taken in Project Spectrum.

Figure 3.1 illustrates a high-level architectural view of Project Spectrum. This figure shows the relationship between the current BJC facilities information systems (source data systems) and the Spectrum enterprise-wide clinical data repository.

The architecture illustrated in Fig. 3.1 highlights two critical organizational assumptions:

• The Spectrum architecture permits each facility to make autonomous decisions about upgrades to existing systems or acquisition of new systems depending on the unique business and operational needs of the facility. Project Spectrum's only demands on future procurements are that new systems be TCP/IP network-aware and that an HL7 Version 2.2 standard interface be supplied by the vendor. We believe the continued decision-making autonomy of the facilities has resulted in a high level of cooperation among the facility-based information systems staffs and the Project Spectrum team.

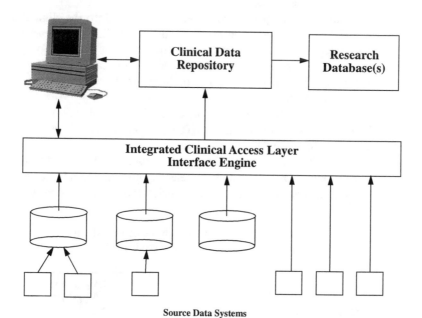

FIGURE 3.1. High-level architecture of the Clinical Information System component of Project Spectrum. Canisters represent centralized hospital information systems, squares represent interfaced or stand-alone specialized systems. Figure used by permission of the author.

- The Spectrum architecture permits each facility to continue to supply mission-critical CIS functionality using existing facility-based systems as Project Spectrum is developed. Thus, our enterprise-wide development schedule does not impede or compromise the CIS services of each facility.

Although our design imposes an additional technical challenge, organizationally it has been an easy model to promote among a wide variety of information systems constituencies and environments.

One possible interpretation of Fig. 3.1 is that all data currently stored in all existing clinical systems will be moved into the clinical data repository. However, as noted in the description of the Spectrum data repository given earlier, "only *key* data elements with *lasting* clinical and administrative value" are stored. Table 3.3 illustrates some crude 'back-of-the-envelope' calculations for the amount of digital data that could be generated each year at just one BJC hospital, Barnes Hospital, which is the largest BJC facility (with 1000 licensed beds). Although the figures in this table have not been adjusted for data compression or other space-saving techniques, even if the estimates were reduced by 100-fold, no organization could afford to keep *all* the data *forever*.[4] Recognizing this fact, BJC must now address a number of critical questions:

- What data are to be migrated from a facility system into the clinical data repository? Only data with enterprise-wide value should appear in the enterprise-wide database. For example, although the microbiology system maintains a record of which laboratory technician read the antibiogram each morning, this information is not likely to be required outside a particular institution.
- Who decides what data have enterprise-wide value? Different physician constituencies are likely to have different data needs. How are these differences to be resolved?
- How long are data to be kept? Do all data stored in the repository need to be kept forever? Or can a policy of selective abstraction and purging be applied as data "age" over time? Can hourly blood pressures be replaced

TABLE **3.3.** Rough estimates of the volume of digital data created at Barnes Hospital and Mallinckrodt Institute of Radiology each year.[4]

Clinical data	7.5 gigaytes
Financial data	9.0 gigabytes
"Real-time" signals	2 terabytes
Digital still frame images	30 terabytes
Non-OB/GYN ultrasound (5 minute clips)	24 terabytes
OB/GYN ultrasound (5 minute clips)	36 terabytes

by daily or weekly high, low, and average blood pressures sometime after hospital discharge?

- Not all BJC facilities have the ability to record the same clinical data. Thus, some patient data may be available from one location but not from another. Can these differences be eliminated by the BJC central administration's information procurement priorities? If not, how can a physician distinguish nonexistent data (not captured at a facility) from nonrecorded data (not entered into the facility system)?
- How is the physician to be made aware of data that may be missing, purged, or modified?

The existence of data repository that unifies data currently scattered among independent systems raises questions about patient confidentiality, privacy, and access. Each facility currently establishes its own data confidentiality policy. However even within the same facility, different policies many be present depending on the access controls available on different hardware platforms, operating systems, or applications. A recent survey of five BJC facilities revealed markedly different policies regarding the automatic expiration of user passwords, automatic logoff on inactive terminals, logging of user activities, and dial-in security. The goal of Spectrum is to enable care-givers from any location within BJC to examine patient-specific data gathered at any other BJC facility. The issues surrounding confidentiality and privacy within a single institution are well recognized[5]; numerous additional concerns arise when data from multiple institutions are combined.[6] For example, what if a patient seeks an independent second opinion and wishes to keep knowledge of this encounter from his primary physician? If both physicians are part of the BJC network, the second-opinion encounter data will be available to the first physician as part of Project Spectrum.

The software technology used in Project Spectrum provides the capability for a wide range of security, access, and privacy policies. BJC has yet to establish an enterprise-wide security and access policy. When queried, physicians raise significant concerns about data security, but they also will not tolerate any impediment to data access.

As Project Spectrum begins to raise these tough organizational questions, BJC has had to form new multidisciplinary advisory committees. To date, many of the questions remain unanswered.

The Technical Challenge of Data Integration

For enterprises that choose to integrate rather than to replace disparate systems, there are two approaches are possible:

- Combine information from disparate data sources only at the time a query is made. We term this approach *dynamic integration*.

- Combine information from disparate data sources into a common data repository as new data are generated. Use the data repository directly to respond to a query request. We term this approach *static integration*.

As illustrated in Fig. 3.1, BJC has chosen the static integration approach.

There are compelling arguments for and against both dynamic and static integration. Static integration requires data to be stored twice (in the original data source and the data repository), requires mechanisms to ensure that changes made in the original system are promptly propagated to the repository, and requires that all queries be processed by the same database engine. On the positive side, network access must be ensured only to the repository, data stored in the repository are independent of the data purging policies of the source systems, and the response time for queries is more predictable.

Dynamic integration does not require redundant data storage, ensures that the returned data are the most current, and distributes to a large number of systems the task of responding to a query. On the negative side, dynamic integration requires live network links to all relevant systems at all times, has access to data only for as long as the source system saves the data, and provides a response to a query only as fast as the *slowest* queried system. Enterprise-wide data security and real-time clinical decision support are more difficult to implement with dynamic integration. Although the dynamic integration approach was developed first, more solutions based on the static integration approach are appearing as prices for electronic mass storage fall rapidly. As a sweeping generalization, it may be concluded that dynamic integration favors the rapid storage of data and static integration favors the rapid retrieval of data. Thus, settings in which data are frequently changed but infrequently queried are better served by dynamic integration; settings in which data are infrequently changed but frequently queried are better served by static integration. In Spectrum, we anticipate that data will be queried much more frequently than data will be changed.

Four critical components of the Project Spectrum architecture are illustrated in Fig. 3.1:

- The existing facilities' information systems;
- the interface engine;
- the data repository; and
- the end-user workstation.

Existing facilities' information systems consist of multiple applications running on multiple hardware platforms located in different facilities connected by separate networks (Table 3.2). Some systems have interfaces for data transfer; most do not. Even those systems with existing interfaces may have significant limitation; for example, only a restricted set of data may be available via the interface or timely data availability may be lacking (e.g., nightly batch transfer only). Not all systems can have network-aware, real-time interfaces. In the worst case, data are available only by electronically emulating an end-user terminal session and picking off the desired data elements using techniques called screen-scraping. The interface engine serves to buffer differences in interface capabilities and formats. The interface engine is responsible for accepting the facility system's messages in their current format, for reformatting the messages into a standardized format (HL7 Version 2.2),[7] and for guaranteeing the delivery of the messages to the repository using store-and-forward message transmission techniques.

Message formats and communications between existing facilities' systems and the interface engine are dictated largely by the capabilities of the source systems; communications between the interface engine and the data repository are based on two national standards: TCP/IP for networking protocols and HL7 Version 2.2 for message formatting rules. Despite standardizing data exchange based on widely published standards, a significant investment has been required to define the BJC implementation details of the HL7 Version 2.2 messages. Over 520 hours have been expended on an initial enterprise-wide definition of only eight HL7 segments. These eight segments contain 176 fields, some of which are complex entities requiring component-level definitions. In addition, 28 tables, which specify allowed values for various fields, had to be proposed, reviewed, and approved for enterprise-wide adoption. Even with this extensive level of effort, approximately 60 fields were not defined because they are not contained in our current Phase One data requirements.

The data repository is the focal point for enterprise-wide data integration. Its data model and structure must capture the key features of clinical data. Given the rapid changes in clinical care and the longevity of the data we wish to store in the repository, the data model must not become carved in stone. Yet designing a data model for unanticipated changes in medical practice and newly evolving medical concepts, while preserving access to historical patient data, is a formidable "cutting-edge" challenge. In Project Spectrum our approach has been to make extensive use of generalization and abstraction in our data model to keep the resulting structure flexible and robust while accommodating unique differences in stored entities and concepts.

To model the data elements contained in Phase One (Table 3.1), the current Spectrum extended entities-relationship (EER) data model contains 28 major entities, 41 relationships, and 230 attributes. A team of three data modelers and three physician experts have invested approximately 1000 hours creating the core EER model.

The clinical workstation is the ultimate "face" of Project Spectrum to the clinical community. No matter how good the underlying infrastructural technology, if the user interface does not meet end-user functional and usability needs, Project Spectrum will fail. Because of the high stakes involved in this component, significant resources have been devoted to this task. A cross-sectional end-user physician group from the six BJC facilities in Phase One has been formed. Using the technique of contextual analysis, over 300 hours of study and 1300 hours of secondary analysis have resulted in a 125-page detailed requirements and usability document. Not surprisingly, end-user demands are quite high — current technology cannot provide the entire set of 542 requirements. However by ranking requirements and carefully setting expectations with multiple milestones and prototypes, we are developing a workstation that meets the key clinical needs of a diverse set of demanding physicians.

An enormous task faced by data integration teams is the resolution of disparate vocabularies. Two systems may use the same term for completely different concepts; likewise, systems frequently use different terms for the same concept. More difficult to resolve are cases in which two systems use the same terms for similar but not identical concepts. For example, each of five hospitals in BJC has modelled the concept of a laboratory test called a complete blood count (CBC), yet *no two* of the hospitals include the same set of hematologic measurements within that test. Given these differences, what is the right "integrated" enterprise-wide definition for a CBC — the union or intersection or some other combination of measurements?

Many efforts to identify or construct a comprehensive standardized clinical nomenclature have been described.[8] At present, no single standard vocabulary is sufficient to describe detailed clinical findings. Our current starting vocabularies are SNOMED International,[9] and the Unified Medical Language System.[11]

Even standardized vocabularies do not solve the problem of standardized concept representation. For example, Evans illustrates the following four valid methods for encoding the clinical concept acute appendicitis in SNOMED[12]:

- DS-46210 — Acute appendicitis, NOS
- DS-46100 — Appendicitis, NOS
  G-A231 — Acute inflammation, NOS
- M-41000 — Acute
  G-C006 — In
  T-59200 — Appendix, NOS
- G-A231 — Acute
  M-40000 — Inflammation, NOS
  G-C006 — In
  T-59200 — Appendix, NOS

These differences in vocabulary codes and structures make it more difficult to integrate similar data from sources that may be using slightly different coding schemes and encoding rules.

Project Spectrum and Community Health Information Networks

In the absence of Project Spectrum, BJC Health System would need to invest significant resources to integrate its clinical information systems to generate CHIN-related data. When the Project Spectrum integrated infrastructure is in place, the generation of the administrative and clinical data usually shared within a CHIN will become markedly easier. By focusing BJC information system resources on the development of a comprehensive integrated information system infrastructure, Project Spectrum has ensured that participation of BJC in a CHIN will require only a marginal effort using the enterprise-wide clinical data repository. No claim is made that the Spectrum approach is either cheaper or easier than a more restricted approach to meeting CHIN data requirements. However, once the system is in place, the unified integrated data in the repository will enable aggressive strategic initiatives in clinical decision support, clinical process reengineering, outcomes measurement, and technology assessment. Thus, although the initial investment most certainly will be larger than that required to respond only to the needs of a CHIN, BJC Health System, Washington University and the Project Spectrum industry partners believe that the final return on this strategic investment will be far greater than that of a single-objective CHIN-based program.

Our ultimate return on investment will be based not only on the quality and quantity of data entered into the repository, but also on the quality and flexibility of the tools provided to explore those data and on BJC's commitment to exploit the results of studies that use these data. Information systems infrastructure and technology alone will never ensure the success of enterprise-wide integration. Only the sustained commitment of leaders, planners, and implementors to achieve true enterprise-wide clinical data integration will ensure success in providing high-quality efficient clinical care.

Acknowledgments. I wish to acknowledge the comments and critiques provided by members of the Section on Medical Informatics at Washington University, members of Project Spectrum, and the editors. Although I didn't use all of their comments — and they gave me more than I had hoped — those that I did use greatly improved the paper. This work was supported by Grants R29-LM05387 and U01-LM05845 from the National Library of Medicine and Grant U01-CA60267 from the National Cancer Institute.

References

1. Fritz KA, Kahn MG. Project Spectrum: An eighteen hospital enterprise-wide electronic medical record. In: Waegemann CP (ed.). *Toward an Electronic Patient Record '95: Eleventh International Symposium on the Creation of*

Electronic Health Record Systems. vol. 2. Orlando, Fl: Medical Records Institute; 1995:59–67.

2. Dick RS, Steen EB. (eds.). *The Computer-Based Patient Record: An Essential Technology for Health Care.* Washington DC: National Academy Press; 1991.
3. Kahn MG. Desktop database dilemma. *Acad Med.* 1993;68:34–37.
4. Kahn MG. The computer-based patient record and Robert Fulghum's sixteen principles. *MD Comput.* 1995;12(4):253–261.
5. Safran C, Rind D, Citroen M, Bakker AR, Slack WV, Bleich HL. Protection of confidentiality in the computer-based patient record. *MD Comput.* 1995;12(3):187–192.
6. Donaldson MS, Lohr KN. (eds.). *Health Data in the Information Age: Use, Disclosure, and Privacy.* Washington DC: National Academy Press; 1994.
7. Fitzmaurice JM. Health care data standards are required for medically effective use of workstations. *Int J Biomed Comput.* 1994;34:331–334.
8. Friedman C, Huff SM, Hersh WR, Pattison-Gordon E, Cimino JJ. The Canon Group's effort: Working toward a merged model. *JAMIA.* 1995;2(1):4–18.
9. Cote RA, Rothwell DJ, Beckett RS, Palotay JL. *SNOMED Internanational— The Systematized Nomenclature of Human and Veterinary Medicine.* Northfield IL: College of American Pathologists; 1993.
10. Rothwell DJ, Cote RA, Cordeau JP, Boisvert MA. Developing a standard data structure for medical language—The SNOMED proposal. In: Safran C (ed.). *Proceedings, Symposium on Computer Applications in Medical Care.* ACM Press; 1993:695–696.
11. Lindberg DA, Humphreys, BL, McCray AT. The Unified Medical Language System. *Meths Inf Med.* 1993;32(4):281–291.
12. Evans DA, Cimino JJ, Hersh WR, Huff SM, Bell DS. Toward a medical-concept representation language. *JAMIA.* 1994;1(3):207–217.

4

Patient-Computer Dialogue and the Patient's Right to Decide

WARNER V. SLACK

I had the good fortune to spend the 1960s at the University of Wisconsin in Madison. A wonderfully radical atmosphere—an atmosphere of strong social conscience and progressive ideology—pervaded the campus, and remarkable science was being done as well. Gobind Khorana was synthesizing a gene in a test tube, Howard Temin was postulating reverse transcriptase in RNA viruses, Milton Yatvin was gaining new understanding of the hormonal control of genetic expression, Harry Harlow was elucidating the psychological bonds between mother and infant, and Carl Rogers, in a small, two-story cottage on University Avenue, was evolving his theory of nondirective psychotherapy.

It was in this environment of receptivity to thinking that departed from the traditional that two ideas evolved in my mind. The first was that the computer could be used wisely and well in the practice of medicine. With its capacity to hold large amounts of data and execute multiple complex instructions with great speed and accuracy, the computer, I reasoned, would find an important role in both diagnosis and treatment. Wisconsin was an ideal place to pursue this line of reasoning. Investigators in a few institutions had begun to explore using the computer in diagnosis,[1-4] but using the computer in medicine under any circumstances was a radical departure from tradition, and concern about dehumanization and the demise of the art of medicine was expressed across the land.

The second idea, which I called "patient power" in the vernacular of the times, was based on the view that patients who want to should be encouraged to make their own clinical decisions.[5] For centuries, the medical profession had perpetrated paternalism as an essential component of medical care and thereby deprived patients of the self-esteem that comes from self-reliance. The assumption was that "the doctor knows best." I questioned this assumption. Why should the physician's perspective be considered superior to the patient's? Clearly, patient and physician may disagree on matters of politics and religion. Why not on matters of health and disease? Suppose they differ in personal values? As Shaw once said,

"Do not do unto others as you would that they should do unto you. Their tastes may not be the same."

If, I reasoned, physicians were willing to let go of the notion that they were responsible for controlling their patients, if they were willing to present possible plans of action in a step-by-step manner, patients could make informed decisions based on their own values. The clinician's province would then be the art and science of medicine; the patient's province would be the right to decide. I suggested that physicians stop thinking in terms of compliance, recognize the right of patients to make their own medical decisions, and help them to do so.[6]

Like computers, the idea of patient power was highly controversial for the times, and debates were frequently lively, among friends and enemies alike. In 1961, during a visit to our home in Madison, my brothers Charles took me to meet Carl Rogers, who had helped Charles in his work with violence among teenage gang members. This meeting was one of the turning points in my life. Rogers had introduced client-centered therapy to clinical psychology, and his support of patient power was the reinforcement I needed to persevere.

I had an opportunity to test these ideas in clinical practice at the University Hospitals in Madison, during neurology residency, and at Clark Air Base Hospital, during 2 years in the Philippines. Tentatively at first, and then with increasing enthusiasm, I shared my write-ups and notes with patients and encouraged them to join me in making medical decisions. I was convinced that medical records were much improved with patients' input. With license to write behind a patient's back, as is the tradition in Western medicine, errors that the patient could correct go uncorrected; furthermore, there is a natural tendency to find fault with the patient when difficulties arise—diagnoses such as "inadequate personality" would have disappeared quickly if patients had seen them early. It was also clear to me that decisions about diagnostic procedures, some of which were draconian in nature (the pneumoencephalogram, for example, was a common procedure in those days), and decisions about treatment were better made with patient input.

Out of the Air Force and back in Madison, I resumed my interest in clinical computing. (It did not occur to me then that the computer in medicine and patient power would become integrally related in my work.) My goal was to use the computer in diagnosis and treatment, but if the computer was to be of any help, good information—that is, from the medical history, the physical examination, and diagnostic studies—would have to be collected. My officemate, Philip Hicks, was working to automate clinical laboratories; I decided to start with the medical history. With Hicks, Lawrence Van Cura, and other colleagues, I hypothesized that we could program a computer to take a medical history directly from a patient. Our motivation came in part from the questions, Can a computer model the physician? Can it actually interview a patient? There were also practical motives. For the busy clinician, particularly in medically underserved areas, there was barely enough time to ask "Where does it hurt?," let alone all the other questions in the standard interview. In America, taking medical histories is a time-consuming and expensive process; in medicine, talk is not cheap.

At the time, self-administered paper questionnaires were being used with some success; the Cornell Medical Index[1] and the "multiphasic" questionnaire of the Permanente Medical Group provided standardized, consistent, and inexpensive methods of taking medical histories.[4] And many good self-administered questionnaires are used. Questionnaires, however, cannot be tailored to the individual situation because they permit no interaction. They provide no mechanism to clarify the patient's meaning or qualify answers about symptoms. If the patient answers "yes" to the question, "Have you ever coughed up blood?," this could mean a speck from the nose 10 years ago or a massive hemoptysis last week. The patient may misunderstand a question (and thereby give an erroneous answer), inadvertently skip a question, or lose one or more pages of the questionnaire.

After considering the attributes of the available questionnaires and the problems of the physician as a history-taker, we decided to embark upon our computer project. Our idea was to incorporate into the program some of the advantages of the physician interviewer: the ability to explore abnormal findings in detail and to personalize the interview in an appropriate, dignified, and considerate dialogue with the patient. At the same time, we wanted the advantages of the questionnaire: completeness, standardization, and economy. We hoped that individual computer-based histories would be helpful to patients and their physicians; we hoped that the computer would be of interest to patients (perhaps even enjoyable); and we hoped that the pooled responses to the interviews would help us learn more about the medical history and the process of clinical interviewing.[7,8]

In spite of the homage paid to the medical history, there has been little research on the subject. Neither the method of history taking and recording nor the reliability and usefulness of the data collected have been studied thoroughly. We hoped that the computer could help.[7,8]

Beginnings of the Computer-Based History

Preliminary Research

Some of our colleagues considered the idea radical. Those who questioned the use of computers in medicine under any circumstances were particularly concerned about the use of the computer to take a medical history. Some said it could not be done. Others wondered if it *should* be done; still others said that patients would find the idea offensive and would refuse to be interviewed by a computer, regardless of the nature of the program.

When I discussed the idea with patients, however, they were enthusiastic.

"It sounds like fun" and "I'd like to try my hand with a computer" were typical responses, particularly if (as was most often the case) they had never seen a computer. Their one concern was that the computer might try to do an "intelligence" test; they didn't like intelligence tests. I assured them that I didn't either, and that I certainly did not want our computer to do intelligence testing. If anything, I wanted the computer to *do away* with intelligence testing.[9] They seemed relieved.

We decided to start with allergies for our first computer-based history. This seemed a neutral, inoffensive subject for a computer; furthermore, it is a subject of great medical importance and diagnosis relies heavily on the medical history; finally, our allergist consultant, Charles Reed, gave his enthusiastic support. We also thought (mistakenly) that an allergy history would be short. By the time we called a halt to expansion (Charles is very thorough), there were over 500 questions in the program.

It was Philip Hicks who suggested that we use the laboratory instrument computer (LINC) for our study. He was already using the LINC to develop his programs, the first of their kind, for use in the clinical laboratories at the University of Wisconsin Hospitals.[10] This small, general-purpose digital computer was developed at the Massachusetts Institute of Technology in 1962 by Wesley Clark, Charles Molnar, and their colleagues[11]; it was a pioneering machine, and in many respects the forerunner of today's personal computers.[12] Flexibility and ease of operation were stressed in the development of the LINC; and the individual user could exert maximum control over the computer—a major departure from the batch-processing brontosaurs of the day. Designed to interact with the environment, the LINC was equipped with relays, sense switches, sense lines, analog-to-digital conversion channels, toggle switches, cathode-ray oscilloscope, typewriter keyboard, and teletype printer; thus, it was well suited for "online" collection and "realtime" processing of experimental data. It was widely used in neurophysiological laboratories where it could be pro-grammed to initiate stimuli, receive responses, and then alter subsequent stimuli contingent upon the responses received. This was a "hands-on" computer; the wires were all hanging out, so to speak. There were no computing committees or subcommittees, no director of computing (or in modern, military-like parlance, chief information officer), no Mr. Binary telling you to keep out or not to touch. Users loved it!

Our plan was to program the LINC to communicate with the patient by means of questions, explanations, requests, and comments displayed on the cathode-ray screen; the patient, in turn, could communicate with the computer by means of the typewriter keyboard. The LINC had a very small memory by today's standards—1024 12-bit words—barely enough to hold the text for one question, together with the instructions in the program that told the computer what to do. (The off-the-shelf PC of today brings with it about 4000 times as much memory as the LINC.) Two magnetic tape drives, which could turn equally well in either direction, provided storage space for text and instructions that were not in use, and these could quickly be called into memory when needed.

The LINC was slow by today's standards, and the time between iterative instructions within the computer to display a character on the screen — time in which the computer was executing other instructions, such as commands to display other characters — resulted in a flicker that became increasingly noticeable as the number of characters increased. There was reason, therefore, to keep the questions short, and this electronically imposed succinctness had a beneficial effect on the quality of our prose.

We used one of the original LINCs, which had been brought to the University of Wisconsin's neurophysiology laboratory by Joseph Hind. The machine was in great demand, and programming time during the day was scarce; we did most of our work between 10 at night and 8 in the morning. Within a few months we had the program written and working well, but we found ourselves continuing to make revisions. Most of these were minor and, in retrospect, inconsequential, and eventually I had to own up to the fact that I was procrastinating. It had been fun to talk about a computer that could take a medical history, to shock the traditionalists, and to argue with the skeptics, but to try it with a real patient — that was another matter.

The time came, however, when I decided it was now or never. I approached one of our medical interns, who seemed amused by the idea; he had been deprived of sleep, and the thought of being replaced by a computer, at least at night, had a distinct appeal. He suggested a patient who might be willing to help, an elderly man who was recovering from a heart attack and was now up and about, getting ready to go home. I went to his room, introduced myself, told him the general idea of the project, explained that I didn't know how well it would work, and asked if he would give us a hand. He replied that he would try anything once, and walked with me to the medical sciences building, where the LINC was housed. (Fortunately, there was a free hour at lunchtime for us to try our first interview. Game as he was, I couldn't have expected our volunteer to "talk" to the computer at 2 in the morning.) I turned on the machine, spun in the program from tape, turned off the lights (the dim characters on the screen were easier to read in the dark), pressed the start button, and stepped back to observe.

The tapes churned, and "HAVE YOU EVER HAD HIVES?" appeared on the screen. The characters flickered, the lights on the console flashed on and off, and the LINC's speaker emitted an eerie, high-pitched sound. On the other side of the sheetrock partition, people were walking in and out, and a cat was meowing (we had the computer, but its owners were still doing a cat brain experiment). It was somewhat like Kafka's *Castle* or Koestler's *Darkness at Noon*. Clearly, these were not optimal circumstances for a medical interview.

Yet my new-found friend seemed oblivious to his surroundings. He got going at the keyboard, responding to the questions appropriately, and after a while it became clear that there was (I could think of no other word for it) *rapport* between man and machine. He laughed out loud at some of the comments from the computer. (Some I had intended to be funny; some I hadn't.) And he talked out loud to the machine, sometimes in praise and sometimes in criticism. "That was a dumb question," he noted with a chuckle, "You already asked me that!" He was right, of course; it was my error (although I rationalized that we could use the results to check for test-retest reliability), yet he never would have said this to me face to face, a doctor with a white coat and Bakelite nametag.

For most patients, even today, the physician seems an authoritarian figure. By contrast, the computer did not seem at all authoritarian to this man, who was comfortable with it and felt free to be critical. At the conclusion of his interview, he turned to me and said, "You know, I really like your computer better than some of those doctors over in the hospital." Surprised, I asked him why. "Well, for one thing, I'm sort of deaf and have trouble hearing them," he answered.

For each of the possible responses to the computer's questions, we had developed phrases that could be printed when applicable. (To appease those who clung to professional mystique, we converted words such as "hives" and "hay fever" to "urticaria" and "allergic rhinitis.") The computer was programmed to print these phrases—in a legible but otherwise traditional format—as a summary for use by the physician. When our first patient had completed his interview, I was relieved to hear the teletype chatter as it began to print; the summary program was working. The patient then turned to me and said, "What's happening? May I read that?" I could not think of any reason why he shouldn't. Once again, the computer was helping him to assert himself as a patient. As he started to read, he commented suddenly, in reference to some details about his hay fever: "No, that's wrong; I didn't mean that," and he then proceeded to pick up a number of other errors. Clearly, there were mistakes in the interview. Yet if he hadn't asked to read his summary, I never would have known.

We learned our lesson, and since that time have asked our patients (whenever they are willing) to read their summaries and help us edit their medical histories and improve our computer-based interviews. And patients' criticisms have been most helpful over the years. With the computer as well as the doctor, it is demeaning to patients to write about them behind their backs, and when we do so we perpetuate errors that could be corrected.

Encouraged by the results of this first interview, we did a more formal study.[7] Fifty hospitalized patients volunteered to have their allergy histories taken. In each case, the results of the computer's history as printed out on the teletype were compared with the allergy history recorded in the hospital chart by the medical student, intern, and resident attending the patient. There were no false negatives with the computer interview. None of the patients' charts mentioned an allergy that was not also described by the computer. For patients whose charts gave no indication of allergies, the computer elicited 2 cases of asthma, 7 cases of hay fever, 12 cases of hives, and 1 case of allergy to penicillin. (In this instance, a mention of rash in association with penicillin was tucked away in the medical student's work-up but was impossible to find unless the entire work-up was read; the intern's note said "no allergies.") In another case, the mention of "penicillin allergy" in the chart was insufficient to determine whether an allergy actually existed, whereas the computer described the single reaction in detail and left no doubt that a serum-sickness type of reaction had occurred. All drug reactions were described in more detail by the computer than by the students and physicians. On the other hand, the computer elicited and printed out some false positive information, such as an allergic reaction to phenobarbital that was later described by the patient as "excessive grogginess."

As we had hoped, almost all of the patients found their interaction with the computer interesting and enjoyable. When asked to compare the computer with physicians in their experience, 20 patients had no preference, 12 indicated a preference for physician-taken histories and, to our surprise, 18 indicated a preference for the computer-based system.

Subsequent Studies

Heartened by these early results, we continued to study computer-based medical histories in our laboratories at the University of Wisconsin and then at the Beth Israel Hospital in Boston. We developed and evaluated a general review of systems (in French and Spanish, as well as English) and histories for patients with problems such as uterine cancer, epilepsy, and headache.[13-16] We also ventured into a field that was somewhat more controversial: We developed a psychiatric history, designed as a general review of behavioral problems, and gave it to 69 volunteers who had been scheduled for psychiatric evaluation.[17] As with other computer histories, the patients reacted favorably. Once again, slightly more patients preferred the computer as an interviewer to physicians (some patients, however, responded "yes" to preferring the physician *and* "yes" to preferring the computer, apparently not wanting to hurt the feelings of either and nicely demonstrating that human beings are not always Aristotelian in their logic). They generally found the computer to be more thorough.

A finding of great interest to us in those early days of patient-computer dialogue,[18] one since corroborated by further study,[19-26] was that patients often were more comfortable in communicating information to the computer about potentially embarrassing matters such as sexual activity and emotional problems than they would have been in talking to their physicians.

During this period, others were also working actively in the field. A general medical history, with emphasis on the review of systems, was developed at the Mayo Clinic, and both patients and physicians reacted favorably. The computer obtained 95% of the information about symptoms recorded in the traditional medical record.[27] Another general medical history was developed at the Massachusetts General Hospital, where patients also reacted favorably.[28] Physicians' attitudes were mixed, but the computer's summaries were in good agreement with the physicians' own findings. A general medical history was also tried at the LDS Hospital in Salt Lake City.[29] With this history, Bayes' theorem was used to make diagnostic suggestions on the basis of patients' responses to the computer. Meanwhile, other investigators were developing and evaluating histories in specialty areas, such as psychiatry and psychology,[30-33] nutrition,[34] headache,[35] venereal disease,[36] and allergy.[37] The field of computer-based interviewing remains active today.[38-47]

Patient Power and Dialogue with a Computer

The Debate

The idea of a computer taking a medical history can evoke worrisome thoughts: *2001: A Space Odessey, Terminal Man, Invasion of the Body Snatchers,* Orwellian thought control. Yet the experience of our first patient (and the majority of patients who have subsequently engaged in dialogue with our computers) was the opposite of what some had predicted. This man had *gained* control, not lost it. For the first time in his role as a patient, *he* was in charge; he was master of his own history. And in his world of deafness he could communicate particularly well with the machine.

In the spring of 1970, I presented my ideas on patient power to the "Second Conference on the Diagnostic Process," held at the University of Michigan in Ann Arbor.[3] Those in attendance were divided in their reaction, and the ensuing debate was heated. The moderator, John Romano (Chair of the Department of Psychiatry at the University of Rochester) staunchly defended the right of the physician to direct the patient ("patients want to be told what to do"); on the other hand, Leonard Savage (Professor of Statistics at Yale) said that he "was particularly pleased to hear the bold and radical defense of the thesis that medical values should be those of the patient."[48] The debate was to continue through the 1970s — Franz Ingelfinger, editor of the *New England Journal of Medicine,* rejected my article, "The Patient's Right to Decide," making it clear that he strongly disagreed with my position. On the other hand, Ian Monroe, editor of the *Lancet* (to whom I will be forever grateful), sent me an encouraging letter of acceptance and published my article forthwith. During those decades of debate, all agreed that when it came to dialogue between patient and computer, the patient should be in charge. Ironically, it was easier to transfer control to the patient by means of an automaton than by means of the physician.

The Computer as a Patient's Assistant

In my view, the largest, yet least used health care resource worldwide is the patient or prospective patient, and the interactive computer can be used to enlighten patients and empower them in the health care process, thereby improving the quality of care while reducing the cost.[49,50] There are a number of common important medical problems, such as sore throat and urinary tract infection, that patients could manage alone if they were provided with the clinical information to do so. Whether clinical management, preventive or remedial, is the responsibility of the clinician or the patient is often dictated by forces of supply and demand. If, for example, the biochemistry of insulin or the physiology of the pancreas were such that a child with juvenile diabetes needed only one insulin injection per year, it is likely that an academic endocrinologist in a teaching hospital would give the injection, and at considerable expense. If the child needed an injection every 6 months, the pediatric diabetologist would give it; if every 3 months, the primary care physician; and if once a month, the nurse practitioner. But because the child needs the insulin at least once a day, the parent or child is responsible for administering the injection, without assistance. And the parent or child usually does this skillfully, conveniently, and at low cost.

In our laboratory in the Center for Clinical Computing, at Harvard Medical School and Boston's Beth Israel Hospital, we have studied the use of the interactive computer as a patient's assistant in a variety of health-related areas. In psychiatry and psychology, where schools of talking therapy generally consider the doctor-patient relationship to be essential to the therapeutic process, my brother, Charles Slack, and I and our colleagues have demonstrated that people will speak to a computer, in the absence of a therapist, about matters of importance to them and in some instances feel they have benefitted from the experience.[19] When we programmed a computer interview to facilitate soliloquy, we found that when encouraged by the computer, subjects talked easily into a microphone, first about anxiety-provoking circumstances and then about relaxation.[25] As an indication of the effectiveness of the program, both mean heart rate and state anxiety scores of the 42 volunteers fell significantly from the beginning to the end of the interview.

In the field of nutrition, we developed a three-part dietary counseling interview that asked questions about general dietary behavior, elicited details of food intake on an average day, and planned with the patient a weight-reducing diet of approximately 1500 kcal.[51] During the interview, the program offered dietary suggestions and, on completion, generated a printed summary for use by patients and nutritionists. In a study with 64 volunteers (32 men and 32 women), each with the diagnosis of simple overweight, the automated counseling interview was found to assist patients in organizing their thoughts about eating and in planning their own dietary behavior, and to assist nutritionists when they subsequently met with the patients.[52] In addition, patients found their time with the computer to be pleasant and personalizing. An updated version of the program is currently in routine use in Beth Israel Hospital.[53]

We have also developed a program to assist women in caring for an uncomplicated urinary tract infection. The program takes a history of the present illness (e.g., "Are you bothered by pain or burning when you urinate?"), performs a review of systems, interprets laboratory data, suggests referral when additional medical problems are indicated, tests the reliability of important questions by repeating them, resolves uncertainties that the patient may have (e.g., when the patient does not understand a question), advises about diagnosis and treatment,[54] explains the therapeutic options in the order of importance to the patient, offers opportunities to review information previously presented, offers the opportunity to decide about therapy (e.g., whether to start with sulfa immediately or to wait until the results of the urine culture are available), writes a prescription, prints a progress note for the chart and reminders for the patient, schedules follow-up visits, conducts follow-up interviews, and helps to guide the progress of therapy. In a randomized clinical trial, the program performed well, to the satisfaction of the patients who volunteered to participate and the clinicians who designed the study. In particular, patients liked being able to make their own decisions about treatment, even though most of their decisions conformed to what a physician in a traditional setting would have recommended.

We also developed a computer-administered health screening interview for the employees of Beth Israel Hospital.[50] The interview is part of the integrated Center for Clinical Computing (CCC) clinical information system used throughout the hospital, and it is available on any of over 3000 terminals. Conducted in private and with protection of confidentiality, the interview seeks information on medical problems and patterns of living for which behavioral change is considered desirable and offers suggestions and advice on matters of health and illness. The interview begins with words of welcome, information about how to proceed, a brief discussion of the purpose of the program ("We hope we can help you discover how your life style affects your health and what you can do to improve your health"), and assurances that all responses will be kept in confidence and made available to clinicians only at the employee's request. Next there is a series of frames that teach the inexperienced user how to operate the computer terminal, how to change answers and back up to previous questions, and how to indicate uncertainty—by choosing "don't understand" or "maybe (don't know)"—and reluctance to respond—by choosing "skip it." The interview itself begins with a section that elicits demographic information, with emphasis on the circumstances of each participant's employment at the hospital. The computer then lists the seven sections of the interview (General Medical History, Nutrition History, Exercise Patterns, Habits, Safety, Environment, and Stress) and offers participants the opportunity to select sections in order of personal preference.

As each section is completed, the program offers to display a summary of the information provided, and at the end of the interview, the program offers a clinical evaluation of problems that could be favorably influenced by changes in behavior. In addition, en route through the interview the program offers information about referral services. If, for example, a person indicates that he or she is depressed, the program provides the names and telephone numbers of places to turn to for help—the Employee Assistance Program, the Samaritans, and the hospital's emergency room.

Over a 5.5-year period ending in November 1995, 2586 employees completed the interview. Eighty-five percent of the employees expressed an interest in the health-related programs offered by the hospital: 73 percent were interested in the fitness center, and 38 percent in the stress-reduction program. Stress and unhappiness were common: 57 percent of the employees reported high levels of stress, and 43 percent reported feeling sad, discouraged, or hopeless in the previous month; 6 percent indicated that life sometimes did not seem worth living. These are difficult times for many people in this country, as illustrated by these findings. We hope these employees moved quickly to avail themselves of the opportunity offered by the computer-based interview to obtain help for their problems.[50]

The Patient in Control

Over the years, we have incorporated into our programs a number of provisions designed to yield control to the patient in dialogue with the computer. In a typical interview, we request permission to proceed (e.g., "May we call you by your first name?" and "Would it be OK with you if we asked a few questions about your emotions?") and do our best to respect the patient's priorities, to respect the patient's right to decide (by offering sufficient alternatives), to respect the patient's right *not* to decide, to help with uncertainty (by offering "don't know" and "don't understand" options, with explanations when appropriate), and to respect a reluctance to respond. Communication between patient and computer (and patient and doctor, as well) should not be used to persuade the patient to answer questions the doctor deems important; rather, it should be used to outline the medical reasons for the questions so that patients can decide for themselves whether they wish to answer.[6,8] Patients should not have to answer questions against their will. In Wisconsin, we incorporated a "none of your damn business" option into the questions. We have since toned it down to "skip it," better accepted in Boston. An expanded set of responses to yes/no type questions—(1) yes, (2) no, (3) don't know (maybe), (4) don't understand, and (5) skip it—enables patients to indicate uncertainty and lack of comprehension, to request clarification, and to bypass questions they don't care to answer. This reduces the number of uninformed responses and the coercion that may lead to inconsistency, subterfuge, and decreased validity. Most of our computer-based interviews also employ, to some extent, other mutually exclusive numbered choices, multiple choices with more than one acceptable response, and free-text responses.[8]

Conclusion

If patient-computer dialogue is eventually demonstrated to be useful in health care (and I hope that it will be, among people of all socioeconomic backgrounds), it can be made available to patients at school, at work, and at home, in addition to physicians' offices and clinics. The chess program in use at the University of Wisconsin[55] and the outreach program at Case Western Reserve University in Cleveland[56] are excellent examples of the helpfulness of interactive computing for patients with serious chronic problems, such as breast cancer and AIDS.

Our experience suggests that concern about the computer as a depersonalizing influence in dialogue with patients[57] is unfounded.[7,8,17,18] Computer interaction thus far has been pleasant, interesting, informative, and empowering for most patients, and it has been effective in helping them both to help themselves and to help their doctors.[58]

References

1. Brodman K, Van Woerkom AJ, Erdmann AJ Jr, Goldstein LS. Interpretation of symptoms with a data-processing machine. *Arch Intern Med.* 1959;103:776–782.
2. Warner HR, Toronto AF, Veasey LG, Stephenson R. A mathematical approach to medical diagnosis: Application to congenital heart disease. *JAMA* 1961;177(3):177–183.
3. Jacquez JA. *The diagnostic process: Proceedings of conference held at the University of Michigan.* Ann Arbor, Mich: Malloy Lithographing; 1964.
4. Collen MF, Rubin L, Neyman J, Dantzig GB, Baer RM, Siegelaub AB. Automated multiphasic screening and diagnosis. *Am J Public Health.* 1964;54:741–750.
5. Slack WV. Patient power. In: Jacquez JA (ed.). *Computer diagnosis and diagnostic methods: The proceedings of the second conference on the diagnostic process held at the University of Michigan.* Springfield, Ill: CC Thomas; 1972:3–7.
6. Slack WV. The patient's right to decide. *Lancet.* 1977;2:240.
7. Slack, WV, Hicks GP, Reed CE, Van Cura LJ. A computer-based medical history system. *N Engl J Med.* 1966;274:194–198.
8. Slack WV. A history of computerized medical interviews. *MD Comput.* 1984;1(5):52–59.
9. Slack WV. Measurement of intelligence: Misplaced trust and the lure of

prophecy. *MD Comput.* 1985;12(5):363-372.

10. Hicks GP, Gieschen MM, Slack WV, Larson FC. Routine use of a small digital computer in the clinical laboratory. *JAMA*. 1966;196:973-978.

11. Clark WA, Molnar CE. A description of the LINC. In: Stacy RW, Waxman BD (eds.). *Computers in Biomedical Research*. vol. 2. New York: Academic Press; 1965:35-65.

12. Bleich HL. Wesley A. Clark, Charles E. Molnar, and the LINC. *MD Comput.* 1994;11(5):269-270.

13. Slack WV, Van Cura LJ. Computer-based patient interviewing. Parts I & II. *Postgraduate Med.* 1968;43:68-74 and 115-120.

14. Peckham BM, Slack WV, Carr WF, Van Cura LJ, Scultz AE. Computerized data collection in the management of uterine cancer. *Clin Obstet Gynecol.* 1967;10:1003-1015.

15. Chun RWM, Van Cura LJ, Spencer M, Slack WV. Computer interviewing of patients with epilepsy. *Epilepsia.* 1976;17:371-375.

16. Bana DS, Leviton A, Swidler C, Slack WV, Graham JR. A computer-based headache interview: Acceptance by patients and physicians. *Headache.* 1980;20:85-89.

17. Maultsby MC, Slack WV. A computer-based psychiatry history system. *Arch Gen Psychiatry.* 1971;25:570-572.

18. Slack WV, Van Cura LJ. Patient reaction to computer-based medical interviewing. *Comput Biomed Res.* 968;1:527-531.

19. Slack WV, Slack CW. Patient-computer dialogue. *N Engl J Med.* 1972;286:1304-1309.

20. Van Cura LJ, Jensen NM, Greist JH, Lewis WR, Frey SR. Venereal disease: Interviewing and teaching by computer. *Am J Public Health.* 1975;65:1159-1164.

21. Lucas RW, Mullin PJ, Luna CBX, McInroy DC. Psychiatrists and a computer as interrogators of patients with alcohol-related illnesses: A comparison. *Br J Psychiatry.* 1977;131:160-167.

22. Greist JH, Klein MH. Computer programs for patients, clinicians, and researchers in psychiatry. In: Sidowski JB, Johnson JH, Williams TA (eds.). *Technology in Mental Health Care Delivery Systems.* Norwood, Conn: Ablex; 1980:161-182.

23. Carr AC, Ghosh A, Aneill RJ. Can a computer take a psychiatric history? *Psychol Med.* 1983;13:151-158.

24. Millstein SG, Irwin CE Jr. Acceptability of computer-acquired sexual histories in adolescent girls. *J Pediatr.* 1983;103:815-819.

25. Slack WV, Porter D, Balkin P, Kowaloff HB, Slack CW. Computer-assisted soliloquy as an approach to psychotherapy. *MD Comput.* 1990;7:37-58.

26. Locke EL, Kowaloff HB, Hoff RG, et al. Computer-based interview for screening blood donors for risk of HIV transmission. *JAMA.* 1982;268:1301-1305.

27. Mayne JG, Weksel W, Sholtz PN. Toward automating the medical history. *Mayo Clin Proc.* 1968;43:1-25.

28. Grossman JH, Barnett GO, McGuire MT, Swedlow DB. Evaluation of computer-acquired patient histories. *JAMA.* 1971;215(8):1286-1291.

29. Warner HR, Rutherford BD, Houtchens BA. A sequential Bayesian approach to history taking and diagnosis. *Comp Biomed Res.* 1972;5:256-262.

30. Greist JH, Klein MH, Van Cura LJ. A computer interview for psychiatric patient target symptoms. *Arch Gen Psychiatry.* 1973;29:247-253.

31. Greist JH, Gustafson DH, Erdman HP, Taves JE, Klein MH, Speidel SD. Suicide risk prediction by computer interview: A prospective study. *Am J Psychiatry.* 1973;130:1327–1332.
32. Coddington RD, King TL. Automated history taking in child psychiatry. *Am J Psychiatry.* 1972;129:52–58.
33. Angle HV, Johnsen T, Grebenkemper NS, Ellinwood EH. Computer interview support of clinicians. *Prof Psychology.* 1979;Feb:49–57.
34. Evans S, Gormican A. The computer in retrieving dietary history data. *J Am Dietet A.* 1973;63:397–407.
35. Stead WW, Heyman A, Thompson HK, Hammond WE. Computer assisted interview of patients with functional headaches. *Arch Intern Med.* 1972;129:1–12.
36. Van Cura LJ, Jensen NM, Greist JH, Lewis WR, Frey SR. Venereal disease: Interviewing and teaching by computer. *Am J Public Health.* 1975;65:1159–1164.
37. Gottlieb GL, Beers RF, Bernecker C, Samter M. An approach to automation of medical interviews. *Comp Biomed Res.* 1972;5:99–107.
38. Erdman HP, Klein MH, Greist JH. Direct patient computer interviewing. *J Consult Clin Psych.* 1985;53:760–773.
39. Quaak MJ, Westerman RF, Schout JA, Hasman A, van Bemmel JH. Patient appreciations of computerized medical interviews. *Med Info.* 1986;11:339–350.
40. Houziaux MO, Lefebve PJ. Historical and methodological aspects of computer-assisted medical history taking. *Med Info.* 1986;11:129–143.
41. Linberg G, Seensalu R, Nilsson LH, Forsell P, Kagar L, Nkill-Jones RP. Transferability of a computer system for medical history taking and decision support in dyspepsia: A comparison of indicants for peptic ulcer disease. *Scand J Gastroenterol.* 1987;128:190–196.
42. Haug PJ, Warner WR, Clayton PD, et al. A decision-driven system to collect the patient history. *Comput Biomed Res.* 1987;20:193–207.
43. Pringle M. Using computers to take patient histories. *BMJ.* 1988;297:697–698.
44. Slack WV, Leviton A, Bennett SE, Fleischmann KH, Lawrence RS. Relation between age, education, and time to respond to questions in a computer-based medical interview. *Comp Biomed Res.* 1988;21:78–84.
45. Lutner RE, Roizen MF, Stocking CB, et al. The automated interview versus the personal interview. Do patient responses to preoperative health questions differ? *Anesthesiology.* 1991;75(3):394–400.
46. Hasley S. A comparison of computer-based personal interviews for the gynecologic history update. *Obstet Gynecol.* 1995;84(4):494–498.
47. Wald JS, Rind D, Safran C, Kowaloff H, Barker R, Slack WV. Patient entries in the electronic medical record: An interactive interview used in primary care. In: Gardner RM (ed.). *JAMIA: The Proceedings of the Nineteenth Annual Symposium on Computer Applications in Medical Care.* Philadelphia: Hanley & Belfus; 1995:147–151.
48. Savage LJ. Diagnosis and the Bayesian viewpoint. In: Jacquez JA (ed.). *Computer Diagnosis and Diagnostic Methods: The Proceedings of the Second Conference on the Diagnostic Process Held at the University of Michigan.* Springfield, Ill: CC Thomas; 1972:131–138.
49. Slack WV. Patient counseling by computer. In: Zoog S, Yarnall S (eds.). *The Changing Health Care Team.* Seattle: Medical Communications and Services Association; 1976:108–111.

50. Slack WV, Safran C, Kowaloff HB, Pearce J, Delbanco TL. A computer-administered health screening interview for hospital personnel. *MD Comput.* 1995;12(1):25–30.
51. Witschi J, Porter D, Vogel S, Buxbaum R, Stare FJ, Slack W. A computer-based dietary counseling system. *J Am Dietet A.* 1976;69:385–390.
52. Slack W, Porter D, Witschi J, Sullivan M, Buxbaum R, Stare F. Dietary interviewing by computer: An experimental approach to counseling. *J Am Dietet A.* 1976;69:514–517.
53. Witschi JC, Kowaloff HB, Slack WV. An interactive dietary interview for hospital employees. *MD Comput.* 1993;103:815–819.
54. Fisher LA, Johnson TS, Porter D, Bleich HL, Slack WV. Collection of a clean voided urine specimen: A comparison among spoken, written, and computer-based instructions. *Am J Public Health.* 1977;67:640–644.
55. Gustafson DH, Bosworth K, Hawkins RP, Boberg EW, Bricker E. CHESS: A computer-based system for providing information, referrals, decision support and social support to people facing medical and other health-related crises. In: Frisse ME (ed.). *AMIA: Proceedings of the Sixteenth Annual Symposium on Computer Applications in Medical Care.* Baltimore;161–165.
56. Brennan PF, Ripich S, Moore SM. The use of home-based computers to support persons living with AIDS/ARC. *J Commun Health Nurs.* 1991;8(1):3–14.
57. Weizenbaum JE. *Computer Power and Human Reason.* San Francisco: WH Freeman; 1976.
58. Slack WV. The computer and the doctor-patient relationship. *MD Comput.* 6(6):320–321.

[From the Center for Clinical Computing, Harvard Medical School, Beth Israel Hospital, and Brigham and Women's Hospital, Boston.

I am indebted to my many colleagues at the Center for Clinical Computing, Harvard Medical School, Beth Israel and Brigham and Women's hospitals, and the University of Wisconsin, who have been so helpful to me over the years.]

[Adapted in part from the *New England Journal of Medicine* (174:194–8, 1966), Zoog S, Yarnall S, eds. The changing health care team: improving effectiveness in patient care (Seattle: Medical Communications and Services Association, 1976, 108–11), *The Lancet* (July: 240, 1977), *M.D. Computing* (1:52–9, 68, 1984 and 12:25–30, 1995), and CyberMedicine (Jossey-Bass, in press) with the permission of the publishers.]

Section II

Linking Organizations

For Section II, we enlisted authors associated with some of the very first information networks that tie together the organizations in the health care field. These authors tell of the unexpected pitfalls and the successes that they encountered in their groundbreaking work. Their experiences can guide those who follow them.

At first, it seems intuitively obvious that physicians, hospitals, pharmacies, and insurers would want to share information more freely. They need information from each other to carry out their roles. Now that the technology for establishing computer networks has matured, there is no question that the players in the health care field can network; the question has shifted to how and to what ends they will network.

In Section II, the authors outline the basic issues facing any group that is developing a CHIN, and the drawbacks and advantages of the various approaches. The issues are basic indeed: What information should be shared in a CHIN? Who will be the information providers, and who will be the information users? How will security be ensured? How will organizations request and retrieve information? How can computer systems that were not designed to communicate with each other be made to do so quickly? Even the user interface—the way the computer screen appears— must be designed in a way that is acceptable to a large number of users with diverse preferences.

Moreover, there are several very basic business decisions when a CHIN is established. Who will own the CHIN? The authors in Section II contrast CHINs that are run by consortia of private organizations and those that are run collaboratively by private firms and governmental agencies. A more basic question facing any new CHIN is, what does ownership entail— simply ownership of the physical networking equipment, or the right to determine who participates in the CHIN, and what information is made available at what time?

Section II begins with descriptions of the approaches taken by the Wisconsin Health Information Network and the Washington State Community Health Management Information System, two of the earliest community health networks. In some ways, the developers of the two systems arrived at similar conclusions: Development of the networks proceeded most smoothly when it took into account the needs and opinions of the participants who were financing the system. A relatively slow, incremental approach to development worked best.

The remainder of Section II discusses how information networks can change the way health care organizations collaborate once the linkages are in place. Chapter 7 shows how public health workers who are geographically dispersed and working within different specialties can collaborate when they are electronically linked. Networks like CDC WONDER, INPHO, and SCARCNET have enabled public health workers to coordinate their responses to many problems, ranging from natural disasters to teenage smoking.

Chapter 8 describes the way computer networking has fundamentally changed the way many cities have organized their drug abuse treatment systems. Where once drug abuse treatment facilities competed for patients and seldom shared data about patients' prior treatments, now their efforts are coordinated by a central intake facility. Since patient data is readily available through a computer network, patients can be quickly referred to the most appropriate treatments. Information networks have fundamentally changed the community-wide approach to drug abuse treatment, and have the potential to impact the community-wide approach to many other health issues.

5

Information Infrastructure for Health Communities: The Wisconsin Health Information Network

Kim R. Pemble

Community or Regional Health Information Networks are being discussed, evaluated or implemented in many communities across the country. Regardless of the name, the challenges to successful implementation as well as the benefits that may be realized are similar in all communities. This chapter presents the Wisconsin Health Information Network (WHIN) as a successful model of a Community Health Information Network (CHIN). Specifically, issues including the conceptualization of a CHIN, ownership models, implementation challenges, security and benefits are presented, and lessons learned and special projects in which WHIN is participating are discussed.

Problem Definition

Our society has become more fluid in many respects. People change employers more frequently, moving constitutes city to city or even state to state as often as across town. To address changing requirements, health care and otherwise, and better manage resources, employers change health care plans, which means that employees change providers. Regrettably, where the patient goes, the medical record does not necessarily follow. Further, demands for more convenient and more easily accessible care, combined with the migration towards ever-increasing outpatient services, are making accessible medical information increasingly important at the very time that it is becoming more difficult to access and integrate.[1] Wilensky and Rossiter noted in 1983 that 90 percent of all health care costs are the consequence of physician decisions (56 percent in ambulatory settings).[2] This ambulatory figure has certainly risen substantially in the past decade. Yet according to a 1992 Arthur D. Little study, as much as 30 percent of the diagnostic data and information required by the physician is unavailable prior to or during any given office visit.[3] This frequently results in repeated tests, as well as delays for physicians and patients while data are gathered. Online access to hospital-based information systems would facilitate communication of data to resolve this problem. However, patient information is usually not limited to a single hospital source but originates from numerous sources, accessed through traditional, cumbersome methods (e.g., courier services, postal services, fax or a variety of system interfaces). Many of these traditional approaches perpetuate the problems by taking computer based information and printing a report to mail or fax. Regional or Community Health Information Networks (RHIN/CHIN) are positioned to assist in facilitating access to and integration of a wide variety of information sources. Wisconsin is a leader in successfully implementing a cross enterprise CHIN, the Wisconsin Health Information Network.[1]

The Wisconsin Health Information Network: The Beginning

WHIN began as a joint venture of Aurora Health Care and Ameritech in 1992. Before this, Aurora Health Care (AHC) was involved in several early projects providing physicians remote access to Aurora-affiliated hospitals' information systems. These projects focused on providing access to clinical information management systems in 1983 and, through a proprietary software application, to hospital information system data including transcription and laboratory results in 1985.[4] In the late 1980s, AHC and Ameritech conducted surveys to explore the evolving requirements of physicians and their office staff who were accessing the Aurora systems. These surveys identified two common requirements: improved response time and on-line access to data from hospitals at which they practiced, outside the Aurora enterprise. Other members of the healthcare community (e.g., employers, payors, pharmacies) were also surveyed, to gain a perspective on their information communication requirements and willingness to participate in a state-wide network. A distillation of the information from these surveys laid the foundation for the Wisconsin Health Information Network (the "Network"). To provide an overview of the Wisconsin environment, Fig. 5.1 summarizes the state's demographics.

Original access to the AHC Hospital Information System (HIS) was through a proprietary software product that provided a hospital to physician link through personal computers, modems and dial connections. The only information services available through this link were from the Aurora Healthcare HIS. Although this interface addressed Aurora-based patient results, a large portion of patient records and, indeed, medical information in general was not available. Access to other information sources required additional system interfaces, each through a proprietary interface, or reliance on delivery of paper reports.

Patient information may be conceptualized as reflecting the continuum of care that a patient receives over his/her life. This continuum may not and frequently does not exist in relationship to one physician or enterprise.

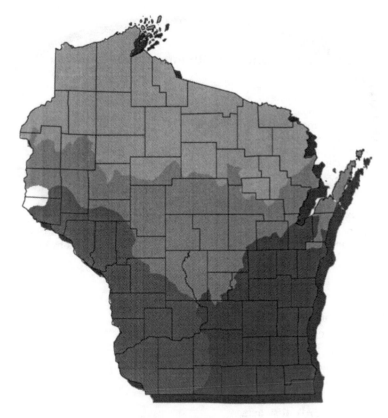

- 64% Urban, 36% Rural
- 1994 Rose Bowl Champions
- 72 Independent Counties
- 154 Hospitals
- 8,700 Physicians

FIGURE 5.1. Wisconsin demographics.

Rather, there is a larger community of information (Fig. 5.2). To augment this information, there is a need for ongoing education, exchange of information between sources other than physicians and hospitals, access to medical information resources and communication with colleagues. Access to the additional information sources is what differentiates a Community Health Information Network (CHIN) from a proprietary physician-to-hospital link. Use of such community based electronic communications has the potential of reducing health care costs by $30 million annually.[2]

Information and services currently available through the WHIN include:

- Patient eligibility verification
- Benefits review

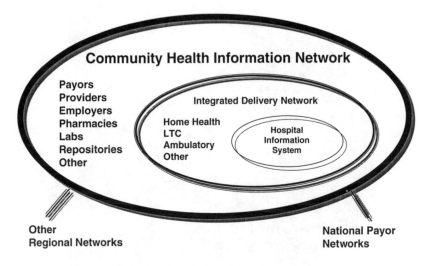

Community Health Information Network

Payors
Providers
Employers
Pharmacies
Labs
Repositories
Other

Integrated Delivery Network

Home Health
LTC
Ambulatory
Other

Hospital
Information
System

Other
Regional Networks

National Payor
Networks

FIGURE 5.2. Strategic network planning.

- Prescription refill authorization
- Electronic mail services
- Recent ED visits
- Patient census by physician/payor
- Patient demographics
- Third party transcribed documents
- Medical records abstracts
- Claims submission
- Electronic mail
- Document image retrieval/viewing
- Consultation/referral authorization
- Electronic signature
- User-defined templates in e-mail
- Claims status reporting
- Listing of physicians on a case
- Hospital-transcribed documents
- Hospital pharmacy patient orders
- Hospital lab results
- Reference lab test results
- Previous care highlights
- Patient education
- Prescription submission

Within the healthcare information systems environment, there is increasing interest in what is referred to as an "integration engine." Within the hospital, this "integration engine" refers to a system used to establish interfaces between diverse systems that exist (e.g., laboratory, radiology, transcription, pharmacy, scheduling, admission). The advantage is that each system needs to establish only one interface with the "integration engine," rather than multiple interfaces with numerous systems. For example, a patient admission system currently interfaces with laboratory, pharmacy and scheduling. With an "integration engine" the same admission system has only one interface to the "engine", which provides transaction interfaces to the other systems. Should any one system be upgraded or replaced, the need to rewrite several system interfaces is overcome by the "integration engine." The new system need only interface with the "integration engine," while the remaining interfaces are the responsibility of the "engine."

Community Health Information Networks are the "integration engine" for the flow of health care information within a given community. Each participant in the network establishes a single interface with the CHIN, which provides integration with the community. The benefits of participation increase as the number of participants increases. (Fig. 5.3).

In addition to providing information integration services, the WHIN is positioned to serve as a posting and distribution point for a wide variety of information that is typically mailed to customers, including:

- Physician directories
- HMO/PPO pharmaceutical formularies
- Announcements for seminars
- Medical society announcements

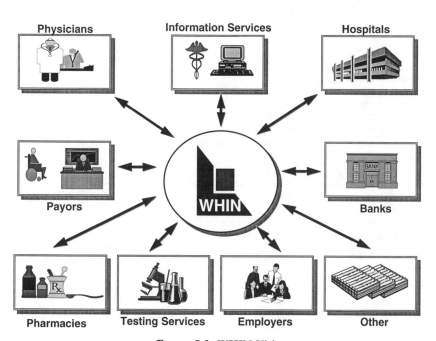

FIGURE 5.3. WHIN Vision.

TABLE 5.1. WHIN current participants.

---

16 Hospitals
  Children's Hospital of Wisconsin
  Community Memorial Hospital (Menomonee Falls)
  Froedtert Memorial Lutheran Hospital
  Hartford Memorial Hospital (Hartford)
  Lakeland Medical Center (Elkhorn)
  Milwaukee Psychiatric Hospital
  St. Luke's Medical Center
  St. Mary's Hospital of Milwaukee
  St. Mary's Hospital of Ozaukee (Ozaukee)
  Sheboygan Memorial Medical Center (Sheboygan)
  Sinai-Samaritan Medical Center
  Trinity Memorial Hospital (Cudahy)
  University of Wisconsin Hospital and Clinic
  Valley View Medical Center (Plymouth)
  Wausau Hospital (Wausau)
  West Allis Memorial Hospital (West Allis)
1300+ Physicians
8 Clinics
  Dean Medical Center (headquarters in Madison)
  Falls Medical (Menomonee Falls)
  General Clinic of West Bend (West Bend)
  Hartford Parkview Clinic (Hartford)
  Medical Associates (Menomonee Falls)
  The Sheboygan Clinic (Sheboygan)
  Two Rivers Clinic (Two Rivers)
  West Bend Clinic, S.C. (West Bend)
7 Insurance organizations (state-wide services)
  First Health
  Medicaid
  The Alliance
  Wausau Insurance
  Wisconsin Education Association Insurance
  Wisconsin Physicians Service Commercial
  Wisconsin Physicians Service Medicare B
Other participants (state-wide services)
  Bayshore Clinical Laboratories—reference lab services
  Community Physicans Network (CPN)
  F. Dohmen—pharmaceutical services
  HDX—Shared Medical Systems based payor network
  Omnimed—transcription services
  System One (National payor network)
  Visiting Nurse Association—home health agency
  Wisconsin Department of Health and Social Services, Disability Determination Bureau

---

(All sites are Milwaukee area unless otherwise noted).

- Grand rounds presentations
- Professional opportunities

WHIN Participation/Ownership

Although the various ownership and operational responsibilities of CHINs have been discussed longer than they have been implemented, "open" needs to be the operative concept. While there are advantages and disadvantages to the variety of models defined, including vendor, community coalition, physician group, government, consumer group, payor and others,[5,6,7,8] a network that is "open" to all wishing to participate is most likely to succeed.

WHIN is currently owned by the original investors, Aurora Health Care and Ameritech. Other equity ownership is available to healthcare organizations within the Wisconsin region. Being a participating member in the WHIN is not dependent on ownership and vise versa. Participants in the WHIN are defined through two main categories:

1. Information providers—sites that make information in their systems available to the "network." These include hospitals, clinics, reference laboratories, payors, physician offices, pharmacies and others.
2. Information users—sites that access information through the "network." These include physician offices, hospital departments, clinics, reference laboratories, payor departments, pharmacies and others.

Note that the roles of information provider and information user are not exclusive.

Perhaps the single most important point regarding ownership and participation is the value that participation brings. As previously noted, a broad base of participants is required to establish a successful community network. More extensive participation by the medical information community in a CHIN creates a broader base of available information from which participants may benefit. Since its inception, the WHIN has been working to bring a wide range of various medical information providers to the network. Initially, the WHIN pilot involved two hospitals and six physician offices. Current participants in the Wisconsin Health Information Network are listed in Table 5.1. Each of these participants is either in production on the network or in various stages of integration. While specific purposes for joining the network vary from client to client, the overwhelming reason is a vision of shared communications, intra- and inter enterprise, through a common network infrastructure whose cost is shared by participants. With the belief that such shared resources bring benefits to the community as a whole. In a community network, "open" applies not only to the technology, but also to the acceptance of new participants. For example, participation of a provider does not imply exclusion of a competitor.

This shared network infrastructure that integrates the requesters of information and the providers of information (Fig. 5.4). Shared expenses and resources include:

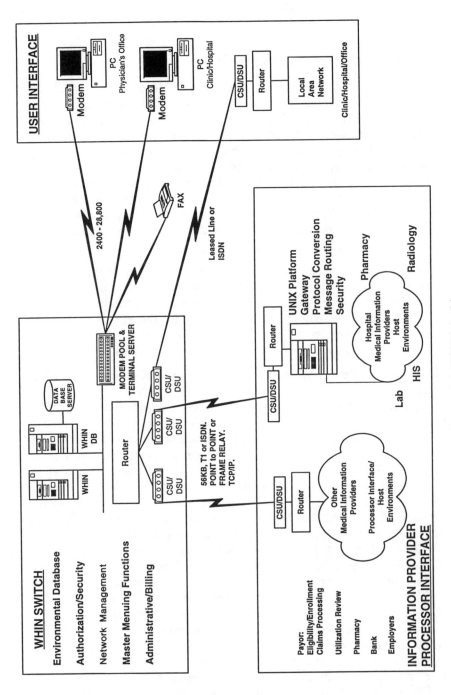

FIGURE 5.4. WHIN Architecture.

1. Software that manages system integration, provides security, routes requests and responses, delivers messages and maintains a full activity log for each information provider.
2. Hardware that provides and maintains a full modem pool, systems to operate the switch services (e.g., request/response, store and forward, and others) and network components to integrate wide area network components.
3. Services that include training, 24-hour-by-7-day customer support, router configuration and management support and full network management services.

WHIN Model

Three main components form the conceptual structure for the WHIN:

1. Information providers;
2. Information Users; and
3. WHIN switch—a community integration engine (switch as in switching requests/response pairs and delivering store and forward messages).

These components provide three main information integration services:

1. Request/response—This process begins when a user requests data related to a specific patient or group of patients. Requests may be made directly to a host or to a stand-in database (discussed later) populated with information provided by a host system.
2. Event driven—This process begins when a host system recognizes an event (e.g., admission, discharge, completion of a lab test, emergency room visit) and passes a message or file to the WHIN host for distribution. This process may be viewed as a store and forward function.
3. Host to host—This process provides the means for movement of data from one host environment to another. An example might be the transfer of patient demographics from a hospital to a physician billing service.

User Interface

In all cases, the need for data to be viewed transparent from its source is accomplished through the 'network'. This allows a physician or office staff to review patient demographics, evaluate lab results, verify pharmacy orders, establish eligibility of a patient, submit referral requests, review transcribed documents prior to signing, submit claims to any payor and communicate with colleagues through electronic mail. All these functions are completely independent of the source system applications.

In the case of the request/response and event driven models, the WHIN User Interface (WHIN UI) is the common link to the network and, subsequently, all information sources. The user sees only the WHIN login screen, navigates only WHIN screens and is able to retrieve information from a wide spectrum of sources. The WHIN UI provides access to clinical as well as financial data and the integrated WHIN electronic mail package. The other half of this host system integration equation is software that interfaces with the information providers' host systems. This software is referred to as a processor interface and is discussed later.

Addressing the common denominator of technology in the physician office, the UI was initially developed in a DOS environment, capable of running on 286 class personal computers. Currently, the Microsoft Windows™ version of the UI is gaining popularity and will, through the graphic capabilities it brings, support enhanced services such as graphic images (e.g., ECG, radiographic images), provide the capability to display trends in numerical results, and provide access to education and information services developed in a graphic multi media environment.

Serving as a client to the WHIN switch server, the User Interface software incorporates communications as well as application components. Requests for information are constructed in a consistent message format, independent of the host site that will respond. Some requests require additional parameters beyond a patient identifier to narrow searches and responses. For example, a pharmacy order search requires date ranges to search, and laboratory results require identification of a time range (e.g., today, last 48 hours, all). Responses to requests are presented using a common interface. Some responses are formatted with discrete data elements, such as patient demographics, while transcribed results are returned as blocks of text with no data element definition. The format of some responses depends on the format from the host. For example, normal ranges and test code names for laboratory results may vary from site to site. There is no WHIN-based nomenclature to which these elements are mapped. If a host is unable to provide a data element as a response (e.g., pediatric patients do not have employers) the field is indicated as not having data available, avoiding confusion with responses that may have a blank field as a valid response.

The User Interface also incorporates a pass-through feature, allowing remote client software to be executed as if the user were directly connected to the host application. This allows a remote clinic access to centralized clinic management software at the enterprise's centralized data operations center. A similar feature allows for a separate Windows™ client function to access a remote host.

By its nature, the UI client software provides additional security to the WHIN. Being resident on the user machine, the UI may temporarily disallow the use of disk, diskette or printer functions, restricting the ability to save or print the data viewed on a screen. This is discussed further in the section on security.

Network connections from the UI may be established in a variety of ways.

- Asynchronous dial connection with supported speeds of 2400 to 28,800 baud, through either direct connect modems or NASI compliant modem pooling.
- ISDN dial connection, offering speeds of 64K and 128K bits per second.
- Direct network connection utilizing TCP/IP protocol.

A UNIX version of the UI is also available, meeting the needs of sites where the practice management system is based on a UNIX platform. To date, these practice management systems have supported primarily dumb terminal interfaces. However, this platform will not support the wide range of applications planned for WHIN in the future. Additionally, price/performance considerations support migration of some dumb terminals in such an environment to personal computers supporting terminal emulation and providing a fully functional PC for other purposes such as connection to a CHIN, and PC based applications over a UNIX based user interface.

Processor Interface

This software is the other half of the equation providing host independent user interface functions. The processor interface communicates messages from the WHIN to the host system(s)/network(s). For the purposes of discussion, this section focuses on the hospital as an information provider. However, the concepts presented apply equally to all medical information providers, including payors, hospitals, clinics, reference laboratories and others.

In a hospital setting, a variety of application systems are typically sources of data. These include admitting, pharmacy, laboratory, radiology, orders, scheduling, transcription and certainly medical records. Depending on a wide range of conditions, these applications may be executing on one or several processors, each of which may be supporting a different operating system and/or network protocol. The proof of this condition is left to the reader. In some institutions, an integration engine may be implemented to simplify internal system interface issues. This may also serve as the connection point to the WHIN, providing a single connection to all these systems. Other enterprises may have a repository, or fully computerized patient record, that contains all the data to be made available to the network. Evaluation of these conditions determines how the 'network' will access the various data sources to submit requests for data and accept responses.

Within the 'network', TCP/IP is used as the wide area communications protocol. Messages that move from the UI through the WHIN Switch and processor interface are defined within established standards from HL/7 and ANSI X.12. One of the primary roles of the processor interface software is to translate the WHIN structures and protocols to those required by the host environment being integrated. To date this has included SNA 3270, LU 6.2, DECNET and TCP/IP.

Once the network connection is established, interface(s) with host application(s) is/are addressed. These interfaces may be accomplished in any of the following ways.

Peer to Peer

This approach involves development of application programs on the host side of the interface, communicating to the WHIN through either a TCP/IP socket connection or LU6.2. The application programs interface with required databases to retrieve information to satisfy requests from authorized requesters. Event driven functions may also pass data to these applications, which format required messages that are forwarded to identified recipients through the WHIN. If the recipient is not a user of the 'network', the information is faxed through the WHIN.

Screen Scraping

Two varieties of screen scraping are possible within the WHIN. One involves writing host-based applications that read messages from and post messages to a terminal interface (e.g., CICS transactions to a 3270). The other involves navigating standard application menus and sub menus, interacting with the application and applying data to required fields and reading data from other fields. This is a useful tool if there are no development resources available for a given host machine. In some instances, a new application may be written specifically for the WHIN interface. Performance and maintenance are considerations when navigating application screens.

Performance is a function of the number of screens that must be navigated, each adding to the overall response time for an on-line transaction. Additionally, all application and communication error conditions need to be accounted for to ensure optimal functionality.

Maintenance is involved when changes to application menus and screens are made. Screen scraping applications are sensitive to relative positioning of fields on a screen. Changes must be reviewed to ensure continuity with the processor interface, potentially requiring software modifications on the PI. Disaster may ensue if there is a breakdown in communications between the WHIN development team and the host team.

Direct Database Access

Direct database calls, using languages such as Structured Query Language™ or similar database queries may be posted to a host database from the processor interface. These calls may be to a remote system or to a local 'stand-in database' as discussed below.

In some instances, the host system may be unable to accept a direct on-line connection with the 'network' because of performance limitations or the absence of on-line transaction processing capabilities. In these instances, data may be forwarded to the 'network' either in a batch or on-line mode to be stored on a temporary 'stand-in database'. This stand-in database is a duplicate version of a full database at a host site. It may represent eligibility information from a payor system or lab results from a laboratory information system. In this implementation, requests for information that would typically be routed to a host site are instead directed to the stand-in database for responses. Access to these stand-in databases is achieved transparent to the requester, as if the transaction were actually being responded to by a remote host.

This stand-in database may be updated (i.e., replaced) with a new version on a regular basis (weekly, monthly) depending on the dynamic nature of the data. Alternatively, data may be passed to the 'network' to be added to a stand-in database, with older data automatically deleted. It should be noted that the WHIN is neither the owner nor the manager of the data in these stand-in databases. The provider of the data remains the owner and maintains all authority to determine who has access.

Stand-in databases have been used for hospital laboratory information systems (result reporting), transcription systems (transcribed documents) and payor databases (e.g., eligibility and benefit plan detail). In all cases, there were systems that because of performance or processing limitations could not accept direct connections to the WHIN. A stand-in database is established through key fields that are agreed upon by the information provider and the WHIN. These fields are passed along with the general data to be posted to the stand-in database. For example, a transcribed document may include an identification block in a specific location in the document. The data in the identification block (e.g., patient name, patient number, document type, date, physician) is used to build specific indexes in the stand-in database.

Typically, implementation of a stand-in database is rapid because little coordination of programming effort is required between the host and the 'network'. A disadvantage of this approach is that the data may become outdated between versions of the database that are forwarded to the 'network'. Feedback from users of this information have indicated that this risk is minimal in comparison to not having the data available at all.

Identifying and Integrating a New Participant

This section discusses identifying and integrating a new participant to the WHIN. Participants are information providers and information users, though, as previously presented, these categories are not mutually exclusive. For example, a hospital may be an information provider, while several departments in that institution are using the 'network' to access information.

Information Provider

Integration of a new information provider involves coordination of numerous resources. Beginning with contacts established through the sales team, presentations are made to executives of a potential information provider, including the chief executive officer, chief financial officer and chief information officer. The goal is to establish an understanding of WHIN and create sufficient interest to develop a plan for integrating systems. Potential information providers sites are identified in part through recommendations from existing participants in the WHIN, either providers or users of information.

Determination of the method for integrating a new client systems with the network is one component of the Statement of Work process. How, and what data is to be shared are determined. The Statement of Work process involves meetings with Information Services staff, as well as management and/or staff representatives from application areas including Medical Records, Laboratory, Radiology, Transcription, Pharmacy and others. Typically, these meetings occur over a 2 to 3 day time frame, allowing for detailed discussions and optimizing time investments. It is important to determine the data that a client wishes to provide to the network. This is typically dependent on what data is available electronically and which systems are in a state allowing them to be included in interface development. For example, a lab system that is due to be replaced in nine months may not be included in the initial interface development; rather, inclusion of laboratory data is delayed pending implementation of the new system.

Depending on the resources available at a client site, the development of a processor interface (PI) (described earlier) may emphasize WHIN or client resources. The PI may be developed to meet 'standard' WHIN specifications, requiring the majority of the application work to occur within the client environment. Or, software may be developed within the network environment to meet the requirements of the host environment. Typically, PI development involves some effort from both parties. Staff from a third party, such as the client's host system(s) vendor(s), may also need to be involved. This is the responsibility of the information provider.

A comprehensive test plan, including system, acceptance and pilot level testing, are outlined in the Statement of Work, along with a comprehensive list of equipment requirements. This document, which provides an overview of system integration readiness and full integration plan, then becomes part of the contract for the customer.

Assuming agreement to proceed with the integration plan, final detailed design and PI development begin. Parallel efforts are undertaken to establish the physical network connection. This involves placement of a router at the client site and establishment of a leased line (or other communications line) between the client site and WHIN. Execution of the PI software may occur on a machine located at the client site or on hardware located at the WHIN data center. Determination of which model is most appropriate depends in part on the network environment being integrated. An environment homogeneous with that of the WHIN will most likely have the PI executing at the WHIN facility. Purchase of all hardware is the responsibility of the client, with specifications provided by the WHIN team in the Statement of Work. For client convenience, the WHIN Technical Services Team may act as purchasing and installation agent for hardware and network services integration (e.g., IP address acquisition, router configuration and management).

Once development and system level testing are completed, the phases of acceptance testing and pilot testing begin. In acceptance testing, staff from the member site, working with WHIN staff, validate the accuracy of information displayed through the network. Acceptance testing is completed with sign-off by the information provider indicating that all integration services are functioning appropriately.

The final stage of testing involves pilot offices selected jointly by the information provider and WHIN. Pilot participants include existing and new users on the 'network'. They thoroughly review all functions for the new information provider, providing feedback on functionality and any errors encountered. Pilot sites are typically chosen for their relationship with the information provider and willingness to work with new concepts. Existing clients provide experience, while new clients provide a perspective specific to the new information provider. Regardless of the source, feedback on new information services is valuable to all parties involved. Additionally, ideas for expanded network services frequently come from pilot sites through their experience in working with the information provider and the WHIN.

Information User

Use of the network is determined in part by which information providers have authorized access to a user. When a new information user joins the network, information provider sites to which they are requesting access are identified. These sites are contacted by the WHIN staff to obtain approval for access. When a new information provider is coming 'live' on the WHIN, the sales team works closely with the information provider team to identify potential users to access that site. This includes reviewing current users and identifying new users the information provider would like WHIN to contact. Typically, for a hospital, this would include staff, referring and consulting physicians.

Once a new information user is identified, they are added to the WHIN Environmental Database, a centralized database of all network users and their privileges on the network. For each information user the medical information providers to which access has been granted, what functions are allowed at each information provider, as well as related user specific security information are identified. Sensitive information, such as passwords, is kept confidential and is not accessible by the WHIN staff.

Users of the WHIN may also take advantage of hospital-independent functions on the network, including electronic mail, referral processing, claims submission, eligibility verification, electronic bookshelves (e.g., storage of HMO formularies, education materials, bulletin board services) and other information services.

Access to the network requires a copy of the WHIN User Interface Software. This software is typically installed at the User office by a member of the WHIN Client Services Team. WHIN provides minimum and recommended hardware configurations for executing the WHIN UI, however, the client is responsible for providing the hardware. Minimum configurations for the WHIN for Windows™ software includes a 486-based PC, with 8 MB RAM and a 14,400 baud modem. Recommended configuration includes a Pentium,™ 16 MB RAM and a 28,800 baud modem. Installation may be on a standalone PC or local area network. The connection to the network may be through a dial modem, direct leased line or ISDN connection.

If a client is interested in using WHIN for submission of electronic claims, the Client Services Team works with the office and their practice management vendor to facilitate this. Steps include determining the location of the claims to submit and defining the format in which claims will be sent to the network and the mapping functions to translate this format to a standard claim format. Claims may be imported through the UI software, or in the case of a UNIX environment, brought into the network through a UNIX communications protocol.

Customer Support

The Client Services Team at WHIN is involved in a wide range of activities, including testing new UI software, working with pilot offices, installing WHIN UI software and training users on the software. Additionally, this team is responsible for staffing the WHIN Solution Center, maintaining the WHIN Environmental Database (EDB, source of all authorized network participants and their privileges), publishing the WHIN Advantage (the WHIN quarterly newsletter), and facilitating the WHIN User Group meetings.

The Client Services Team installs UI software for all clients, trains clients and coordinates "train the trainer" programs. They prepare all materials and present classroom and/or onsite training. Installation and training costs are included in the one time charges for each new information user on the network.

Additionally, the Client Services Team is the focal point for troubleshooting all problems related to the WHIN User Interface software. Given the wide range of environments and variety of platforms in which the WHIN UI may be installed, this team must respond to and resolve a wide range of problems. They include problem-solving in areas such as modems, network software, compatibility and integration with practice management systems and file transfer functions.

Twenty-four hours per day, 365 days per year, the WHIN Solution Center is available to all clients through an 800 number. The Solution Center maintains full records on problems, their resolution, requirements for follow up training and call.

Security

Ownership, integrity, availability, utility, source control, errors/omissions and leakage are among the issues related to confidentiality and security of patient medical records.[9-11] Although computer networks may create new challenges to the confidentiality of patient records, they also have advantages over traditional paper records.[10] Maintaining confidentiality and privacy of the data moving through the Wisconsin Health Information Network is paramount. To accomplish this, WHIN has implemented a wide range of security measures, both procedural and technical/physical. Figure 5.5 outlines the elements that compose the WHIN security infrastructure. Several of the steps discussed involve functions controlled by the WHIN Environmental Database (EDB).

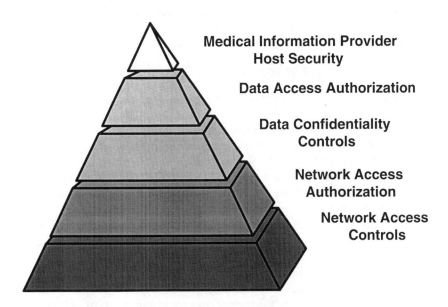

Medical Information Provider Host Security

Data Access Authorization

Data Confidentiality Controls

Network Access Authorization

Network Access Controls

FIGURE 5.5. WHIN network security.

Network Access Controls

Control over access is the foundation layer in the security pyramid. To access network services, a copy of the UI software must be present. The User Interface serves as the client process to the WHIN switch, controlling functions of dialing the network and making the initial login to the switch. A unique serial number associated with each copy of the software is passed to the host upon connection. This is used later to verify the software and the relationship between the user and the software package. The UI software issues an initial 'login' to the network, identifying version number for control over version specific functions and to trigger electronic download capabilities.

Dial-back modems have been identified as a means of adding an additional layer of security.[10] However, with call forwarding, this security feature may be compromised, and the additional delay in connection time is unacceptable to most clients. Therefore, WHIN is not utilizing call back modems. Another security feature, allowing hardware key based authentication of a user prior to allowing connection to the 'network', is currently being investigated.

Physical access to the network also occurs on the information provider side of the equation. This connection provides the host network interface and may also serve user interface connections across a network connection. Routers in place at all client sites and at WHIN allow the establishment and management of route filters, permitting only known traffic to enter the network connection. Information provider sites typically have a leased line connection to the network, preventing public access to the communication lines. Other sites transmit batch data to WHIN through dial connections initiated by the network to preestablished numbers.

Network Access Authorization

The final step in the connection process is for the user to identify herself/himself to the WHIN application. User ID and password are used to accomplish this. This password is established by users and are required to be changed every 60 days. With passwords stored in encrypted forms on the EDB, no one on staff at WHIN knows a user's password. Additionally, single use password tokens are available to any WHIN client. Such tokens generate a new password every 60 seconds through an algorithm synchronized with the host processor.

With completion of the dial connection and user authentication, user-specific information is downloaded from the Environmental Database to the user interface software. This indicates which information providers have granted access privileges and which transactions are allowed. Connection to the WHIN does not automatically grant the user access to resources on the network. Rather, each information provider (e.g., hospital, payor, laboratory, etc.) is responsible for establishing this authority. When new clients are added to the network, they are asked which network services they wish to access. This request is taken by the WHIN staff to those facilities for approval in writing. Only sites that have granted access will appear as choices for the client. As with other user parameters, this information is stored in the EDB.

All sites have the potential for staff turnover. To address this, procedures are in place with all client offices to notify the WHIN Solution Center when an employee leaves the office. This notification results in the removal of that employee's User ID and network privileges.

Date Confidentiality Controls

When a client signs a contract with WHIN, it includes a section that reviews the sensitive nature of the data the client will be accessing while using the network. It emphasizes that the network contains sensitive, confidential and proprietary information that must be protected against unauthorized disclosure, release modification or other action. The contract further states that all federal, state and local laws (including laws requiring exercise of due diligence to prevent unauthorized disclosure or improper use of this information for any purpose not specifically intended by this system) are to be complied with. Each access to the WHIN requires the user to again accept these conditions electronically. The applicable laws include the Wisconsin Computer Act.

Data are encrypted in the network. This encryption includes all requests and responses traveling on dial lines. A copy of the WHIN UI software is required to break the encryption.

Some health information networks maintain repositories of patient information passed through the network. For example, they may extract patient-specific information from claim forms to build and maintain a repository of patient information. The WHIN does not store or aggregate such patient-specific information.

Data Access Authorization

As a function of network access authorization, access privileges are granted by the information provider to specific clients. This access is not universal for all information at that site. For example, information providers may elect to further restrict information access to physicians of record for a given case. To date on the network there have been three versions of "viewing rights" granted to authorized users by information providers:

- Physician of record only;
- Right to view based on staff privileges at an institution; and
- Right to view until the case is abstracted, then restriction to physicians of record only.

Which of these options is implemented is decided solely by the information provider. Obviously, the information provider must have procedural and system functions in place to provide accurate and timely tracking of physicians of record. The degree of success in implementing these contributes to the viewing rights decisions an institution makes.

An institution may also select, on a per user basis, which data types a particular user is allowed to access. Establishing access to a facility does not open all doors. For example, one user may be allowed to view all types of information while another may be restricted to patient demographic information.

In addition, some sites may choose to restrict access to specific data types. For example, a hospital may restrict access to laboratory test results related to sexually transmitted diseases.

Nonphysician users of WHIN (e.g., physician office staff) are able to act on behalf of the physicians for whom they work. These staff members may however, have further restrictions on what data they may access, view or print. For example, a physician may be allowed to view data a staff member is not allowed to see, or a physician may be allowed to view, save, and print data a staff member may only be allowed to view.

Other nonphysician users of the network are restricted to what data they may access. Billing agencies acting on behalf of a physician, or ambulance companies that have transported patients to a hospital may be allowed to review patient demographics and insurance information for billing purposes, but they will not have access to any clinical data.

Medical Information Provider Host Security

In addition to all the security provided by the WHIN, host systems have extensive security functions inherent. Working with the information provider, many of these security functions may be passed along to the requester of information. For example, if the host environment requires a login to obtain certain information from an application, the password for this functions may be kept in the EDB and passed to the application when a request for that information is made. This allows the host security to be enforced, while requiring only one login by the end user.

Audit trails of all accesses to the network are maintained on a per user basis. Reports of activity are available to the user accessing the network, as well as to information providers. These reports outline the facility accessed, date and time of activity, and the type of information retrieved. As an element of security, WHIN does not "open" any of the messages that pass through the network. This prevents reporting of the which patients' data that has been accessed.

Other Security Topics

CHINs are thought by some to create environments where antitrust issues may be involved.[12] This is particularly true for CHINs that function as repositories for prices charged by physicians, hospitals, HMOs and others. WHIN does not broadly provide access to such information, nor does it archive this information. Any access to information at a site is determined solely by that information provider.

In addition to security on the network, several measures have been taken at the WHIN office location. These include proximity card readers and motion detectors to protect the space and network cabling.

Implementation of comprehensive security functions should be measured against the usability of the services and utility of the data. Any secure network has the potential of being breached through the actions of an authorized user acting unethically.[13]

Challenges, Advice, and Outcomes

Health information, by definition, has many aspects that are private, confidential, and, in some instances, involve a proprietary element. As a result, security was an initial barrier to community networks. The competitive nature of health care institutions requires that there be no unauthorized access to any given institution's information. In fact, although a computer network facilitates access to records from a broader range of geographic sites, such a network provides more security than the traditional paper record system. For example, an authorized copy of a medical record may be copied and mailed to dozens of addresses, with no record of the activity at all. The same process on the network would generate an audit trail of electronic mail messages being sent.

To learn from those using the WHIN, client satisfaction surveys were conducted in 1994 and 1995. The mailed surveys were designed to gain an understanding of client perceptions of the WHIN staff's service and benefits from use of the network. Overall client satisfaction in 1994 was above average with a rating of 90 out of 100 percent in a scaled satisfaction index. In 1995, there was an increase in satisfaction with a rating of 93 out of 100 percent. Respondents reported time saving through the use of WHIN functions in a variety of areas including clinical and administrative information as well as information sharing.

To objectively assess these benefits, the University of Wisconsin Milwaukee was contracted to conduct an impact study.[14,15] Visits to physician offices, clinics, and hospital departments were made to conduct interviews and gain an objective measurement of the actual and potential benefits. In addition, this opportunity was used as a means to again study information requirements and flow at these sites, in an effort to see where new application efforts should be focused. The study covered 21 provider sites including physician offices (specialty and primary care), hospital departments, home health agencies and other sites.

Although the specific benefits recognized in any given physician office, clinic or hospital department vary depending on the implementation and usage of the tools provided, real benefits are attainable in all locations. Examples of the benefits observed and reported include:

1. *Information provider* (hospitals) — Historically, information requests from outside the hospital came through Medical Records and were handled individually. A $5.10 savings is projected for the Medical Records Department for each information request handled through the WHIN. Effective use of the WHIN virtually eliminates use of traditional methods of information exchange such as fax, mail and phone. Depending on the volume of requests responded to, this represents an annual savings of $375,000 to $1,000,000.[14]
2. *Information user* (physician office and others) — In general, savings include $1/electronic referral request, in excess of $2.50/clinical information request and additional savings from electronic claims processing. Again, depending on volume in an office, savings will vary. Annual savings potential for physician practices, depending on volumes of usage, is $17,000 to $68,000 or more. Additional benefits may be realized from electronic referral and claims processing.[14]

Realized savings occurring as a result of changing the model for communication of health-related information is directly proportional to the volume of usage. The greater the number of physicians accessing any given hospital through a network such as WHIN, and the greater the number of sites from which these physicians may retrieve information the greater the savings for all parties. Additional benefits reported included:

1. More rapid response to requests; minutes rather than hours and days.
2. Decreased patient stays due to more timely information exchanges. For example, a home health care agency involved in the study reported an average of 2 to 3 patients per week experienced extended stays due to untimely information exchanges.[14,15]
3. Recovery of previously lost charges due to procedures missed in billing and missed program filing deadlines.

One message was particularly striking in the impact study. Community Health Information Networks need to add value to be competitive with traditional means of communicating health information. It is this added value, such as a community wide electronic signature application or a community repository of patient indexes, that will assist in breaking people's ties to traditional means of accessing information. To change habitual practices, people need to have a threshold of volumes exceeded. Once passed, the new becomes standard and the old the exception. In the case of eligibility checks, if less than 30 percent of covered lives may be checked electronically, there may not be a change in practice in how these checks are performed. If 60 percent of covered lives may be checked electronically, this may facilitate change.

There needs to be a common focus on the added utility of information in an electronic form. If medical informatics is to reach the next level, where the broad benefits of electronically available medical information are recognized, the process of resorting to printing and mailing or faxing of reports needs to be reduced or eliminated. This process perpetuates reliance on the paper medium. Functions and processes facilitating separation from the paper security blanket need to be identified if we are to realize genuine changes and benefits in medical information and consequently medical care.

Special Projects

Society is becoming more fluid and the need for integration of health care information is increasing. In no instance is this need greater than when a patient is brought into an emergency department (ED). Someone vacationing far from home is involved in a traumatic accident and brought to the ED unconscious with no means of obtaining medical information such as allergies, current medications or diagnoses, or identifying the primary care physician. The ED physician has never seen this patient before, yet must deliver urgent care to save a life. Access to any information related to the patient would significantly benefit this physician and the patient.

WHIN is a member of a consortium of companies that is currently working on a project that is funded in part by the Advanced Research Projects Agency. Titled the National Information Infrastructure Health Information Network, the project seeks to establish community or regional repositories for an Essential Emergency-Department Data Set (EEDS), and to define and implement the message and communications infrastructure for inter-CHIN communications to facilitate access from outside a given region. These regional repositories will be populated from ED systems as well as from hospital based systems (e.g., laboratory, ADT).

Future Projects

To further expand the functions available through the network, the WHIN staff and clients are involved in identifying new applications. Currently, projects being investigated include telemedicine server/education, multimedia education services, community based repositories (e.g., minimum emergency department data set, immunization records, global participant index) and expanded use of INTERNET/INTRANET services. In all cases, the goal is to improve the efficiency with which quality medical care is delivered and increase the value of participation in the network and the utility of information available through the WHIN. Health care information may have a variety of faces. For example, a county may be involved in tracking offenders of statutes prohibiting driving while intoxicated. A network such as WHIN may be useful in moving the paperwork related to treatment plans, court mandated follow up and related issues. These and other projects will establish a new structure and standard for the integration and communication of diverse health care and health related information, within a given region and across the country.

Author's Addendum

In 1996, WHIN has entered another phase of evolution. Over the past three years, as WHIN has grown and client server applications have become more commonplace, the technical infrastructure of WHIN has evolved to support communication of other client/server pairs (Fig. 5.6). This model allows point to point protocol communications as well as direct network communications to occur at a separate level, where network services route the traffic to the requested server based on user identification/authentication and server granted privileges. This model provides a single point of communication to multiple servers while integrating the protection of a firewall. This single communications point provides for easy integration of applications at the client workstation. In Fig. 5.6, bold lines indicate links that have been completed at one or more locations, light lines indicate efforts that are underway and dashed lines indicate concepts under investigation. The frequent user of a given client software package is allowed access through that client, as well as through the common user interface of WHIN when needed. For example, one physician may be experienced in using the client software for a hospital based CPR system, while another with less exposure to that CPR system may prefer a common user interface. With this model, both user requirements may be addressed with a single point of connection. Business partnership conversations are in process to bring global participant index, telemedicine and community based ordering applications to the community health information network model at WHIN.

Acknowledgments. I would like to take this opportunity to recognize my colleagues at the Wisconsin Health Information Network.

Michael C. Jordan, President and General Manager
Rhonda C. Nelson, Vice President Sales
Janet E. Pachmayer, Manager Finance
Kim R. Pemble, Vice President Operations and Development
Marsha M. Radaj, Business Manager
Collin M. Chaffin, Software Engineer
Lori A. Dupont, Project Manager
Stephanie E. First, Account Executive
Cora V. Fisher, Client Services Analyst

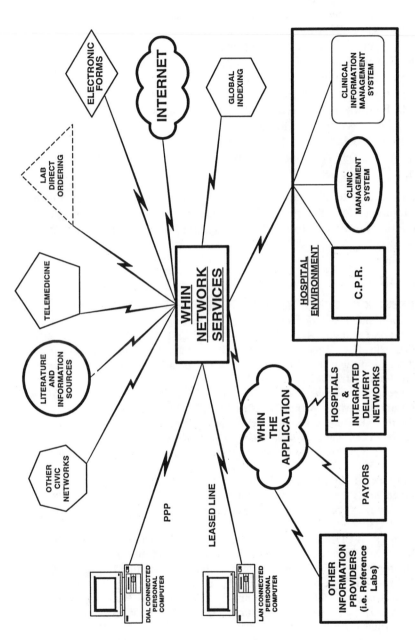

FIGURE 5.6. WHIN network overview.

Paula J. Grintjes, Account Executive
Chuck A. Hill, Network Manager
Diana L. Kane, Systems and Database Engineer
Linda L. Kimball, Administrative Assistant
Kurt R. Knipper, Account Executive
Dodie Kovac, Solution Center Analyst
Rebecca Maldonado, Receptionist
Susan M. Ouellette, Project Manager
Brenda Panawash-Bielinski, Client Services Analyst
Dee Piziak, Account Executive
Colleen K. Shields, Client Services Analyst
Gayle A. Stoffer, Account Executive
Marian G. Tate, Senior Project Manager

A special note of thanks to Frank T. Hoban, Director of Business Development for Ameritech Health Connections, for the insight and foundation he brought to WHIN as General Manager during our first three years.

References

1. Pemble KR, Regional Health Information Networks: The Wisconsin Health Information Network, A case study. *Proceedings of the 18th Annual Symposium on Computer Applications in Medical Care*, November 1994:401–405.
2. Wilensky GR, Rossiter LF. The relative importance of physician induced demand in the demand for medical care. *Milbank Memorial Fund Quarterly/ Health Society*. 1983;61(2):252–277.
3. *Telecommunications: Can It Help Solve America's Health Care Problems?* Cambridge, Mass: Arthur D. Little, Inc., 1992.
4. Pemble KR. Remote access: Meeting the requirements. *Proceedings of the Sixth Annual Conference on Computing in Critical Care*. February 1986.
5. Wakerly RT. Info networks to be integral in reform. *Modern Healthcare*. 1993; Oct:54–56.
6. Korpman R, Blevins LF, McChesney J, Hanlon P. Which CHIN ownership model holds the promise for long-term success? *Infocare*. 1994;April:26–27.
7. Morrissey J. Control, cost top issues facing CHINs. *Modern Healthcare*. 1995; Feb:74–80.
8. Zinn TK. A CHIN Primer". *Health Management Technology*. 1994;Feb:28–32.
9. Kabay ME. Information systems security and management in today's healthcare environment. Presentation at Fifteenth Annual Association for Applied Clinical Information Systems Conference. March;1995.
10. U.S. Congress, Office of Technology Assessment. *Protecting Privacy in Computerized Medical Information*, OTA-TCT-576. Washington, DC: U.S. Government Printing Office; 1993.
11. Lawrence LM. Safeguarding the confidentiality of automated medical information. *Journal of Quality Improvement*. 1994;20(11):639–645.
12. Waller AA, McDevitt DD. Playing the CHIN game: Avoiding antitrust pitfalls. *Health Management Technology*. 1994;Dec:28–36.

13. Wetzlink JP. Make it a C-CHIN instead: Extending the utility of community health information networks., *Infocare*. 1994;Sept:20–24.
14. Lassila KS, Cheng RH. Wisconsin Health Information Network: Impact Study. Executive Briefing; 1995.
15. Lasilla KS, Cheng, RH. Taming the RHINO: Interorganizational implementation issues of regional health information networks. *Proceedings of the Inaugural America's Conference on Information Systems*. 1995;Aug:25-27.

6

CHMIS Evolution: The Metamorphosis of a Community Health Information Movement

RICHARD D. RUBIN and MEGAN C. AUKEMA

Long-distance runners use the term "hitting the wall" to describe that point when the mind is still willing but the body is out of gas. When you hit the wall, despite a good strategy and the best of intentions, you cease to make progress because the resources you need simply are not there.

Over the course of the last two decades, many of those involved in trying to solve the manifold problems of the American health system feel as if they have been running a marathon. Billions of hours, words and dollars have been invested in this long-running competition. However, despite good ideas, conscientious effort, and much skill and determination, health reformers have hit the wall. There are many reasons why various policies have had difficulties in solving the health system problems they were designed to tackle. A major hurdle that crops up consistently is the absence of information needed to execute policy. Examples from the past few years are plentiful:

Policy: *Contract with the most cost/care effective providers.*
Reality: We don't always know *what* is care/cost effective, let alone who does it best.
Policy: *Buy based on value, not just price.*
Reality: We still struggle to measure cost. Assessing quality (the other half of value) is even more problematic.
Policy: *Manage care. Deliver the best outcomes for the lowest price.*
Reality: Measuring, let alone managing, outcomes is more a hope for tomorrow than something routinely accomplished today.
Policy: *Provide access to needed care for those without insurance coverage.*
Reality: We cannot easily identify those without coverage, their unmet health needs, or the services that will most effectively address their needs.

As Samuel Taylor Coleridge wrote in "The Rime of the Ancient Mariner," "Water, water, everywhere, not any drop to drink." Ironically, health data abounds. We are drowning in data, yet desperate for information. Health data resources are largely fragmented, incompatible, and inaccessible. The content and the infrastructure needed to transport data and assemble information are inadequate to the task.

The health information deficit was even more pronounced a few years ago than it is today. In 1990, a small group of people, having suffered, on multiple occasions, the bruises and frustrations that come with hitting the data wall, decided to tackle the problem. The John A. Hartford Foundation (a private philanthropy based in New York City) and a few pioneering community organizations created the Community Health Management Information System (CHMIS) movement (see Table 6.1).

In the early 1990s, the Hartford Foundation funded seven community groups to work toward meeting the shared health information needs of their communities. In 1994, the Hartford Foundation also funded the Foundation for Health Care Quality to serve as the CHMIS Resource Center and provide information, technical assistance, and tools to interested communities. In addition to the "Hartford seven," other community organizations around the country have participated in selected CHMIS activities.

The initial vision guiding the CHMIS pioneers in 1991 was:

- Providing access to aggregate health information;
- Delivering management information, electronically, at the point of service;
- Implementing standards for electronic handling of common administrative transactions;
- Linking trading partners through electronic networks; and
- Creating partnerships to govern and apply the information.

To execute this vision, CHMIS initially adopted a "top down" approach because CHMIS developers perceived the need to "wire-up" the community

TABLE 6.1. Establishment of CHMIS

Community	Name of Organization	Type of Organization	Date of Hartford Funding
Washington	Foundation for Health Care Quality	Purchaser-initiated partnership	January 1991
Iowa	Iowa CHMIS	Public/private consortium	June 1991
Ohio	Ohio Corporation for Health Information	Purchaser-initiated partnership	January 1993
Vermont	Vermont Health Care Information Consortium	Public/private consortium	January 1993
New York	State of New York Department of Health	Public agency	May 1993
Minnesota	Minnesota Institute for Community Health Information	Public/private consortium	August 1993
Memphis, TN	MidSouth Health Care Alliance	Purchaser-initiated partnership	October 1991

and centralize access to data. The early CHMIS model featured the following components:

1. *The Transaction System.* CHMIS was designed to cost effectively aggregate health information by means of a comprehensive electronic transaction system or network. The hope was that the costs of data collection could be rationalized to the industry by piggy-backing on value-added business transactions, such as electronic transmission of claims. Business transactions were also to provide the revenue stream to sustain the CHMIS organization and data repository.

2. *The Data Repository.* The overriding rationale for CHMIS was to provide broad access to information. The administrative efficiencies gleaned from electronic transactions were seen as secondary, albeit valuable, benefits. A central data repository would aggregate and store data, and a broad spectrum of community users would have varying levels of access to the repository, depending on authorization policies. The concept of a blended data set was key to the perceived value of the repository. Traditionally, claims data had formed the bulk of health information available for analytical purposes. CHMIS strongly urged that claims data be enhanced by blending it with person-centered survey measures, clinical information, and demographics.

3. *The CHMIS Organization.* At the heart of the information infrastructure lay the CHMIS organization. To ensure community control and the capability to address shared health information needs, CHMIS advocated a coalition model of governance. The exact mix of stakeholders varied across communities, as did the convening entity. In all cases, however, the CHMIS organization reflected a diverse mix of providers, plans, purchasers, consumers, and public sector representatives.

Many CHMIS concepts are now embodied in the CHIN movement, the managed care revolution, and other broad-based industry trends. CHMIS encouraged the health industry, information technology vendors, and policy makers to consider the advantages and commercial opportunities of broad-based electronic community networks. The CHMIS organization has provided a model for many of the coalition-style CHIN groups.

While the CHMIS vision has remained stable, the methods and strategies for executing the vision and the participants in the process have changed. The initial CHMIS concept came under significant criticism as soon as a description was published.* The main criticisms of the CHMIS concept were:

---

*The description of the initial CHMIS vision was presented in the *CHMIS Specifications,* published by the Hartford Foundation in 1991 and then revised in the fall of 1992. Both versions were prepared by Benton International, a New York based consulting firm, with input from CHMIS sites.

- Financial feasibility: How will it all be paid for?
- Redundancy: Is CHMIS needed if enterprise efforts are already under-way?
- Control: Can a coalition get this complex job done?
- Value added: Will CHMIS services meet immediate business needs?
- Standards: How can implementation proceed in such a diverse environment?
- Privacy, confidentiality, and proprietary information: How will person/provider identified data be protected?

As CHMIS developers in different parts of the country attempted to implement their vision, they encountered resistance usually based on some combination of the factors listed above. Some of the seven Hartford funded sites persevered with the original approach or made only minor changes. Other sites made significant changes in their approach, or ceased operation. By 1996, only four of the seven original Hartford funded sites—Minnesota, Ohio, Iowa, and Washington—continue to pursue CHMIS activities.

Observing how CHMIS adapted to a changing environment offers useful guidance in considering a wide range of health information issues. The sections that follow describe key aspects of the CHMIS experience over the last five years.

Organization and Structure

Collaborative activities begin with a joining of diverse stakeholders interested in exploring the feasibility and desirability of a shared venture. Some form of organization is required for any such venture. Typically, CHMIS and CHINs have, from the earliest stages of organization, emphasized how they are unique. Regrettably, this emphasis on distinguishing identifies has had a pernicious tendency to polarize constituencies, until the terms CHMIS and CHIN have reached a point where negative connotations often obscure their substance. The emphasis on what divides health information advocates and who is "right" has obscured the similarities among the different initiatives. Too much time has been spent disputing which acronym is best.

Some in the CHMIS and CHIN movement are now trying to deemphasize the acronym and focus on the common qualities of all those seeking to improve the health information infrastructure. After all, a group attempting to "wire up" a diverse delivery system faces many of the same challenges as a group trying to develop a community infrastructure. Perhaps the best way to view the CHMIS organization is as a community health information partnership, sans acronym.

The strength of a partnership comes from the participation of a broad mix of stakeholders working to meet their shared health care information needs. This collaborative activity can be facilitated through a variety of organizational and governance options. Finding the right arrangement requires consideration of three key issues:

- *Neutral Ground.* To achieve the cooperation of all stakeholders, a health information partnership must be perceived as belonging to all stakeholders and serving all their information needs equally well. No single party can be in a position to co-opt the organization. The primary strategic asset of the organization is its status as neutral ground.
- *Operational Effectiveness.* The partnership must add value to the community by "doing something." The organization and governance must enhance, not restrict, operational effectiveness. This usually means empowering management and avoiding micromanagement by the Board. It also suggests the importance of a clearly defined mission and operational focus.
- *Unique Environments.* Successful social engineering requires attention to the peculiar nuances that make each community unique. Each organization must be custom built. Although CHMIS sites share common objectives, the means they employ and the structures they use to realize these objectives vary as much as the communities themselves.

Although the precise nature of the partnership organization will vary, certain similarities appear across communities:

Not-for-Profit Status

The community mission of the partnership and its broad mix of stakeholders tend to be incompatible with a for-profit status. Most partnerships are 501 c-3 organizations, permitting stakeholder contributions to be tax deductible and grants to be accepted from foundations. However, 501 c-3 organizations are not allowed to lobby. On occasion, a partnership may be structured as a 501 c-6 to permit lobbying activities to be conducted, particularly at the state level.

Stakeholder Governance

Common to most partnerships is governance by a balanced board of health care stakeholders. The key stakeholders typically are:

- providers
- health plans
- insurers
- private employers
- consumers
- government officials.

Most sites tend to seek some balance between health industry groups (plans, insurers, and providers) and nonhealth industry groups (purchasers, consumers, and government). This balance is critical in light of the fact that most partnerships go beyond electronic networking and also focus on assessment. The various stakeholders within the industry and nonindustry groups will not concur on all issues. The industry groups tend to see more immediate return from the networking projects, whereas the nonindustry groups are more interested in the assessment work. Having a good governing balance ensures that both will be pursued aggressively.

Committee Structure

Governance is exclusive by nature. No organization can hope to involve more than a tiny fraction of its constituents at its Board level. Yet to be effective, a health information partnership must engage its customers. The solution is an inclusive committee structure. While a Board is likely to be limited to 15–20 people, committees may involve hundreds of stakeholders. At the committee level, constituents with specific interests (e.g., confidentiality, technology, data analysis) can become engaged and invested in the process. Effective committee work helps the community see the products of the partnership as "ours" rather than "theirs."

Health information partnerships across the country feature a number of organizational and structural arrangements. There is no one *right* approach. The two key questions to ask in designing the organizational architecture for a partnership are these:

• Are the key customers (as opposed to just staff and other "believers") engaged and invested in the outcome of the process?

• Operationally, can the partnership accomplish the tasks at hand?

If the answer to both questions is yes, the organizational approach is likely to succeed. If the answer to either question is no, the organizational approach is likely to fail.

Technological Approach

If a word could summarize the initial CHMIS concept, it would be "centralized." While this was viewed as desirable by some in the policy-making community, to most others it was not a positive appellation. The centralization of data and network services meant a loss of control. Enterprise and integrated delivery system developers did not want to depend on a broad-based coalition to build, operate, and control an information infrastructure they viewed as critical to their success. They believed they would be more likely to meet their needs in a timely manner if they did it themselves.

The centralized approach was also inconsistent with industry trends. Automation continues to expand rapidly at all levels of the health care industry. From individual enterprises to large integrated delivery systems, networks and data bases were, and continue to be, developed and installed. As automation efforts matured, it became increasingly obvious that the community was being wired from the "bottom up." Thus, it was difficult to justify the concept of a top down, centralized development effort when much of the same capability was being deployed on a decentralized basis.

The trend toward a decentralized health information infrastructure was accelerated significantly by the growth of managed care. Most managed care plans view health information systems as a critical component of success. Those communities with the greatest managed care penetration tend to have the most emphasis on decentralization, and they tend to be most resistant to centralized systems.

CHMIS partnerships in strong managed care markets were the first to address concerns about centralization. The CHMIS architecture was modified from a single central network to a decentralized "network of networks" model. Similarly, the central repository evolved into a "virtual repository," which assumes that "minirepositories" will be created by the integrated delivery systems. Selected data could then be extracted from these decentralized repositories and aggregated to provide answers to community questions.

The decentralized approach to addressing community health information needs has proven to be much more politically acceptable to health industry participants. It eliminates concerns about centralized control and redundancy, and links existing community capabilities instead of replacing them.

In pursuing implementation of a decentralized system, partnerships have chosen different approaches that reflect the unique characteristics of their communities. In Ohio, a number of CHIN projects are underway, as the Ohio Health Information Corporation (OCHI) has positioned itself as the "CHIN of CHINs." OCHI will offer services to enhance connectivity among and between the Ohio CHIN networks. In Minnesota, the Minnesota Health Data Institute has developed MedNet, the classic network of networks. It is a "neutral" value-added network that links competing enterprise and integrated delivery system networks. In Washington, the Foundation for Health Care Quality is working to link the four proprietary EDI networks already deployed in the community. This linkage will create a single "virtual" network of networks.

While decentralization has proven more attractive to key stakeholders than a centralized system, there are still significant feasibility problems. To be successful, the decentralized components must have significant market penetration and be technologically sophisticated enough to link to the common network and data base. This has not often been the case. In fact, other network developers are now encountering many of the same challenges in developing a health information infrastructure as the early CHMIS sites. In most communities the system integration task is formidable. It is very expensive to deploy technology, train participants, and link disparate systems. To truly add value, a network must have a critical mass of subscribers and offer transactions that meet current user needs. Inability to achieve this critical mass of subscribers creates a vicious cycle. The absence of subscribers limits perceived utility, which limits market penetration. Limited market penetration constrains revenue, which in turn limits funding to deploy new functionality and attain critical mass. As the health care value-added network movement painfully attempts to grow, a new phenomenon, the Internet, is causing some partnership sites to reevaluate their basic strategy once again.

The explosive growth of the Internet is well documented. There is a vigorous debate currently underway as to whether the Internet will ultimately be *the* community health information network. Some partnerships are asking the following questions:

- Can undercapitalized, not-for-profit community organizations solve the health information system integration challenge?
- Is the proprietary VAN approach, either centralized or decentralized, the best place for the partnership to be?
- Should the partnership shift its emphasis to the Internet?
- Should the partnership "forget" about building networks and facilitating system integration, assume the Internet will "win," and concentrate on the development of content and the naming and authorization functions needed to exchange this content securely among Internet users?

The answer to these questions is not yet clear. However, the questions suggest the possibility of a third shift in CHMIS implementation strategy, from a centralized VAN/repository model, to a decentralized VAN/repository model, to the Internet and a focus on content and naming/security. An implementation strategy that makes use of the Internet may be the most feasible and appropriate role for broad based, neutral community organizations.

The Business Case

Initially, the CHMIS and CHIN concepts were considered to be intrinsically great ideas. How could one not support a means to solve all the health information woes in one fell swoop? Add in concepts like community and collaboration and it was hard to miss. Unfortunately, interested parties began to ask some challenging questions such as:

- "What will it all cost?"
- "Who is going to pay for it?"
- "What's in it for me?"

The original CHMIS concept ran into trouble when it could not satisfactorily answer these questions or identify a viable financial strategy for capitalizing and operating the system. The original financial strategy assumed vendors would build the system on a risk basis, and the community would flock to use it. The Memphis partnership put out an RFI to this effect. However, the vendors were not willing to provide capital for anything without clearly identified paying customers attached to an ongoing revenue stream. The response to the RFI was lackluster and the Memphis partnership eventually failed. The need to make a sound business case continues to haunt community health information network developers.

All of the CHMIS partnerships have wrestled with this issue as have most CHINs. Their deliberations have highlighted two key concerns: focus on your customers and be incremental.

Customer Focus

Many stakeholders will benefit from, and participate in, a community health information activity. However, to get a partnership off the ground and reach any kind of critical mass, the needs of paying customers must be given primary consideration. Public data dollars are drying up; there is not a public sector entity in the country that can finance large scale health information infrastructure projects. Therefore, paying customers will be calling the shots. A customer has needs they are willing to pay to meet. Other stakeholders may also have wants they would like to address. The ability to distinguish wants from needs can be the difference between success and failure.

A classic example of this phenomenon was the Washington State Health Services Information System (HSIS). HSIS was mandated in the health care reform bill passed by the Washington state legislature in 1993. It was a mandated CHMIS/CHIN. HSIS called for comprehensive data collection and a broad range of electronic capability. As part of the planning process, a needs assessment was conducted. The outcome of this assessment was a vast collection of stakeholder preferences, expectations, and desires. Unfortunately, the stakeholders were not constrained by willingness to pay. The system that emerged from the design process never got off the ground. It was too unwieldy and lacked support from the people expected to finance it. Legislative mandates will not get systems built. Expecting private customers to pay to build a system that is controlled by the public sector and designed to meet primarily public policy objectives is a recipe for failure.

To focus on customers is not to say that only the private sector, or only the health industry will get their needs met. The public sector is a large potential paying customer as are other stakeholders. The key is to identify a means to add enough value to attract funding from a broad range of sources. Common needs are the perfect opportunity to partner; unique needs and/or wants, likely will be pursued independently. In this customer-driven model, it is vital for those customers who care most about open access to data and improving the health of the community to participate in the effort. These customers must be forceful in ensuring their needs do not become overwhelmed by the business needs of the industry customers.

Focusing on customers suggests a new model for public/private collaboration. In the past, the public sector has mandated or contracted with the private sector. The private sector has been the contractee and the target of the mandate. Now both parties are on the same footing as customers. This means a greater sharing of control. It will be a challenge for both sectors to learn to do business in this manner. However, it will ultimately be more rewarding and is likely the best approach to leveraging private capital to achieve public policy objectives.

Figures 6.1 and 6.2 illustrate the distinction between the "big bang" approach to achieving a community health information vision and a more incremental, value-added approach. The vision of a fully integrated health information network provides great added benefit to all potential custom-

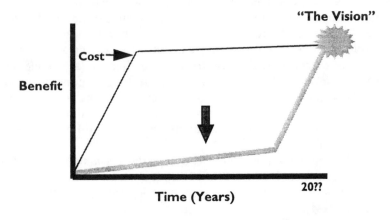

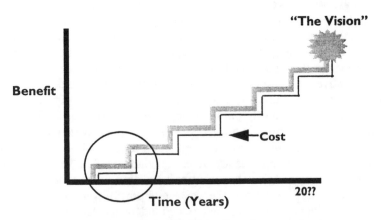

FIGURE 6.2. Value-added incremental approach.

ers, but it lies far in the future. The "big bang" approach (Fig. 6.1) incurs significant costs from the beginning but adds little value until several years out. This model fails the business test. It will fail to attract savvy investors or paying customers. The incremental model (Fig. 6.2) builds toward the same vision. However, it adopts a phased approach, matching cost incurred with value added. This appears to be the most successful approach.

The area in the circle in Fig. 6.2 represents the key challenge for most partnerships, choosing the initial functionality to be deployed. Answering this question correctly is mandatory to building critical mass and achieving long-term success.

Figure 6.3 illustrates an approach to phasing in functionality in a community system. The services have been parsed to allow high value, less costly, less threatening functionality to precede more complex offerings. This model is by no means the only approach and it may not even be the best approach. As partnerships confront rapid changes in technology and the marketplace, the question of initial functionality largely boils down to what business the partnership wants to be in and which customers it will serve.

Even with the best business planning, proceeding with a health information project will, to some extent, require a leap of faith. Cost and benefit data are largely unavailable and there are few successful models to emulate. A pioneering spirit is a necessary accompaniment to sound business planning.

Health Information Studies

As the name implies, the CHIN movement focuses on networking. It revolves around technology. CHMIS partnerships have another dimension, an interim low-tech strategy for adding value in the absence of a comprehensive electronic infrastructure. While the ultimate CHMIS concept envisions using electronic health information systems to aggregate data for analysis and reporting back to the community, it will be a long time before such capability exists in most communities. The CHMIS partnerships have elected to move forward with a variety of health information studies using more low-tech methods to acquire data.

Minnesota has recently completed an extensive consumer satisfaction survey, covering public and private health plan enrollees and measuring several dimensions of satisfaction. Of particular relevance to MHDI's community mission, extensive effort was applied to the dissemination phase of the project. Approximately one million copies of the study were distributed through newspaper inserts. This study was a separate effort from MHDI's MedNet initiative. The network was not employed to gather data, though the results have been made available on the partnership's WEB site.

In Washington, the Foundation for Health Care Quality has conducted a

---

Type 1

Provide access to general information about individual entities and processes
- that is not considered propriety by the data supplier,
- that is needed by multiple parties,
- that requires little or no added processing, and
- that has limited privacy concerns
  e.g., provider directories, drug/drug interactions, medical research data bases, clinical practice guidelines, health education, etc.

Type 2

Provide access to both general and unique information about individual entities and processes
- that is not considered propriety by the data supplier,
- which is needed by multiple parties,
- which can be produced with minimal additional processing, and
- which has more advanced privacy considerations
  e.g., community master entity indices [patients, providers, plans, etc.], provider credentials information, provider drug dispensing licenses and authorizations, authorized referral lists, child immunization history, current patient medication usage, patient-specific allergies and adverse drug reactions, etc.

Type 3

Provide access to unique information about individual entities and processes
- that is produced through complex valued-added processing applied to both general and unique information obtained from multiple entities (both proprietary and non-proprietary),
- which is needed by multiple parties, and
- which has significant privacy considerations
  e.g., coordination of benefits priority determinations, balances payable by secondary payers or by the individual, practice protocols, disease management guidelines, critical patient health history and conditions, clinical outcomes assessment data sets, etc.

FIGURE 6.3. A phased approach to implementation.

number of outcome studies. For example, the statewide Obstetrics Review and Quality System (StORQS) project compares the performance of all hospitals in the state that deliver babies. The Foundation is also engaged in outcome projects related to coronary artery bypass grafts, low back pain, and a project to supplement HEDIS measures with selected clinical outcome data. These projects are conducted in collaboration with researchers at the University of Washington, Washington State University, and other stakeholder groups. As in Minnesota, these outcome projects are separate and distinct from the electronic networking initiatives.

The CHMIS partnerships interpret their mission as meeting community health information needs, with or without electronic solutions. This tends to distinguish the CHMIS partnerships from some of the more traditional CHIN efforts. Community health information studies are a short-term means to add value, define content, clarify methodological approaches and establish positive working relationships with groups that are also likely to be involved in the electronic initiatives.

Privacy Protection

From the beginning, confidentiality and privacy concerns presented a major stumbling block for CHMIS. The idea of a "giant centralized data repository" worried consumers and privacy advocates. Among providers and health plans, concerns arose about how data viewed as proprietary (e.g., containing plan or provider identifiers) would be used or abused.

The CHMIS partnerships have concentrated more on privacy and confidentiality policies and procedures than on technical security considerations. This is in contrast to many CHINs. Security tends to be of more interest to health industry and information systems personnel than most other community stakeholders. With this in mind, the CHMIS partnerships have attempted to address the privacy and confidentiality issue in a different way than most CHINs.

Legislation

Minnesota has secured the passage of legislation increasing protections for privacy and confidentiality of health information. Washington and Vermont made unsuccessful efforts to pass similar legislation in their states.

Technical Assistance

The CHMIS Resource Center has provided technical assistance, education, and written materials to assist communities in developing confidentiality and privacy policies and procedures.

Consumer Involvement

Washington and Vermont have conducted community forums to elicit concerns and inform grass roots consumer groups. Washington and Minnesota have also convened consumer advisory groups to provide input into the process.

Over time, the partnerships have listened, learned, and modified their approaches to protecting health information privacy. The lessons learned may be summarized as follows:

- The current system for protecting the privacy of personal health information is not adequate to meet the demands of the paper age, let alone the age of electronics.
- Improving the protection of personal health information privacy is an essential priority.
- Automation is a threat to privacy; however, it also offers the best opportunity to improve personal health information security and privacy.

- Greater effort must be made to sell the benefits of automated health information networks outside the health industry. Most individuals perceive the threats more clearly than the benefits.
- The distinctions between person-identified data and aggregate information must be more effectively delineated. The relative threats, opportunities, and requirements for protection and uses of the two data types must be clearly defined and communicated.
- The nature of electronic commerce dictates that a federal legislative solution ultimately will be required to address health information privacy concerns.

As consumers become more involved in partnerships, the importance of the privacy issue increases. For many consumers, this is the only health information issue about which they care strongly. Failure to satisfactorily deal with concerns about privacy and confidentiality are likely to doom large scale data collection efforts.

Engaging Consumers

In its early years, CHMIS, like most of the CHIN initiatives, focused largely on health industry stakeholders. While these groups remain critical to the success of any community health information partnership, consumers are becoming increasingly important. Community health information initiatives will not meet long-term needs if the ultimate consumers are an afterthought.

The move toward managed care makes this all the more important. To many consumers, fee-for-service concerns are related to overtreatment while managed care raises fears of undertreatment. The latter is seen, correctly or not, as of greater concern. Consumers are seeking better sources of information to protect their interests and allow for more effective participation in treatment decision-making.

For the health industry, the proliferation of the Internet, kiosk technology, and computers in the workplace and home offer cost-effective means to disseminate information and deliver health care service. The partnerships are using the increasing involvement of consumers as a powerful argument for ensuring that inter-enterprise capability is present in every community. It is difficult enough to justify juggling multiple proprietary networks, each operated by "closed" managed care systems, to health care industry participants. This approach is impossible to sell to consumers whose needs regularly cross system lines.

The CHMIS partnerships are factoring the demand side customers into their long term plans. Partnerships are making increasing use of consumer advisory boards. Consumer tools like provider directories to help navigate the complexities of managed care are assuming a higher priority in business planning. "Translation" of health information studies also assumes greater prominence. Traditionally, health information studies have been conducted by, for, and of industry stakeholders, and researchers. A plain English translation is needed for everybody else. The same study that reported with pages of data to a health plan quality improvement manager may become a few punchy paragraphs when distributed to a consumer. For health information partnerships with true community orientation, mastering this communication challenge will be a growing priority and opportunity in the years ahead.

Conclusion

The CHMIS model has evolved over the years. The community partnerships have gained valuable insights, made some small progress and learned with the health industry what works and what does not. CHMIS faces two major challenges in the immediate future. The first is to keep the focus on community needs. In trying to build a successful business case, there is a risk that the community partnerships will tilt too far toward becoming "health industry information networks." To lose the community focus is to lose the heart of the CHMIS vision, and the partnerships must be vigilant in this regard.

The second challenge will be to "just do it." Concepts, theory, and lessons learned are all nice, but the real need is for working models. The partnerships need to be able to produce infrastructure improvements, health information products and other concrete achievements. They need to add value in their communities and provide an example to others. The time has come to deliver the goods. Community health information partnerships have a challenging and exciting time ahead.

7

CHINs: A Public Health Perspective

J. Nell Brownstein, Mark W. Oberle, Kathleen R. Miner, Melissa Alperin, Elizabeth H. Howze, and Kevin Patrick

The impact of the information technology revolution, including Community Health Information Networks (CHINs), is just now being felt in the field of public health and has yet to be measured. However, the limited anecdotal information available suggests that technologies will bring profound changes in the way public health is practiced. Two-way and multiway interactive communication will become the norm and will occur in a variety of media—graphics, video, voice, and data on personal workstations at home, school, and work.

Just as in private contexts, three forces are driving these trends: (1) the need for agency accountability and responsibility, (2) explosive changes in the information technology field, and (3) the need for streamlining systems.[1] Enhanced computer networking will directly affect both public health consumers and public health professionals. Ultimately, CHINs will probably completely change the way private and public agencies deliver services to consumers.

The Public Health Approach

The 1988 Institute of Medicine report, *The Future of Public Health*, described the three core functions of public health services as assessment, policy development, and assurance.[2] In 1994, the U.S. Public Health Service prepared an additional statement titled *Public Health in America*, which further subdivided these three functions into 10 essential public health services[3]:

CHINs can enhance and facilitate each of these.

1. Assessment

- Monitor health status to identify community problems.
- Diagnose and investigate health problems and health hazards in the community.
- Inform, educate, and empower people about health issues.

2. Policy Development

- Mobilize community partnerships and action to identify and solve health problems.
- Develop policies and plans that support individual and community health efforts.

3. Assurance

- Enforce laws and regulation that protect health and ensure safety.
- Link people to needed personal health services.
- Assure a competent public and personal health care workforce.
- Evaluate effectiveness, accessibility, and quality of personal and population-based health services.
- Research for new insights and innovative solutions to health problems.

Assessment refers to the ability and capacity of public health agencies to collect data to improve decision-making. It is essential for identifying and solving emerging public health problems. Public health agencies regularly collect, analyze, and disseminate information on the health of their communities, including information on personal and environmental health, community concerns and resources, and the quality and range of health services. Because this assessment function cuts across all aspects of the community and all levels of government, CHINs, which connect these diverse elements, promise to play an important role in supporting public health assessment services. A fully evolved CHIN can link hospitals, managed care organizations, private clinics, hospitals, community health centers, laboratories, and other sources of health-related information. A CHIN can thus increase efficiency and provide public health professionals a far greater wealth of data than any of these resources accessed individually.

The policy development process relies on the ability to access and use data (e.g., published research, surveillance data, expert opinion, and consensus). Enhanced ability to integrate and use multiple sources of information will permit health needs to be defined and ranked by priority, and disease prevention and health promotion interventions to be developed, evaluated, and improved. The ability of CHINs to link relatively small or isolated communities into the larger framework of public health expertise is thus an asset to public health agencies as they seek to develop shared definitions of problems and policy solutions.

Public health agencies also need to ensure that health policies are implemented and that health services and functions are available and carried out appropriately.[4] In some cases, a public health agency may provide a direct service, such as restaurant inspection or family planning services. Here, too, CHINs can play a valuable role, particularly in regard to the growth of managed care. The prevailing forces in health care reform are shifting emphasis toward population-based services and away from services to individuals. It is likely that public health agencies will be asked to monitor clinical treatment and preventive services delivered by the private sector. CHINs can assist public health agencies in this new role by providing data for evaluation of the quality and delivery of services. In some states this type of integrated health system partnership has already been developed.[5]

The Federal Governments Role in Fostering CHINs

In 1994, the Clinton administration initiated the planning process for the National Information Infrastructure (NII), a seamless (compatible), high-speed communications "network of networks" capable of delivering voice, data, and video to people anywhere, anytime.[6] In addition to networking technologies, NII components include data, applications and software, standards, and transmission protocols and people involved in providing development, exchange, analysis, storage, and other services supportive of the NII.

Driving this effort is the vision that the NII will enable federal, state, and local government agencies to exchange databases and to provide information and services to the public 24 hours a day via electronic mail, computer bulletin boards, and computer kiosks. Pilot applications have already been developed. For example, the "Info/California" kiosk program helped Los Angeles County citizens deal with the transportation problems that followed the January 1994 earthquake. Eighty kiosks provided the following online items: rapidly updated maps showing traffic density, registration for ride-sharing, and a mass-transit database from which citizens could print out routes and schedules.[7]

National public health agencies such as the Centers for Disease Control and Prevention (CDC) have taken leadership in the development of the public health component of the NII. A variety of CHINs are beginning to provide critical communication, information, and data linkages among private, local, state, and federal agencies with public health intents. One key public health initiative to coordinate an integrated infrastructure is the Information Network for Public Health Officials (INPHO). Initiated by CDC, the INPHO aims to connect the fragmented public health system and helps states build strategic information partnerships based on modern telecommunications and computer networks. INPHO addresses virtually all aspects of public health services.[8] Most INPHO projects involve public-private partnerships, the coupling of CDC dollars with funds from other state or federal agencies, or both. These partnerships increase the pool of available resources and expand the ownership of the projects to several agencies.

Georgia pioneered the INPHO project in early 1993 with a $5.4 million grant from the Robert W. Woodruff Foundation. The Georgia Division of

Public Health, the Medical College of Georgia, the Georgia Center for Advanced Telecommunications Technology, the Rollins School of Public Health at Emory University, and the CDC collaborated in establishing a statewide public health network.[9] The CDC has provided funding to establish subsequent INPHO efforts in Florida, Illinois, Indiana, Michigan, Missouri, New York, North Carolina, Oregon, Rhode Island, Washington, and West Virginia.

The three basic components of the INPHO effort are network linkages, data exchange, and information access.

Network Linkages

INPHO helps states develop coordinated computer networks and software to link local clinics, state health agencies, and federal health partners, slicing through geographic and bureaucratic barriers to communication and data exchange. Local public health agencies are also developing network links with hospitals, managed care organizations, community health centers, and other health care providers. These networks integrate population-based public health practice with clinical medical practice, building the public health sector's capacity to establish partnerships with private health care providers. These public-private partnerships are expected to lead to collaborative efforts to design and evaluate cost-efficient health services delivery systems.

The Georgia INPHO project contributed significantly to the public health response to the devastating flooding in the southwestern portion of the state during the summer of 1994. One of the most severely affected communities was Albany, where floodwaters left hundreds of families homeless and put public health clinics and the county health department out of commission. Dr. Lynne Feldman, Albany district health director, found that INPHO provided invaluable assistance in the relief efforts:

By using my portable computer and INPHO software, I was able to send detailed reports every day to the state health director, telling him and the state-level public health relief team exactly what we needed, what was working, and what day-to-day problems needed to be solved. We also used INPHO to get fast access to reports from the state office survey on health conditions in the flooded area. Just by itself, the electronic communications feature of INPHO helped us in the field and the state health director's office really function as if we were all right on the site together.[10]

INPHO uses the CDC WONDER (Wide-ranging Online Data for Epidemiological Research) as an online public information system (multiway data communication). CDC WONDER is a software program for microcomputers that creates a fast and efficient electronic link between CDC and public health practioners. CDC WONDER can access CDC datasets; analyze data; create charts, maps, and tables; send e-mail, reports, and guidelines; and transmit secure data files. A closely related Georgia effort was the surveillance system that the State epidemiologist and staff from Albany, Dublin, and Macon health districts set up to identify disease outbreaks and monitor the health impact of the floods. Using CDC WONDER e-mail (see "Data Exchange" section), more than 100 health care facilities in the region sent daily reports to district and state health officials. More than 30,000 reports were transmitted.

Statewide electronic calendars let every public health worker learn about upcoming public health meetings, conferences, and training opportunities. Also, CDC maintains a national training catalogue on CDC WONDER to coordinate satellite broadcasts and other distance learning opportunities. This allows individual employees or agencies to tailor priorities for commitment of staff and economic resources.

Data Exchange

Electronic networks give public health professionals access to federal and state databases for epidemiologic analysis, assessment of the effectiveness of health programs, and comparison of local health status data with state or national averages. For example, health department personnel can reference national and state data on prevalence or risk factors to assist them in setting local priorities for programmatic action. With high-speed data exchange capability, frontline public health practitioners can rapidly assess health problems, including developing epidemics. As in the private care sector, standards and procedures for data exchange are still evolving.

Simple but powerful, e-mail provides the ability to communicate rapidly, expand access to professional contacts, and transmit documents. INPHO uses CDC WONDER, which includes an e-mail system that enables users to communicate with each other and with CDC staff and to attach files to their e-mail, which makes sharing information easier. These networking efforts are expected to reduce costs, increase productivity, improve data and information systems, and enhance communication — all of which are critical to strengthening the public health system.[5]

CDC WONDER also makes information and resources immediately accessible to public health officials and the public worldwide. It gives users easy access to a variety of data sets and CDC and state health department activities. CDC WONDER provides a convenient vehicle for research and surveillance collaboration: data from local providers can be sent to the CDC mainframe or to any local area network-based application, where they are verified, interpreted, and added to centralized databases.[11] No longer must data providers wait weeks for the results of analyses; they are available in minutes. In addition, community public health agencies have found that CDC WONDER affords an excellent opportunity to exhibit their own data.[11] CDC WONDER's public health analytic software allows users easily to create graphs, maps, and tables and to export results for various applications.[11] The data sets are heavily used.

Electronic reporting of infectious disease cases and other morbidity data speeds recognition of outbreaks and health risks and helps local and state staff respond quickly to community health emergencies.[12] Similarly, exchanging laboratory results over high-speed networks helps local authorities and practitioners take rapid action and monitor the spread of drug-resistant organisms.[13] For example, an INPHO-based system to improve hospital reporting of notifiable diseases is being developed by the Georgia Department of Public Health (GDPH) and the Medical College of Georgia (MCG). Their goal is to enable emergency department physicians to report notifiable disease cases electronically as they gather, and record routine information on patients. GDPH is designing reporting templates to match its disease notification requirements. MCG will coordinate those templates with clinical software to capture disease reports and forward them to GDPH for verification. Once verified, cases of notifiable diseases will be reported to CDC electronically and trigger action by state and local public health agencies. Additionally, GDPH is exploring electronic disease reporting by health maintaince organizations and private hospitals.

CDC WONDER also provides electronic access to the CDC Prevention Guidelines Database (PGD). PGD is a central, accessible, up-to-date repository of relevant protocols for handling cholera, disaster response, dengue fever, suicide attempts, malaria, lung cancer, and other health problems. The PGD meets the information needs of public health officials by providing a single point of access to the most current guidelines and recommendations issued by CDC. PGD was designed to solve a common problem: lack of access to guidelines for the direct provision of public health services.

Information Access

The INPHO puts health publications, reports, databases, directories, and other resources into electronic formats, giving public health practitioners access to current information in many areas of interest.[14] States that have INPHO are developing electronic editions of publications and reports for local and state network users. Executive Health Information Systems (EHIS), an electronic reporting system, lets front-line health professionals and top public health directors keep close tabs on health conditions, community trends, and other social and political issues in formats they construct for their specific purposes. EHIS allows public health workers to monitor frequently updated databases that are maintained in clinics and local and state health departments, making it possible for local and state public health professionals to coordinate the preparation and dissemination of health communications for public advocacy campaigns.

Through electronic publications health care agencies can access the latest public health research and interpretations, whatever their proximity to medical library facilities. *CDC's Morbidity and Mortality Weekly Report,* for example, is electronically accessible days before the mails can deliver the paper report. Other publications, including *Electronic Prevention Guidelines and Resource Directory,* provide state-of-the-art protocols for personal protection, public safety, and public information and are accessible through local and state computer networks for immediate use in clinical settings. When a local health department encounters a potential disease outbreak, the staff have immediate electronic access to appropriate protocals. The 1995 online debut of a new CDC scientific journal, *Emerging Infectious Diseases,* will build an international network of researchers who can rapidly exchange infectious disease information.

At the state level, the CDC Resource Center for Health Systems Reform provides a forum, via CDC WONDER, for sharing ideas, innovations, and strategies and for building networks, and thus strengthens public health officals' planning ability. This electronic forum allows users to keep abreast of public health reform activities in other states and learn how other health departments are adapting their structures and services. This linkage serves to build capacity in states and communities with little experience in the health reform area. New Jersey, for example, passed a law in 1994 requiring that all health care providers cover 14 key prevention items in annual "prevention exams," which will replace annual physical exams. Information about New Jersey's law may spur other states to give more serious consideration to preventive health services.

The Georgia INPHO project demonstrates the benefits of network linkages, data exchange, and information access. Access to electronic networking via CDC WONDER has allowed public health workers in Georgia to practice more productively and efficiently. One Georgia community has private physicians linked into its system, which allows the physicians to readily access immunization data. One rural community efficiently contained an outbreak of Shigellosis because it had instant access to CDC information and was able to immediately initiate appropriate protocals. Through INPHO, Georgians can be linked statewide with national and international agencies. This will make it easier for Georgians and others to form partnerships and coalitions between the private and public health sectors and to work to improve health care delivery. Other public health agencies are providing similar access to client educational materials, administrative forms, and other information.

Nongovernment CHINs are well suited to serve public health policy development and advocacy functions. For example, electronic communication and data retrieval and reporting have become increasingly important to states and local communities that are struggling to prevent and reduce tobacco addiction. CDC WONDER and specialized tobacco control net works, such as SCARCNET (described below), facilitate the flow of information to and from state and local levels. The state networks often reach from health departments to coalitions of community voluntary organizations, hospitals, health care providers, university researchers, police, elected officials, parents, teachers, and youth.

SCARCNET is a private, nonprofit computer communications network devoted to tobacco control advocates, including grassroots organizations, national voluntary groups, state and local health departments, and federally funded grantees. In addition to providing up-to-date information in the form of daily bulletins, action alerts, and directories, SCARCNET provides a forum for tobacco control activists to share information and strategies and build skills promoting clean indoor air, restricting advertising and promotion, and restricting tobacco industry access to youth.

The benefits of CHINs to the tobacco control movement are considerable. Information about the availability of resources, advice, and news about current events are rapidly and widely shared and can be stored for future reference. Users find CHINs invaluable in facilitating collaboration, because they can post a question and quickly receive advice or answers. Information on pending national events is shared in a timely fashion, allowing users to involve their local coalitions to bring in local press in a related story. Transmission of electronic documents that can be localized reduces the staff time needed for projects. CHINs also cut program costs by reducing postage and staff travel. In addition, CHINs have helped the tobacco control movement mobilize people on the community level behind a common goal and with a united voice. In Georgia, the Atlanta Tobacco Control Coalition has set up electronic communications among its 25 member organizations through CDC WONDER. Minutes of meetings and relevant documents are exchanged among coalition members, reducing the number of face-to-face meetings needed without diminishing the quality of the communication.

Other nongovernment CHINs are also furthering the interests of public health. The International Network for Interfaith Health Practitioners (IHP-NET) links public health practitioners all over the world. Online, they collaborate on projects, share valuable resources, contacts, ideas, and practical and policy strategies, and gain peer support (especially important for those working in isolated rural areas) on a wide range of topics. Information for State Health Policy Program (InfoSHP), established by the Robert Wood Johnson Foundation in 1992, assists states in their policy-making efforts through sharing data across state programs, agencies, and private partners; 10 states are currently partners.[15] In addition, South Carolina has been funded " to link patient and program-specific data systems with vital records to create a comprehensive patient-centered data base. When stripped of identifiers, the data base will be used by policy makers for planning and assessment purposes."[15, pp. 7–8]

Consumer-Health Information

Among the tasks that have traditionally fallen to the public health community is provision of health information to the public — from information about the safety of foods to the need to become immunized against polio, measles, or influenza. As with other traditional roles in public health, CHINs and the broader NII of which they are a part have a role to play in restructuring the delivery of and access to health information.

Consumers need various kinds of health information, ranging from information on what they should do to keep themselves and their families healthy to how to access the health care system. As part of the recent NII, representatives from federal agencies involved in health-related programs proposed the following definition for *consumer health information (CHI)*:

CHI is any information that enables individuals to understand their health and make health-related decisions for themselves or their families. This includes information which supports individual and community-based health promotion and enhancement, self-care, shared (professional-patient) decision making, patient education and rehabilitation, how to use the health care system and select insurance or a provider, and peer-group support. From the perspective of the consumer, CHI can be actively sought or it can be provided to them through public or private education campaigns which target specific health issues (e.g., media efforts aimed at cholesterol reduction). CHI encompasses a wide range of information, essentially the "who, what, how, why, where, when and how much?" of health information. The nature of CHI can be economic, technical, logistical and/or qualitative. It is available in health care settings as well as such locations as homes, schools, libraries, work-sites, stores and other arenas open and accessible to all.

To be effective, CHI must be tailored to the interests, literacy, language, cultural background, emotional state and desires of its user. From the standpoint of providers of CHI, effectiveness may be measured both by how rapidly and completely desired messages are communicated and by how completely changes in behavior occur. Ultimately, for both producers and consumers of CHI, effectiveness will be measured by individual and population improvements in health status and quality of life.[16, p. 1]

The NII promises to change substantially our approach to CHI. Health-related decision-making depends in part on having correct information on hand. Information provided previously through general public service announcements on broadcast radio or television will be increasingly available in media that enable it to be tailored to individual behavioral or information consumption patterns. In-home health and medical information systems, as stand-alone devices or connected via cable or telephone line to information or service providers, will play a major role in providing this kind of information.

Public health agencies are beginning to form innovative CHIN partnerships to provide information and deliver services to underserved and special populations. One such partnership is envisioned between San Francisco's public library and the San Francisco City and County health departments. The vision of the San Francisco library is to have a "portal" to the "information superhighway" in every home, school, and workplace in the city by the year 2000. In its assessment of consumer interest, the library found that health information was among the most desired type of information. The health department sees this as an ideal opportunity to provide CHI of the city on everything from immunizations to violence prevention to environmental health. The health department also plans to use this cooperative relationship to help provide coordinated community services to city residents. Although funding constraints and other issues may slow attainment of the vision, this is a good example of the kind of interagency partnering fostered through the most broad-based definition of a CHIN.

For public health agencies to ensure comprehensive health coverage, barriers to access to health care—geographic, logistic, economic, attitudinal, and cultural—must be overcome. Dr. Walt Cairns and other researchers affiliated with the San Francisco Heart Institute have developed an innovative "smart telephone"—based case management approach to post-hospital cardiac rehabilitation and are using it in rural western Michigan. Designed to replicate a hospital-based rehabilitation program, the "smart telephone" approach allows individuals to be monitored at home by case managers, to input information on vital signs, to access by means of a touch screen on their telephone information about their condition 24 hours a day, and, in general, to receive all of the elements of support that they would in a hospital-based program. This program is delivered at roughly one third the cost of traditional cardiac rehabilitation and encompasses state-of-the-art medical knowledge not previously available in rural western Michigan. If successful, the program could revolutionize postdischarge medical practice, because today public health patients, as well as private care patients, are discharged from medical facilities while still under medical treatment.

Not all NII-related approaches to public health problems are based on so—called "high-tech" approaches. Strategies such as the Cleveland Telephone Medicine program, developed by Dr. Farouk Alemi, can give public health clients such as medically indigent and homeless persons access to health care providers through a simple voice mail system. Once seen for a problem, persons served by this system can call in from any telephone and, through their unique identifier number, obtain test results, find out if they need a follow-up appointment, connect with peers with similar health concerns, or receive specific advice directly from their health provider.

Community Services Networks

Another important NII approach to public health concerns is embodied in the Community Services Networks (CSNs) project being piloted in Washington, DC. CSNs are based on personal computer "workstations" located in the offices of any health and human service provider willing to become a part of the network. They make possible a collaborative working environment that supports integrated, "one-stop-shopping" for clients of these services because the information technology of a CHIN allows a "virtual record" of each client to be accessible instantaneously to all members of the health care provider network. Use of CSNs will enable public health agencies to ensure that at least a minimum level of health services are available to their clients. The ability of these systems to centralize client data makes it possible to provide quality client assistance in an efficient, timely manner because each client receives as many services as possible in one visit rather than requiring multiple visits spread over several days.

Similar CSN integrated information systems are already operating. The Cornerstone (Casey Project) in Illinois also offers a model "virtual one-stop shopping" that will sustain an integrated health service delivery system. The Missouri Health Strategic Architectures and Information Cooperative (MOHSAIC) allows for the exchange of information among public and private providers and health and human services agencies, thus improving client triage. For example, a local health department or collaborating health care agency can access a child's immunization status independent of the agency housing the record.[16] Georgia's Health Outcomes and Services Tracking System (H.O.S.T.) is a client-based approach that will improve service delivery by health departments because it tracks "direct delivery of heath care services to individuals using a single point of data entry."[16]

Adaptable to differing configurations of service providers in urban or rural settings, CSNs are the kind of sophisticated applications likely to be "running" on CHINs in the near future. A multitude of organizational, political, and financial issues must be worked out to make this possible, but such challenges have always been a part of public health and will likely be for the foreseeable future.

Demand Management

One of the fastest growing uses of telecommunications for health, and one from which considerable cost savings are likely to occur, is in the area of "demand management"—reducing the burden on health care providers by providing information about self-care and alternatives to medical care in the home. Important distinctions can be made between "need" for medical care and "demand" for medical care services. Effective medical care, (e.g., prenatal care and immunizations) is needed to prevent illness and optimize health status. On the other hand, much of the "demand" for medical care stems from unrealistic expectations about what "modern medicine" can provide. Unneccessary medical care—for example, visits for antibiotics for simple viral infections—consumes professional services, is unlikely to improve health status or outcomes, and may even result in additional health problems. Demand management is the process by which health care systems prevent these unneccesary health care visits. The timely provision of health-related information to individuals at the time they are making decisions about seeking medical treatment can yield more informed and satisfied individuals. Self-care guided by print media has gained considerable credibility over the past decade as a tool for demand management.[17,18] Advanced communication technologies promise to provide more powerful and effective means of accomplishing this, including network-based consultation with interactive reference materials through a computer to "real time" interaction with a health care provider over a home personal health information system wired through the local cable or telephone network.

It remains to be determined which parts of the consumer health information and demand management marketplace will end up in CHIN environments. This is an area in enormous flux, as corporate information service providers—ranging from AT&T to Reuters to Microsoft to Time-Warner—struggle to find their appropriate role in the provision of all kinds of information to individuals, families, and communities. One thing is clear: the notion that entertainment will drive everything in the NII is probably inaccurate. Health information for the public will be an important dimension of CHIN activity in the future.

Public Health Data Exchange

Data exchange is another important function of computer networks in the provision of public health services. For example, CDC is providing $25 million annually in pilot grants to develop state immunization registries that will allow public and private clinicians to update or download patients' immunization files. These registries will provide information on which immunizations a person might currently need and avoid duplicative immunizations and associated costs. Some states are working on a freestanding application; others are integrating the immunization registry into a multipurpose client database.[19] For both approaches, most states are developing capability for access for clinical providers via computer networks, modems, or fax. The Robert Wood Johnson Foundation is funding the development of a similar computerized record at several U.S. sites to allow clinicians to access daily tuberculosis treatment records immediately. These computerized patient records, accessed from multiple physical locations, are just the beginning of networked clinical applications in public health.

Tracking Performance Indicators

Most U.S. residents do not receive direct clinical services from public health agencies but use private practitioners or health maintenance organizations.

Increasingly, public health officials will be called on to monitor how effectively the private sector is providing clinical preventive services and helping to achieve disease prevention and health promotion goals.[4,20] For example, the Health Plan Employer Data and Information Set (HEDIS) has been developed for health maintenance organizations by the National Committee for Quality Assurance, to provide a common set of performance indicators for health plans.[21] General categories are quality, access and patient satisfaction, membership, use, and finance. The quality category includes several public health measurements, such as use of childhood immunizations, cholesterol screening, mammography screening, and prevalence of low birth weight. Public interest in these types of indicators has been so great that a parallel effort is under way to develop a similar set of indicators for the Medicaid population. At the moment, these and similar indicators are tracked through a series of traditional paper-and-pen utilization reviews and monitoring steps. However, as data systems become more sophisticated, these steps will be computerized.

The Hartford Foundation has launched an electronic approach to tracking performance indicators, funding seven centers in the United States under its Community Health Management Information System (CHMIS). These groups are working with private hospitals, physician groups, insurers, and in some cases, state health agencies for quick and economical management of claims reimbursement information, checking of client eligibility, and provision of a repository and framework for sharing data and accessing information.[15] A stated goal of the CHMIS project—electronic exchange of key public health and performance data—will be accomplished by creating shared community or state databases that will be available to researchers and government agencies.[15] In essence the CHMIS concept is the same as the CHIN concept—partnership for sharing health-related information among all who produce it and all who might benefit from it.

Most public health data transmitted electronically are stripped of personal identifiers, because they are not relevant to a specific surveillance task. However, claims information and some types of infectious disease case reports require personal identification for completion of claims or disease control functions for which the systems were designed. As a result, confidentiality about clinical information has become a public concern. Increasingly, encryption will be used in networked transmissions of clinical information, at some additional cost to the system. Ironically, however, the risk of interception of clinical information may be greater in the current paper system of filing records than in many electronic systems. Further, the insurance industry already shares clinical data among providers, but this practice will receive greater public scrutiny as publicly accountable health agencies become involved in electronic data transmission and information access to ensure that public health goals are met. Public health agencies will be forced to develop "firewalls" around their databases to protect them from unauthorized intruders.[22] However, firewalls and other sophisticated security devices are costly and may stretch the resources of local health departments and agencies.

Implications for Practice

One lesson learned by the tobacco control movement is that the volume of information and "connectedness" can quickly overwhelm receivers. The information collected needs to be organized and its dissemination stream-lined if it is to be of any value to users.[23] Nevertheless, a variety of CHIN users recognize the benefits of the greater openness that now exists. Many types of information are readily available, and distance does not have the same power that it once had, especially to isolate rural health systems and deny a full range of services to rural residents. As Naisbitt points out in *Global Paradox*, "Ignorance is no longer bliss or at least a viable excuse for not taking action."[24, p. 192] He postulates that as technology reduces the effects of distance, it increases the power and response of local communities to take steps to resolve problems.

The Institute of Medicine report, *The Future of Public Health*, raised serious concerns about deficiencies in the public health system.[2] Those that have direct bearing on electronic technology include lack of skill and consequent need for training of the public health workforce. Local and state public health officials are overwhelmed by the amount of national data made available to them. Public health workers who have not been trained to collect and handle data are faced with unfamiliar and often complicated tasks. Untrained local-level workers who can now access national data may not be able to manage the data. Some have had difficulty in downloading data (e.g., errors have been made in transcription). In addition, many workers are not sure how to interpret and apply the data locally. Undertrained workers tend to incorrectly extrapolate local implications from national data and therefore draw inaccurate conclusions. The low literacy levels among some workers who will be expected to enter or manipulate data are also a concern.

In a recent Georgia survey of all state and district-level public health employees ($N = 974$), nearly 70 percent of the respondents who used a computer at work indicated that they used computers every day.[25] Their work tasks included both word and data processing; only 16 percent of the respondents, however, reported that they had had any formal instruction in the hardware or software they were using.[25] There was no evidence that they had received training relevant to the use of CHINs. These results show that although computer technology has become prevalent in the public health workplace, employees have not received adequate training in its use. The results also suggest that the development potential for local area CHINs in public health settings in Georgia is limited by the computer expertise of the public health workforce and the literacy levels of employees.

As the public health field steps onto the information superhighway, demands for employee training will escalate. At a minimum, public health workers will need training to:

- integrate computers into their daily work environment;
- redesign their data collection and processing and record-keeping systems;
- expand their use of computers to conduct local area needs assessments, advocacy, and public information programs;
- establish ongoing two-way and multiway electronic communication with other agencies, colleagues, and interest groups;
- access and assess contemporary and relevant information;
- develop long-distance learning programs to improve worker competence; and
- integrate national data with locally collected data.

The gulf between technologically advanced data and communications systems and technically unsophisticated end users must be narrowed. Currently, most of the local and state public health workforce is inexperienced in handling data and lacks the technical skills required to negotiate the available information systems. Insufficiently trained workers are limited to the least powerful capacity of the technology, such as using e-mail functions and reading documents online. At local and state levels the public health infrastructure needs to include resources for training and upgrading computer hardware so that computer networking advances can be successfully implemented, now and in the future. Managers also require education about their workers' need for access to computer networking.

Other steps needed to assist CHIN development and use include: (1) the development of adequate telecommunications infrastructure; (2) reasonable transmission costs; (3) compatible (seamless) systems; (4) support and sense of ownership by community health leaders and end users; (5) formal and systematic evaluation of operating CHINs; and (6) financial commitment.[26] The greatest efforts are needed in rural America: "The best designed systems still face barriers to implementation. While much has been said about building the nation's electronic highway, we in rural America are often dealing with the equivalent of a dirt road."[26, p. 61] CHINs have a vital role to play in public health:

Community health information networks (CHINs) will be the critical link among patients, providers, purchasers, and all other health care constituents. Although it is uncertain at this point how and at what pace the implementation of CHINs will take place, one fact is clear: awareness and positioning in regard to their development and use are vital for organizations that intend to succeed in the new health care marketplace."[1, p. xiii]

Before CHINs achieve their potential, several challenges must be addressed:

The struggle to link diverse data sources for public health use will require major advances in technology, public and private attitudes, and human resources and skills. It is clear that planning efforts to improve the state of epidemiologic computing must consider (a) data content, availability, and quality; (b) computer technology adapted to public health use; (c) human resources and skills for computing; and (d) international cooperation and data exchange in many languages.[27, p. 439]

In addition, the CHIN strategy will not be immediately successful until the conflict between proprietary data ownership issues and community health needs are resolved. For example, CDC's National Immunization Program has encountered resistence on the part of managed care organizations who are not interested in sharing immunization registry type of information that could reveal information on their pediatric coverage to competitors.

Clearly, planning for global health requires vision, linkages, needs identification, and culturally appropriate solutions. Among the many possibilities are: (1) an international electronic database of teaching materials for continuing support of public health workers and managers; (2) international partnerships for using and improving public-domain epidemiological software; (3) a broad, standardized database for use and input by health care providers and others; and (4) a national hospital discharge and medical records data system.[27] CHINs of the future have the potential to provide information on what does and does not work, global disease telemonitoring, online vital statistics and journals, environmental monitoring, and distance learning.

Global public health needs to begin to plan for a public health communication system that can reach all the public health workers in the world. The first step is to network public health workers. It is time for public health to enter the electronic information superhighway.[28, p. 165]

References

1. Wakerly RT. (ed.). *Community Health Information Networks: Creating The Health Care Data Highway.* Chicago: American Hospital Publishing, Inc.; 1994.
2. Committee for the Study of the Future of Public Health, Division of Health Care Services, Institute of Medicine. *The Future of Public Health.* Washington, DC: National Academy Press; 1988.
3. Public Health in America. Essential Public Health Services Working Group of the Core Public Health Functions Steering Committee. Washington, DC; 1994.
4. Oberle MW, Baker EL, Magenheim MJ. Healthy People 2000 and community health planning. *Annu Rev Public Health.* 1994;15:259–275.
5. Baker EL, Melton RJ, Stange PV, et al. Health reform and the health of the

public safety: forging community health partnerships. *JAMA*. 1994; 272:1276–1282.

6. Information Infrastructure Task Force. *The National Information Infrastructure*. Washington, DC: The White House, September 15; 1993.

7. Corbin L. Speeding up the data superhighway. *Govt Exec*. 1995;27:14–22.

8. Baker EL, Freide A, Moulton AD, et al. CDC's Information Network for Public Health Officials (INPHO): A framework for integrated public health information and practice. *J Public Health Management Practice*. 1995;1: 43–47.

9. Chapman KA, Moulton AD. The Georgia Information Network for Public Health Officials (INPHO): A demonstration of the CDC concept. *J Public Health Management Practice*. 1995;1:39–43.

10. Center for Disease Control. *The Georgia Information Network for Public Health Officials: 1993–1994; Second Annual Report to the Robert W. Woodruff Foundation*. Atlanta, Ga; 1994.

11. Friede A, Reid JA, Ory HW. CDC WONDER: A comprehensive on-line public health information system of the Centers for Disease Control and Prevention. *Am J Public Health*. 1993;83:1289–1294.

12. Oberle MW, Kobayashi J. Morbidity, mortality, and modems: Disease surveillance in the computer age. *Washington Public Health*. 1993;11:4–5.

13. Paul SM, Finelli L, Crane G, et al. A statewide surveillance system for antimicrobial resistant bacteria: New Jersey. *Infect Control Hosp Epidemiol*. 1995;16(7)385–390.

14. Freedman FA, Paul JE, Rizzo NP, et al. DATA2000: CDC WONDER information System linking healthy people 2000 objectives to data sets. *Am J Prev Med*. 1994:10:230–234.

15. Public Health Macroview (Newsletter) 1995;7:1–8.

16. Patrick K, Koss S. Consumer Health Information White Paper, Health Information and Applications Work Group, Committee on Applications and Technology, Information Infrastructure Task Force, Department of Commerce, July, 1996.

17. Vickery DM, Fries JF. *Take Care of Yourself: A Consumer's Guide to Medical Care*. Reading, Mass: Addison-Wesley Publishing; 1993.

18. Fries JF, Harrington H, Edwards R, et al. Randomized controlled trial of cost reductions from a health education program: the California Public Employees Retirement System (PERS) study. *Am J Health Promotion*. 1994;8:216–223.

19. Land GH, Stokes C, Hoffman N, et al. Developing an integrated public health information system for Missouri. *J. Public Health Management Practice* 1995; 1:48–56.

20. Washington State Department of Health. *Public Health Improvement Plan*. Olympia, Wa; 1994.

21. National Committee for Quality Assurance. *Health Plan Employer Data and Information Set and User's Manual*. Washington, DC; 1993.

22. *Information Technology Guide: Security*. Govt Exec. 1995;27:16A–20A.

23. Gates, S. Personal communication; Feb. 1995.

24. Naisbitt J. *Global Paradox*. New York: Avon Books; 1995.

25. Escoffery MC, Miner K, Alperin M, et al. An Assesment of Computer

Knowledge and Attitudes of Public Health Workers in Georgia. Presented at American Public Health Association Annual Meeting, Oct. 1995.

26. Puskin DS. Opportunities and challenges to telemedicine in rural America. *J Med Sys.* 1995;19:53–61.

27. Dean AG. Microcomputers and the future of epidemiology. *USHHS Reports.* 1994;109:439–442.

28. LaPorte RE. Global public health and the information superhighway [editorial]. *Brit Med J.* 1994;308:1651.

8

The Target Cities Program: Management Information Systems for Drug Abuse Treatment

D. PAUL MOBERG, DORINE D. FULLER, J. PHILLIP GOSSAGE, PATRICIA S. LITTMAN, KEVIN P. MULVEY, MICHAEL SHWARTZ, and JOHN E. VETTER

The Target Cities Program

The Target Cities Program is a national demonstration program to develop improved substance abuse treatment infrastructures in major U.S. cities. The program is funded by cooperative agreements between the U.S. Department of Health and Human Services, Substance Abuse and Mental Health Services Administration, Center for Substance Abuse Treatment (CSAT); offices on the state level that oversee substance abuse services ("Single State Agencies"); and local city or county governments. The legislative authority for the Target Cities program falls under Section 510(B)(5) of the Public Health Service Act as amended (42 USC 290bb-3), which provides for assistance to cities categorized as "crisis areas" with regard to drug abuse. The program was designed to "improve the quality and effectiveness of drug abuse treatment services in a limited number of cities" that could serve as models to the rest of the nation, and was intended "primarily to enhance and improve existing treatment services, rather than to increase treatment slots." [1, p. 2]

Public Drug Abuse Treatment Prior to Target Cities

The alcoholism and drug abuse treatment system in the United States is bifurcated into systems that treat primarily either publicly funded or privately funded clients. [2-4] The Target Cities Program, while not excluding private-sector providers, essentially addressed the public-sector treatment systems in each of the funded cities. These public systems are typically composed of a mix of government operated and contracted private non-profit agencies.

Prior to implementation of Target Cities programs, clients typically would self-refer to a specific program site because it was close to their home or workplace, or because the program was suggested by associates, friends, or family. Treatment was provided at the discretion of the provider in regard to modality and length of stay, within the range of services available at that site. Individual providers maintained their own waiting lists. In general, assessment of potential clients was idiosyncratic, with each treatment program using its own approach and assessment tool. Services were limited to a circumscribed set of providers, funded under sum-certain contracts or operated directly by a state or local governmental entity. The range of program offerings to public-sector drug abuse clients was narrow, with few specialty or niche services (women, ethnic groups, etc.). Referral networks tended to be informal between providers, with sequential referral of clients in need of further services. Referrals occurred only after the potential services — or funding — at the initial site had been exhausted. Client tracking and a relevant system-wide data base were limited or non-existent.

From the perspective of provider agencies, adequate numbers of clients are a critical organizational resource that enables them to justify contractual funding and/or to bill for services.[5] Thus, there is an incentive to maintain a stable flow of clients and this takes precedence over selection of only the most appropriate cases for the services offered by a particular agency. When a sufficient number of clients is reached, then selection of the most desirable clients becomes operative.[6]

Prior to Target Cities, information on ancillary services available within the community to assist clients with other social (e.g., daycare, housing, legal, employment) and health related problems was typically haphazard and informal within provider agencies. These related issues have frequently presented obstacles to seeking drug abuse treatment, and if not addressed, they interfere with treatment effectiveness.[7]

Thus, prior to Target Cities, client needs were matched with program characteristics only on an informal basis in most public substance abuse treatment systems. The assessment of client needs was unstandardized, the choice of providers and range of services were limited, providers controlled their own intake and eligibility process, and large sums of public money were spent without consistent determination of need. An integrated continuum of care, while often discussed, was rarely a reality, and the interrelationships of substance abuse treatment with other health and human services were underdeveloped. There was typically only a very a limited common database, which was inadequate for management of the public treatment system.

The Target Cities Model

In the systems-oriented treatment improvement demonstration called Target Cities, cities were required to include four mandatory activities to address the problems of the typical service system:

- improved coordination among drug abuse, health, mental health, education, law enforcement, judicial, correctional, and human service agencies;
- establishment or enhancement of central intake and referral facilities, including automated patient tracking and referral systems, and the

development of appropriate computer and management information system capabilities;
- implementation of measures to ensure the quality of services provided; and
- activities in which there is a focus on improving treatment services for at least one of [a specific set of] . . . populations.[1, p.4]

Implementation of the Target Cities program necessitated the development of management information systems (MISs) to coordinate service delivery, to enable operation of central intake units (CIUs) with standardized assessment and tracking, and to facilitate system management, state and federal reporting and ongoing program evaluation. In its early technical assistance workshops, Center for Substance Abuse Treatment (CSAT) spelled out the expectations for the Target Cities MISs. Diesenhaus[8] saw the Target Cities effort as a mechanism to test "the self-correcting treatment system vision" and emphasized the incorporation of "outcome monitoring" in Target Cities information systems and in ongoing local evaluations. As part of central intake, patient tracking systems integral to the MIS were viewed by Jaffe[9] as evaluation tools capable of providing ongoing comparative feedback on patient capture and retention within a system of providers, with the ability to control for differences between providers in the severity of client problems (i.e., case mix).

A recent CSAT publication[10, pp. 8-9] on the Target Cities Program emphasizes the importance of the MIS as "the linchpin of the program," which "enables the project to manage a treatment system rather than merely placing the client in the next available slot." The MIS should be able to "identify:

- whether individuals referred to specific programs are actually admitted to the referral site;
- how long individuals remain in treatment;
- their progress; and
- whether they drop out or are discharged.[10]

The MIS is also expected to "track use and availability of treatment services," monitor alcohol and other drug (AOD) use trends, manage billing data, and facilitate state and federal reporting requirements. The CIU concept is feasible only with an operative MIS.

Beginning with eight awards totalling $29 million in 1990, a total of 19 projects have been funded since the start of the program.[10] Annual funding has been approximately $30–35 million per year; most cities have received funding for 5 years, although the original grants were provided as 3-year awards. CSAT reports costs for MIS development to range from $250,000 to $1 million per project.[10]

This chapter presents case studies of MIS development in four of the original projects funded in 1990—Boston, Massachusetts; New York, New York; Albuquerque, New Mexico; and Milwaukee, Wisconsin. These cities were chosen to illustrate how sites of varying sizes and with differing public substance abuse treatment systems implemented MISs within the frame-work of the Target Cities Program. Cities from the first round of funding were chosen because each has had a full 5 years of implementation experience. Technical details regarding MIS hardware and software, while already reflecting obsolescence at the time of writing, are provided to situate the effort within the evolution of computer technology and to provide an understanding of Target Cities' information network legacy in each city.

Boston

The key substance abuse treatment system enhancements of the Boston Target Cities Program (called BOTI, the Boston Office of Treatment Improvement) were the following: (1) the establishment of a personal computer (PC)-based citywide management information system (MIS) that links PCs at each of 53 programs receiving state block grant funds to a central computer and allows tracking of client admissions and discharges throughout the system; (2) the establishment of three CIUs where clients are assessed and referrals facilitated; (3) the introduction of 66 case managers into the treatment system, most located at the programs, to support client treatment and to address clients' ancillary needs; and (4) primary care assessments, performed at the CIUs, with linkages to primary care sites for those in need of service.

At the core of the Boston program was a commitment to shared decision-making. Providers were actively involved in the design, implemen-tation, and management of the project. Organizationally, the city was divided into three clusters, to a large extent reflecting historical utilization patterns and informal provider collaboration. A CIU site was established and a lead agency identified in each cluster. Overall program management was performed by core BOTI staff, who reported to the director of the city health department. A management infrastructure was established at each cluster, and clusters were given responsibility for coordination among providers within their cluster and cross-cluster collaboration. A represen-tative from the State Bureau of Substance Abuse Services (BSAS) actively participated with core and cluster management on all aspects of the program.

The BOTI Management Information System (MIS)

The decision to use a PC-based system linked through modems to a central server was driven by the desire to improve provider computer infrastructure and allow community-based staff to take charge of their own management information. The central system consists of two high-performance Sun Microsystems SPARCstation 2 servers, networked together, each with 1.3

and 2.3 gigabytes of hard disk storage and 28 megabytes of memory. Each of the central computers supports OS Windows and a bank of 16 dial-up 9600 baud modems. Foxbase database management software is used for creating, querying, and maintaining program database files. Analyses for management reports and evaluation are done using the SAS statistical software system.

The standard provider computer system includes a 386SX microcomputer with a 52MB hard disk, 4MB of memory, dual floppy drives, DOS 4.1, Windows™, and a mouse. On the provider computers are BOTI database software, written in FoxPro, and telecommunications protocol software (PC-TCP) used to communicate with the Central BOTI system over SLIP (Serial Line Interface Protocol). Communication includes both automatic night-time batch uploads and immediate client record transfer.

The main data collection instruments include the State BSAS admission form,[11] which is required for state reimbursement and includes socio-demographic information, education, employment, living situation, treatment/service history, and pattern of substance abuse information; the BSAS discharge form, which includes information on reasons for discharge, referral source, employment status at discharge, social and health services obtained, and client goal achievement; a case management activity log, which records case management activities performed for each client, resources accessed and outcome of each activity; a primary care form, used to record the results of clinical encounters; and a referral log, which tracks the status of clients as they transition from CIUs to treatment. The Addiction Severity Index, a common psycho-social assessment instrument,[12] is used. A slot vacancy notification process and a waiting list monitoring system have been implemented but are still too cumbersome for routine use.

Implementation of Boston's MIS

MIS implementation consisted of three phases. The first phase, the "naive" phase, was shaped by the belief that by the end of the first year of program operation (fall 1991), there would be a reasonably complete functioning MIS. In fact, technical difficulties in software development, telecommunications, form development, and program compliance were all much greater than anticipated. Nevertheless, by mid 1992 (the beginning of the "centralized" phase), most data collection instruments had been automated and compliance with data entry was rapidly increasing.

In addition to continual work on system improvements, data entry compliance, and data integrity, much of the second half of 1992 and early 1993 was spent working with central management and cluster coordinators on developing management reports. Under pressure from clusters and, increasingly, from CSAT, by mid-1993 we were able to undertake significant analyses of system performance and begin to provide management reports. By the third quarter of 1993, CSAT was focusing on continuous improvement activities and, fundamental to that, facilitating direct access to the data. Centralization, with central staff performing analyses at the request of cluster management, was increasingly unable to meet programmatic requirements. Thus began the transition to the third phase — data "decentralization." Working with cluster management, a set of 25 standard tables meeting cluster management needs were developed. Each table, which could be requested as needed using SAS-based menus, had input parameter fields (time period covered, programs of interest, case managers of interest, etc.) that could be varied according to user need. In the final phase of the project, we plan to develop Epi Info-based menus to allow programs the same ability. (EpiInfo is a nonproprietary software package developed by the Centers for Disease Control and Prevention.)

Impact of Boston's MIS

Because an MIS is usually developed to support program activities, it is very difficult to isolate its impact. In terms of impact on clients, the MIS allows immediate transfer of client information and thus reduces the data collection burden as clients move through the treatment system, though this aspect of the system is not yet widely used. At the program level, provision of computers, training in computer skills, and access to database programs and word processing have been of great value. More and more providers are recognizing the potential of data to improve program management and operations. If we are able to nurture and support this interest over the last phase-out year of BOTI, there is the potential for long-term system impact. More immediately, the MIS has allowed programs that were not yet electronically billing the state to do so, improving the timeliness of payment and probably the integrity of the data. Further, by linking providers, it has increased their recognition that they are really part of a treatment system, a perspective that also needs nurturing, but one with long-term potential benefits.

At a system level, the MIS is one of the underpinnings of the CIUs. It has been at the core of our ability to monitor activities and impact, and to make adjustments to improve operations. The MIS has allowed us to demonstrate the significant impact of case management on treatment success, a finding that may have long-term implications for the field. However, much like MIS development, the impact of an MIS is slow in coming and needs continual support to realize its potential.

New York City

The New York State Target Cities Project is intended to improve drug abuse treatment in Harlem and the South Bronx, focusing special attention on addicted women with children, adolescents, medically impaired chemical abusers, and racial and ethnic minorities. The NYS Target Cities project has established a central intake, assessment, and referral process with multiple points of entry, designed to match client's needs with available services and treatment slots.

The New York State Target Cities project has three CIUs, including one in a criminal justice setting. Clients self-present at the CIUs through referrals from hospitals or criminal justice sites and by information gained through word of mouth within the community. Client assessments and case management are performed at all intake sites. Based on client needs identified through the assessment process, clients are matched to services provided by over 70 treatment programs participating in the project.

The cornerstone of the New York State project is automation of the assessment, referral, and matching functions and the subsequent tracking of client admissions, treatment services, and discharges. The system was developed and is managed by the New York State Office of Alcoholism and Substance Abuse Services (OASAS).

The New York State Target Cities System

The broad goal of the automated Target Cities System (TCS) is to provide an information network for participants in the Target Cities initiative. The system was designed as a tool to enable CIU counselors to more appropriately match the individual needs of a client with specific services in the community, while providing functions for tracking and evaluating client progress, program effectiveness, and capacity management.

As a client presents him or herself for treatment, the CIU screens the client to determine needs and make referrals. The matching process is driven by client needs, the client's previous history, including previous assessments performed, service and operational information regarding treatment programs and a tracking process driven by the counselor's entry of the activities occurring on the client's behalf. For more dysfunctional clients exhibiting a variety of social, medical, and/or mental health problems, the central intake staff refer the client to case management staff and continue to monitor, through the MIS, the progress of the client until placed in treatment or terminated.

The TCS provides participating treatment providers with the ability to view assessments performed at CIUs, view clients' previous treatment history at their program and process client admissions and discharges. This provides an up-to-date base of available slots and the ability to maintain and track a client waiting list.

Target Cities project management and NYS OASAS staff are provided online information to manage the project and review effectiveness. The MIS has extensive online query, reporting, and statistical capabilities with which to evaluate client progress and treatment outcomes and system-wide effectiveness. A variety of analyses have been used to review manual procedures and assessment measures, resulting in procedural and systematic changes.

The TCS is the core system on which the NYS Client Reporting System was built, providing online access to NYS treatment providers for entry of admissions, discharges, transfers, and waiting list data. Queries and reports are available to each provider to assist in tracking and monitoring clients in treatment. A capacity management module, which includes each provider's current and historical census and capacity, is maintained and is retrievable through reports and online queries; the database allows demographic breakdown of the client population.

The aim of the TCS is to provide an information network for participants in the project. The TCS was developed as a set of integrated modules providing linkages to all participants as well as other state-funded entities.

The NYS TCS was developed using a UNIX operating system and ORACLE database management software. The application is resident on a UNIX computer located in Albany with a dedicated line connecting to the NYC OASAS office modem bank. The CIUs dial in via modem to the NYC site. Linkages are also provided to over 70 TCS programs with dial-in access to the NYC modem bank. Other NYS funded programs may also elect to enter client information online rather than via paper transmission.

This computer network has allowed NYS OASAS to maintain up-to-date records on available treatment slots and treatment program characteristics, which in turn increases the ability to refer clients to appropriate treatment locations within communities.

Implementation Issues

The NY OASAS approach to implementation and support is comprehensive. Sites are identified for participation in the automation process by word of mouth from current participants, if they receive numerous referrals from CIUs, or through contact with other NYS OASAS projects. As new intake and referral sites are established, programs in the community are solicited for inclusion in the project.

MIS conducts an executive briefing for new programs with an overview and demonstration of the application. Information is provided on equipment and communication software requirements. Hands-on training sessions are conducted with a 2-day training session for intake/referral staff and 1-day training for treatment program staff. The training has been modified over time to include a systems overview to introduce users to the interrelationships of all functions. User reference guides have been developed and are distributed at training sessions, including a quick reference guide that was developed after the original extensive guide was found to be impractical for daily usage. All new functions or modifications to the application are distributed through system broadcast and/or enhancement notices. On an ongoing basis, MIS supports the operation of the application through a help desk. As training and documentation have improved, calls to the help desk have decreased and the timeliness of data entry has improved.

User groups meet on a regular basis to discuss the system's ability to assist users in achieving the project goals as well as hindrances, problems, corrective actions required, and desired enhancements. These groups increase user understanding and investment in the system and help identify system limitations, problems, and required enhancements.

Impact of the New York State MIS

The MIS system has provided tools to more appropriately match client needs to services provided by treatment programs. In the past, clients would self-present at specific programs because they were close to their home or workplace, or because the program was suggested by associates, friends, or family. The treatment provided depended on services available at that site and on slot availability. With the TCS, clients now arrive at a CIU and, based on assessment, the TCS identifies programs with available slots offering services that will most effectively meet the clients' needs. The counselor is also provided with information on examinations, identification, and other requirements of the program prior to admission. These features decrease the chance of losing clients due to delays in admission and loss of motivation.

The TCS also provides the CIU with information on services available within the community to assist clients with other social and health-related problems (e.g., daycare, housing, legal problems). These related issues have frequently presented obstacles for people seeking treatment (e.g., some fear loss of children or unsupervised care if they enter a treatment facility).

Although the impact of the system on clients has not yet been fully evaluated, the general finding is that by better matching client needs with program characteristics, we achieve a better success rate for treatment. The system has also improved the timeliness of submission of data on admissions and discharges, providing online information that makes it easier for caseworkers to place clients in effective treatment. The system also allows counselors who once were engaged in time-consuming paperwork to spend more time with their clients.

As part of our mission, the NYS OASAS has stressed four key concerns facing the field today: assessment of client needs, integration and realignment of the continuum of care, interrelationships of the addictions field and other health and human services, and the role of information in system development. The first three areas are clearly critical to the service delivery system; less obvious but equally important is the accessibility of timely and accurate information on which to base the planning, policy direction, management, and clinical decisions that will shape the future of the field.

The NYS OASAS Target Cities Project and the MIS clearly address these focus areas, and information sharing and network capability have continued to expand to other areas of the state. There are increasing demands for network capability and access as the provider community, counties, and other health and human services organizations gain knowledge of the application and strive for integration of services within communities, consistent with the move toward managed care in New York State. Demonstrations and the distribution of information on the application throughout the state and nationally have created a clear recognition of the significant impact the MIS can have on the effectiveness of the service delivery system.

Albuquerque

Problems associated with alcohol and other drugs have been severe in Albuquerque and the State of New Mexico. Abuse of alcohol has been especially high: the rate of alcohol-related deaths in the Albuquerque metropolitan area is approximately 600 percent above expected mortality rates for cities of comparable size. Problems associated with abuse of drugs, particularly heroin addiction and methamphetamine use, have also been endemic. To address these issues, project planners established four major goals in their proposal to implement systemic treatment improvements within Target City-Albuquerque (TC-A). These were:

1. *Improvements in intake and outreach,* including development of an integrated computer tracking and referral system linking major agencies in the treatment community. A CIU existed at the University of New Mexico's Center on Alcoholism, Substance Abuse, and Addictions (CASAA), the central node in the treatment system, which included nine distinct programs. In addition, a standard decentralized intake process was established at each of the nine partner agencies. These linkages are illustrated in Fig. 8.1.
2. *Improvements in drug treatment center services,* including reestablishing inpatient detoxification; reducing therapist caseloads, while at the same time expanding services; developing an outpatient detoxification observation unit; staffing a laboratory for on-site drug screens; providing child-care services for children of patients while in therapy; and developing an intensive adolescent outpatient rehabilitation program.
3. *Enhancements to community-based residential treatment,* including development of a 12-bed residential facility for postpartum addicted women and their children; development of community-based residential treatment capacity for the homeless and other adults in need of this form of treatment; provision of drug treatment services in youth corrections programs; and provision of case management and aftercare services for adolescents discharged from community-based residential facilities.
4. *Enhancement of drug treatment staff skills, knowledge, and efficiency* through the development of a centralized training unit to support

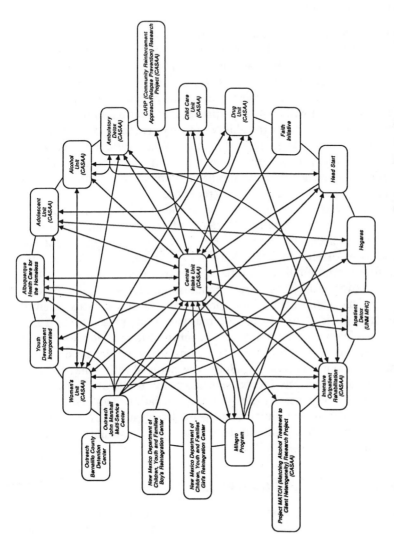

FIGURE 8.1. Referral patterns and linkages established or enriched among the original Target Cities' Service Delivery Units and other agencies as a result of the Center for Substance Abuse treatment sponsored–Target City Albuquerque Drug Treatment Improvement Project.

publicly assisted drug treatment programs and the development of an interactive medical records system to increase the time that clinical staff have available for patient encounters.

Albuquerque's MIS

Albuquerque's MIS—The Substance Abuse Assessment, Tracking, and Referral Network (SAATARN)—was developed to respond to the lack of a sophisticated method for client tracking, case monitoring, and referral, and the lack of precise data on the activities carried out by the treatment system and the scope of drug abuse problems within the community. The primary objective of the SAATARN was to improve coordination among agencies within the system and enhance the ability of the system to track patients and monitor case progress in an integrated manner. What was envisioned was a system through which data from a client's file in one location could be entered into that client's file at another treatment site, establishing a continuous record of services rendered/received.

A second objective of the network was to enhance the system's capabilities to serve patients in accessing a range of treatment and supportive services through electronic referrals. By sharing information about the types of services offered by various agencies, clinicians in different sites would become more familiar with referral sites that would provide the best mix of services for particular patients. In addition, accessing a database of available services would help ensure that all of a patient's needs received attention. It is difficult to address the multiple needs presented by some patients, but reference to the online service information would allow better attention to service availability while recording which service needs would require attention at a later date. Flexibility was planned within the system to allow for easy and relatively inexpensive expansion to a wider network of supportive service providers (social welfare, education, employment and training, and other public and private provider agencies), which would significantly increase the likelihood that needed services would be obtained in a timely manner.

Implementation of Albuquerque's MIS

Many challenges were encountered in establishing a comprehensive management information system for TC-A; some were process-based while others were technical. Not surprisingly, different partners were interested in monitoring different kinds of data. This greatly complicated the efforts of the SAATARN staff to develop a single data base that would properly support differing data needs. But it was technical issues that presented the greatest challenges for the SAATARN staff. In the spring of 1993 (the third year of the project), the TC-A project chose to meet its information needs by adopting the system that had been developed by Target City-New York

City (TC-NYC). Its data system used a database environment and a development toolset from Oracle Corporation that were installed on a Hewlett Packard 9000 series minicomputer. Albuquerque chose to install Oracle on Sun Microsystems hardware. The first decision that had to be made by the SAATARN staff was the degree to which TC-A would remain faithful to the system architecture chosen in TC-NYC. The TC-NYC system was designed in a host/terminal configuration—all processing was done centrally on a minicomputer, with users connecting to that computer via character-based terminals or personal computers (PCs) running terminal emulation software.

For the SAATARN, we decided on a client/server architecture, using the processors in our users' PCs to handle local tasks such as screen generation, data entry, and report generation. This architecture was chosen for three reasons: (1) to take full advantage of the processing power represented in our existing base of PCs; (2) to provide maximum flexibility in the design of user applications, and to allow use of the latest graphical development tools; and (3) to save money on initial purchase and subsequent mainte-nance and to provide an inexpensive path for expansion through the purchase of small UNIX servers. The timing of our Oracle installation confronted us with another choice. In the spring of 1993, Oracle was releasing a major new database engine, *Oracle 7*. The TC-NYC applications had been designed using the older *Oracle 6* software. It was not a hard decision to opt for the newer data environment, especially because Oracle provided fairly good conversion utilities. The major difficulty involved importing the security environment developed by the TC-NYC into the new database. The problems were resolved with the help of Oracle technical support. By choosing the most up-to-date database engine, we were able to take advantage of features unavailable before, and we positioned ourselves well for future technical support and use of the steady stream of improved development tools that Oracle has since produced.

The adaptation and development of the TC-NYC system to meet Albuquerque's needs were also shaped by the feature/performance trade-off involved in choosing between graphic- and text-based development environments. The shift to graphic computing environments over the last several years has confronted application designers with a dilemma: re-taining access to the most advanced tools and techniques dictates shifting away from character-based development, but the resources at hand may not support the memory- and power-hungry requirements of the new software, and performance is often lackluster if the computers or software are inadequate. In keeping with the objectives of providing developers and our users with the friendliest and most flexible computing solutions, we decided to implement graphic solutions in all newly developed applications, re-taining character-based solutions only where necessary (as for dial-up users forced into terminal emulation), or where we have not had time to convert. This decision was possible because we were able to use only relatively new

486 or better PCs in our implementation. However, it has also had significant costs in terms of administrative complexity, slower development, performance difficulties, and immaturity of development tools.

Impact of Albuquerque's MIS

Throughout the grant period, the SAATARN staff were intimately involved in all aspects of service delivery planning and management. This included helping to plan outreach, screening, and assessment; slot management and tracking of treatment events; pharmacy activities; submission of services for payment; and similar tasks. Indeed, at times, the SAATARN staff was so deeply involved with clinical staff that they found it difficult to find the time to develop or modify database software. The power of the data that emerged over the life of the project gave managers insight into their individual programs as well as other partners' capabilities. For example, data from the SAATARN helped managers tailor processes within the CIU that solved a highly problematic "no-show" rate and created a more streamlined screening, assessment, and referral process.

The TC-A project substantially increased access to substance abuse treatment within the Albuquerque metropolitan area. In virtually every aspect of the project, the contributions of the SAATARN and its staff were substantial and direct.

Milwaukee

The Milwaukee Target Cities Project (MTC) developed in two phases. The initial phase (MTC-I; serving clients in 1992 and 1993 after a year of planning) served a restricted geographic area and tested the feasibility of a delivery system using central intake, comprehensive assessment, case management, treatment preauthorization by case managers, and fee-for service (FFS) payments ("vouchers") for treatment services. The goal was to improve treatment accessibility, retention, and outcomes for publicly funded substance abuse clients in central city neighborhoods. In the MTC project, the term "vouchers" was used to refer to centralized preauthorization of a specific number of treatment units in a specific treatment modality, client choice of provider, and FFS payment to those providers. Case managers were central to the project, conducting assessment, facilitating client choice and brokering both ancillary and alcohol and other drug abuse (AODA) services. The project also employed public health nursing and other specialists extensively.

Fiscal, administrative, and case information necessary to operate this program was captured in the project's management information system (MIS). This vouchered FFS managed care system replaced sum certain contracts with providers that the county had historically used to cover substance abuse treatment services for public sector clients. During the initial phase of the project, the two systems ran concurrently, with vouchers replacing contracts only for residents of six zip codes.

The second phase of the project (MTC-II; 1994 on) has been essentially a county-wide substance abuse managed care system for all public sector clients. In this broader implementation, central intake has been redefined as screening and referral (rather than assessment, referral, and case management). Central intake is provided by a contracted organization at two CIU sites, with computer-assisted level of care determination and provider selection; clients are offered a choice of appropriate providers and are referred for assessment and treatment. Case management and other specialist components have been eliminated, and public health nursing services are targeted only to pregnant and postpartum women and to control of communicable diseases. Provider sum-certain contracts have been replaced by the managed care system with FFS reimbursement county-wide.

Milwaukee's MIS

The initial MIS design was primarily oriented to fiscal management of the "voucher" system, rather than clinical and systems management, as in other cities described in this chapter. The major functions of the system were automation of administrative and fiscal details of service authorizations, referrals, voucher and expenditure tracking, and linkages to payment authorization systems, with minimal provision for clinical data. The MIS was grafted onto the county's existing data processing unit, with limited input from treatment providers, minimal data access (beyond data input and service status and fiscal/voucher queries on individual cases) by project staff and management, and no provider access. Thus, the first MIS (MTC-I) functioned primarily as a control and accounting system for treatment vouchers. The main database for this system was appropriately called "Service Case Registry and Integrated Payment Tracking System" (SCRIPTS).

An additional database, the "Clinical/Evaluation Summaries" (CES), was included primarily as a data entry and storage mechanism for clinically relevant client level data. This included detailed client demographics, substance use history, treatment history, diagnostic codes, assessed needs, ancillary services provided and closure data including ratings of success. The data were accessible to project staff only as hard copy once entered into their PCs. CES data were transferred to tape and sent to the project evaluators quarterly for analysis. Case managers were responsible for data entry via on-screen menus. By default, the CES served as the sole systematic source of nonfiscal clinical and evaluative client data.

Operationally, the creation of a valid SCRIPTS record required minimal data, namely the data necessary to authorize and pay for treatment: modality, provider, and units authorized. The MIS was not structured to require capture of the CES data. While not synchronized, SCRIPTS and CES were relationally linked through client ID numbers, but they were merged only after the fact by the outside evaluation team.

Based on the experience gained during the first phase of the project, the MIS was refined and modified for the expanded county-wide implementation. MTC-II includes expanded client registration and tracking capabilities, wait list management, and a structured intake screening protocol, including key items from the Addiction Severity Index. The screening data are processed through an algorithm and decision tree to determine appropriate modality. This is followed by an informational display on potential providers of this modality from which the client can select.

The screening process and algorithm at the CIU are designed only to decide on initial placement (i.e., outpatient, intensive outpatient/day, inpatient, or residential treatment); unlike the CIU assessment systems in other cities, this system does not serve as an in-depth psychosocial assessment. Initial placement is computer-assisted through direct entry of client responses to a structured interview about the client's symptoms, substance use patterns, living and social environment, health issues, and treatment history. Responses are weighted to generate a composite score which translates into a modality recommendation. CIU intake workers are all certified alcohol and other drug abuse (AODA) counselors and have the power to override the computer-assisted recommendations, based on their clinical judgment. An in-depth psychosocial assessment takes place at the provider (SDU) level. The authorized treatment modality may be changed in consultation with the CIU if warranted by the additional information obtained through this assessment.

All elements of the data system are synchronized; a specific variable is entered only once and all cases are opened, updated, and closed on what appears to the user to be a single data system. This MIS allows project management real time data access for analysis and feedback of useful information. In addition, providers will eventually have limited online access to the system, providing data on admissions, discharges, and service changes for their clients.

The present Milwaukee MIS runs on an IBM-compatible Amdahl mainframe using CICs and DB2 software. There are two communication ports with 16 lines each. Reports are generated through the Query Management Facility, with SAS available for statistical analysis. Two database systems run on offsite Sun Microsystems (UNIX) workstations — one documents referrals and serves as a case registry for the entire county human services department, while the second database is an improved version of the SCRIPTS system discussed above. SCRIPTS functional interfaces include client screening, modality selection, and provider selection; provider maintenance; wait list management; voucher management; billing; and check writing (including transfer of data on service units to the mainframe).

These systems are accessed from four sites — two general CIUs, one CIU for intoxicated drivers, and the county systems management unit. The three CIUs use IBM desktop PCs running terminal emulation software; the county systems management staff use Apple-MacIntosh PCs. The two general CIUs are also connected in peer-to-peer local area networks (LANs). Data entry to the client tracking feature is integrated into the screening operation.

Implementation of Milwaukee's MIS

Many participants in the original MIS design process were inexperienced using electronic data and did not fully understand substance abuse services, the project's vision, the management value of data, or evaluation needs. Consequently, the original MIS had minimal provision for usable clinical data. Standardized assessment data, measures of case management intensity, wait list information, follow-up data after referral, objective treatment outcome measures, and key provider characteristics were not included. Although the MIS was able to describe some ancillary services, it could not track them throughout a treatment episode. Public health nurses, a critical project component, used a different and incompatible information system.

While data on a large number of variables were collected in the initial system, use of the data for program management, staff clinical decision-making, and evaluation was hampered by several factors. Data integrity was compromised because information was entered after the fact. The unsynchronized structure of the data system caused many inconsistencies (including huge discrepancies in client counts) between SCRIPTS and CES, and the Query Management Facility (QMF) was unable to generate spontaneous reports from the clinical database (CES). Data on services used were recorded incompletely in both MIS databases, and workers had limited access to full client records. Reporting, management and evaluation functions, and clinical efficiency were impeded by these problems. As an accounting and billing system, however, SCRIPTS was effective in assuring prompt authorization of services and payment to providers.

In spite of the limitations of the data structure, a comprehensive analysis of MIS data from the first 3 years was conducted by the evaluation team. This evaluation suggested the importance of case management, provision of ancillary services, and residential treatment in enhancing short-term client outcomes.[13] The project's county-wide expansion during the final 2 years (MTC-II) was accomplished in the face of budget cutbacks and the related decision to drop case management and screen rather than assess clients in the CIUs. This second iteration of MTC with its volume increases would have been unmanageable without an improved MIS. Many of the problems described above have been mitigated in the revised MIS, although some persist. The public health nursing component is still tracked through an independent system, and technical LAN networking problems exist. While CIU compliance is good due to operationally integrated data entry, provider reporting is problematic (except for billing). The QMF for report production remains very restricted, largely due to the sensitivity of its data configurations and programming language; and there is as yet no arrangement for treatment providers to report ancillary services or access data directly from the system.

Impact of the Milwaukee MIS

Although the initial MIS primarily tracked vouchered services, the system had an under-utilized capacity to record most of the case activities that took place and an unrestricted FFS structure. As such, it functioned with benign neglect: the range and intensity of services recommended depended on case manager skills, and motivated clients were technically unlimited in the amount of treatment they could receive. Unfortunately, this approach affected both clients and providers negatively. First, not documenting client and service data uniformly or completely hindered analysis and feedback, particularly on client outcomes. Clients were denied the benefits of project experience with others having similar profiles, and the county's evaluation and quality assurance activities with providers were not data-driven. Second, without budget allocations by modality, treatment expenditures were not closely monitored, and intake was closed several times due to (apparent) insufficient funds, wreaking havoc on provider organization budgets and depriving clients of treatment on demand. In addition, the MIS did not manage treatment slot availability, with resulting allegations by providers of case manager referral bias or incompetence.

The new MIS implemented during the second phase of the project offers a timely means of allocating and monitoring expenditures, more consistent and synchronized capture of clinical data, and a modality determination and authorization process based on research and experience. The change from a comprehensive, inductive, progressively more trusting relationship between case managers and clients to a brief, weighted computer protocol administered at access sites by contracted counselors dramatically illustrates the changes in decision-making processes and the increasing importance of the MIS in supporting these structural changes. MTC's managed care significantly changed Milwaukee's public substance abuse treatment system by centralizing control and accountability while increasing both the number and range of treatment services available.[5] Access improved and minority representation among AODA providers in the public sector doubled. The modified MIS has set the stage for an ongoing managed care system for public substance abuse treatment in Milwaukee County, and it has been expanded to support multiple program areas within the county human services department.

Discussion

These case studies provide an overview of the MIS design and implementation issues, successes, and impact on clients and systems when complex public human service networks are required to automate and rationalize their processes. Because MIS development was one part of larger system design and management infrastructure changes, it is not possible to isolate the impact of the MIS from that of other changes oriented to "systems improvement." For example, coordination and communication between providers were enhanced in several cities by the Target Cities program, but the role of the MIS in this is unclear—the primary MIS linkage was from individual providers to central intake, and not directly between providers.

While there are similarities between the four systems discussed, the Milwaukee system's orientation to fiscal management was unique. Milwaukee was the only site that emphasized a managed care approach, and the MIS which was developed and refined in Phase Two was integral to this. The other three cities, where provider reimbursement was not based on a fee-for-service model with prior authorization, placed far greater emphasis on capturing clinically relevant and valid data on clients, tracking services provided, and sharing the data with providers. All have provided, or plan to provide, real time network access to provider agencies. Albuquerque has also given special attention to multiple client needs beyond substance abuse and is extending its system to include a wider network of ancillary human service providers.

The systems in all of these sites have improved the process by which potential clients are matched to appropriate services. Each city was required to develop a "central intake unit," and this has been implemented in multiple networked sites in each city. While the screening/assessment process was increasingly rationalized and routinized by these units and the supporting MIS data systems, client choice was also facilitated by providing (where possible) a list of potential service providers from which to choose. However, the CIU may also have been an impediment to access in some settings, as it disrupted traditional referral patterns within communities and added new steps that potential clients had to follow to enter treatment.

The Target Cities program, and the MIS systems essential to them, have also had significant impacts on public service delivery systems. On the positive side, these systems have increased service coordination, improved the flow of data on (sequentially or simultaneously) shared clients, and reduced the paperwork and time delays inherent in paper systems for authorization, reporting, and billing/payment. The MIS also allows for increased centralized control over the public service delivery system. With the availability of data system-wide, a " systems management" function is evolving for which use of data—collected with care and integrity—is critical. There is increased ability to monitor and evaluate the entire system, as well as the effectiveness of providers within the system. The MIS applications increasingly allow decentralized access *to* data by providers, although this is occurring at a slower pace than is data capture *from* providers. The MIS systems have also proven to be transferable—both to broader areas within the substance abuse arena (as in the statewide implementation of New York's system) and to other local categorical human service areas (as in Milwaukee).

Lessons Learned

Significant lessons for the field have emerged from these case studies. The most important lessons identified in each site is the time it takes to implement a MIS. As the Boston team reported, "Whatever time originally anticipated, system design and implementation will be much slower than planned." Similarly, the Albuquerque team reported that "there are no quick fixes," even when an existing system is adapted, updated, and enhanced. The projects studied in this chapter have each spent 5 years as Target Cities and are finding that MIS development is in fact never completed. We need to view the system as subject to continual modification, rather than thinking that a system can be established and then allowed to run in a maintenance mode—as many computer departments have traditionally operated.

Time is also a critical feature in developing the mind-set among administrators and providers to use the data capabilities the MISs provide for program and system evaluation and management. Many administrators are not accustomed to working with client-level data in program decision-making and system management. In each of the cities, we see expanding use of data as a learning process.

Another significant lesson is the need for provider involvement in system design, training, system improvement, and data interpretation. The need to give providers direct access to data on their own clients for their own analysis is becoming apparent in every city. This improves the integrity of the data, as well as the sustainability of the system. New York has found that regular user group meetings are an excellent way to accomplish these ends.

Training of users is a critical feature of MIS implementation. New York found that training that includes a system overview, the "big picture" rather than just technical and functional details regarding data input screens and procedures, significantly improved data quality and compliance. User-friendly documentation and reference guides were also critical.

While provider collaboration and coordination have been stressed as a potential outcome from establishment of the MIS in Target Cities, the systems that have emerged have improved coordination only as mediated by the CIU and systems management node. These systems are structured largely in a hub and spoke configuration, in which providers interact only with the CIU and the central data base, not directly with one another. (This is largely the consequence of strict federal and state regulations regarding client confidentiality in substance abuse treatment.) Thus it is the central system's management authority that fosters cooperative improvements, and that is blamed for any apparent inequities regarding the distribution of resources (i.e., funds and clients) within the treatment network. For example, in Milwaukee a number of providers have experienced significant financial distress as a result of the transition from sum-certain contracts to a centrally managed FFS system in which the provider has little control over the referral network. While providers do not have direct access to data on other providers, suspicions about unfair referral patterns have arisen. In response, Milwaukee is developing output reports summarizing referral flow from the CIU to each SDU and sharing these regularly with all participating providers. Public or interagency sharing of data on individual provider performance is not in place in any of these cities — output reports emphasize overall system performance.

Technical issues related to hardware and software selection are also important. Boston found that a PC-based system improved the provider infrastructure and enhanced local management potential. Albuquerque used a state-of-the-art graphic environment, and the latest version of the software, relying on training at vendor facilities and vendor support to upgrade the system they adapted. None of the projects found it necessary to accommodate to existing hardware and software at the provider level. Typically, the available computers at provider agencies were heavily used for other applications, tended to be nearing obsolescence, and represented a hodge-podge of unstandardized equipment. The cost of new state-of-the-art PCs or terminals for provider agencies was not prohibitive within the context of most Target Cities MIS development and equipment budgets. However, even the equipment purchased under Target Cities funding has become obsolete. We have provided technical details on hardware and software throughout the chapter to situate the Target Cities effort in the evolving world of computer technology, where decisions made today may have serious limitations on what one can do tomorrow. For example, Boston's local PCs (386 SXs, 52 mg hard drives, 4 mb memory) were already obsolete by the end of the five year demonstration period. Nontheless, the equipment purchased under Target Cities funding will likely be in place for quite some time due to funding limitations in public-sector drug abuse treatment.

Finally, there is a personal and attitudinal factor. The design, implementation, and use of an MIS require significant involvement from persons who understand what an MIS is capable of doing, how it will be used, and why. They must view it as a valued feedback loop and management tool, rather than simply as a data storage device to be used sparingly, driven by external accounting and reporting demands.

The Self-Correcting Treatment System?

CSAT's vision of the Target Cities program as movement toward "self-correcting treatment systems" in which central intake and assessment, client tracking, and ongoing evaluative and managerial use of data occur is becoming a reality in these cities. All have centralized and standardized client-level assessment (or at least screening, in Milwaukee), referral and tracking systems, and some level of provider interface active or planned. Tracking of available slots on a daily basis and waiting list management have been less formalized/automated in these systems. All systems now capture NIDA's Minimum Data Set and other state reporting requirements. Use of data at the provider level is in its infancy, but is also beginning to occur, with increasing access to MIS data on an agency's own clients at the provider level. Provider and system manager recognition of the potential of data to improve program management and operations and to analyze system performance grows over time and with reinforcing experience. It takes time and systems-oriented collaborative management teams who are comfortable with data to have a truly "self-correcting system."

The legacy left by Target Cities is likely to be the MIS, expanded to serve larger state, regional, or cross-program needs, and linked to many providers in support of emerging managed care systems. The impact on public systems of substance abuse treatment will include increased ability to centrally manage and evaluate services and clients, decentralized availability of data at the provider level, and potentially improved coordination of care between providers, mediated by the CIU. However, the MIS system may also serve to break down informal communication and networking patterns between providers that in the past were critical to coordination, may further distance public and private sectors of the treatment system, and has the potential to fuel conflict between providers competing for clients and other resources. Whether the "self-correcting treatment system" eventually emerges as a reality depends upon how well the systems management role is enacted in each city, using the analytic and evaluative capabilities afforded by the MIS.

Acknowledgments. Additional contributions and suggestions from Merna Jarvis (Milwaukee Target Cities) are gratefully acknowledged.

References

1. Department of Health and Human Services, Office for Treatment Improvement. Cooperative agreements for drug abuse treatment improvement projects in target cities. Request for Applications OT-90-01. Rockville, MD: DHHS; 1990.
2. Schlesinger M, Dowart R, Clark R. Public policy in a fragmented service system. In: National Institute on Drug Abuse, Drug Abuse Services Research Series: Background Papers on Drug Abuse Financing and Services Research. DHHS #(ADM) 91-1777. Rockville, MD: DHHS; 1991:16-57.

3. Weisner C, Morgan P. Rapid growth and bifurcation: Public and private alcohol treatment in the United States. In: Klingemann H, Takala JP, Hunt G, (eds.). *Cure, Care or Control: Alcoholism Treatment in Sixteen Countries.* Albany, NY: SUNY Press; 1992:223–251.

4. Yahr H. A national comparison of public- and private-sector alcoholism treatment delivery system characteristics. *J Studies Alcohol.* 1988; 49(3):233–239.

5. Littman PS, Moberg DP, Harrell M. *Qualitative Process Evaluation Report: Milwaukee Target Cities Project.* Madison, WI: Center for Health Policy and Program Evaluation; 1993:Paper #93-8.

6. Moberg DP. *The Social Control of Deviance: Intervention with Adolescent Alcohol and Other Drug Users.* Unpublished Ph.D. thesis. University of Wisconsin-Madison; 1985.

7. Gerstein DR, Harwood HJ (eds.). *Treating Drug Problems*, vol. 1. Washington DC: National Academy Press; 1990.

8. Diesenhaus H. Target Cities systems improvement projects as test of "the self correcting treatment system vision." Presented at the Target Cities Technical Assistance Workshop, Los Angeles, CA. August; 1992.

9. Jaffe J. Central intake. Presented at the Target Cities Technical Assistance Workshop, Los Angeles, CA. August; 1992.

10. Center for Substance Abuse Treatment, Division of National Treatment Demonstrations. *The Target Cities Program: Partnerships to Increase Availability of and Access to Alcohol and Other Drug Treatment.* Rockville, MD: CSAT; 1995.

11. Camp JM, Krakow M, McCarty D, Argeriou M. Substance abuse treatment management information systems: Balancing federal, state and service provider needs. *J Mental Health Admin.* 1992;19:5–20.

12. McLellan AT, Luborsky L, O'Brien CP, Woody GE. An improved evaluation instrument for substance abuse patients: The Addiction Severity Index. *J Nervous Mental Disease.* 1980;168:26–33

13. Moberg DP, Littman PS, Connor TG, Lake D, Garb B. Milwaukee Target Cities Project Management Information System Client Data Report. Madison, WI: Center for Health Policy and Program Evaluation; 1995:Paper #95-5.

Postscript for Section II

Sid J. Schneider

The theme running through the four chapters in Section II is that computer networks transform health care organizations, making them more mutually dependent, functioning together as components of an overall community-wide health care delivery system. For example, when clinical laboratories or physicians' offices join the Wisconsin Health Information Network (WHIN; Chapter 5), they must reexamine their missions, not as individual health care organizations, but as users and suppliers of information within their communities. They must determine what information they require from other organizations in the network, and what information they will put onto the network.

WHIN presently links over 1100 physicians, 21 hospitals and clinics, 7 insurers, various pharmacies, transcription services, payers, clinical laboratories, home health agencies, and even the Disability Determination Bureau of the State Department of Health. Kim Pemble (Chapter 5) points out that WHIN can transfer patient information among these organizations more efficiently than couriers, mail, and faxes can. However, more than just adding efficiency, WHIN allows health care organizations to function more easily in concert to deliver what Pemble calls the entire "continuum of care that a patient receives over his or her life."

In Chapter 7 Nell Brownstein of the Centers for Disease Control and Prevention, and her colleagues, show how similar network technology links public health workers in the Information Network for Public Health officials (INPHO). The authors write that "INPHO aims to connect the fragmented public health system and helps states build strategic information partnerships." INPHO links federal and state health agencies, physicians, and clinics, making possible a coordinated, unified approach to public health matters such as natural disasters and infectious disease surveillance.

The Community Health Management Information System (CHMIS) described by Richard Rubin and Megan Aukema in Chapter 6 also links health care organizations to address public health problems. Their chapter emphasizes how a decentralized, incremental approach to building a network can help ensure that the network will be widely accepted and used. The chapter also discusses the role of networks in health care research. CHMIS has already provided data for patient satisfaction studies and outcome studies of obstetrical, surgical, and orthopedic services. Rubin and Aukema point out that it may be a long time before computer databases containing community-wide information are routinely used for research. However, it is easy to imagine the day when the aggregation of community-wide data on CHIN databases facilitate rapid outcome evaluations and comparisons among treatments, as well as epidemiologic surveillance studies.

The Target Cities project (Chapter 8) is an excellent example of a network that alters the function of health care organizations. Prior to the Target Cities project, the drug abuse treatment centers in a city would compete for patients; each center would independently encourage patients to refer themselves for care. Patients sometimes referred themselves to inappropriate centers. Also, treatment centers found it cumbersome or impossible to obtain data about a patient's past treatment at other centers. Some patients took advantage of this fragmented system by surreptitiously enrolling in several methadone programs simultaneously to smuggle methadone.

In the Target Cities program, these problems are diminished. Each city has a small number of central intake units where drug users present themselves initially. The central intake units are connected by a computer network with the city's treatment facilities, and in some cities, with criminal justice agencies. All intake examinations occur at the intake unit, along with a review of any past treatment that the patient has received. Intake examinations may include interviews, psychological testing, drug tests, and medical examinations. The patient is referred to the most appropriate treatment facility based upon the intake findings, a review of the patient's treatment and criminal justice histories, and the availability of treatment slots.[1] With the Target Cities program, treatment centers are freed from much of the burden of doing intake assessments and can devote more of their time to treatment. Patients who attempt to enroll in multiple methadone programs can be easily spotted.

The changes brought about by WHIN, INPHO, CHMIS, and Target Cities will sometimes precipitate disagreements among organizations. In the Target Cities project, the staff at some treatment facilities might conclude that they are not receiving a proportionate number of referrals from the intake center. On a CHIN, one health care provider might wish to avoid sharing data that another organization wants. In Chapter 7 there is an anecdote about an HMO that did not wish to share immunization data that were sought by a governmental health department. The HMO feared that competitors would learn too much about the HMO from the data. Despite these potential conflicts, computer networks allow greater coordination among health care organizations than has ever been possible before.

These chapters show that networks are already having a substantial impact. As an increasing number of health care organizations join networks, more and more health care functions will be changed by network technology. For example, the National Information Infrastructure will allow providers to obtain patient data very quickly. In Chapter 5, Pemble describes how the National Information Infrastructure will permit emergency room personnel to gather accurate medical and demographic data about their patients. In the future, network technology might transform many health care activities that presently have nothing to do with computers, such as partner notification programs.

Partner notification programs (sometimes called "contact tracing" programs) are a long-standing public health approach to controlling the spread of sexually transmitted diseases (STDs) and human immunodeficiency virus (HIV) infection. The concept underlying partner notification programs is simple: the sexual (and, for HIV, needle-sharing) partners of patients with STV or HIV infection are contacted and asked to come in for counseling, testing, and if testing indicates, treatment. Partner notification programs are intended to reach individuals who are at high risk for infection or who are unaware that they were exposed and may be infected.[2-4]

At present, there are several impediments to the success of partner notification programs. Patients are often unwilling to divulge the identities of their sexual or needle-sharing partners. Also, patients often do not know the present whereabouts of their partners. Partner notification programs can require patients to identify partners over the past several years; however, the patients may have only outdated addresses or telephone numbers for their partners. When patients cannot provide useful data about their partners, it can be very difficult and expensive to locate and contact the partners.[5] Even when the partners can be reached, they must be motivated to report for counseling and HIV testing. However, partners often do not report when telephoned by public health workers whom they do not know.[6]

Osborn[7] has argued that present partner notification programs could drive HIV disease underground by discouraging HIV-seropositive people from coming forward when they fear that their seropositive status will become widely known. Therefore, both the American Public Health Association[8] and the Centers for Disease Control and Prevention[9] have argued that partner notification programs must take precautions to guard the confidentiality of patients and their partners.

The new information networks and the National Information Infrastructure might diminish these problems with present partner notification programs. In a computer-mediated partner notification program, patients would not have to divulge the identities of their sexual and needle-sharing partners to another person. Nor would they have to reveal any information about their infection to their partners. Instead, they could provide the needed information through interactions with a computer. Computer-mediated interviews may be superior to face-to-face interviews in eliciting sensitive personal information[10] (see also Slack, Chapter 2, and references 18 through 26 in Chapter 2).

In the future, patients may not need to provide current addresses or telephone numbers for their partners. The National Information Infrastructure may provide a means to locate the patients' partners, even using outdated or incomplete information.

Partner notification could then occur in several ways. Most simply, computer software could generate letters to the partners asking them to communicate with the staff of the partner notification program. Alternatively, software on the network could identify the partners' physicians and ask them to contact the partners. Because the partners presumably know and trust their physicians, partners may be more willing to report for testing and counseling than they would be if they were contacted by public health workers whom they did not know.

A computer-mediated partner notification program must respect the confidentiality of patients and partners to at least the same extent as existing partner notification programs do. The issue of security and confidentiality on computer networks is addressed specifically in Chapter 16. Pemble (Chapter 5) makes the point that computer networks may be better able than paper medical record systems to ensure confidentiality. As computer networks are increasingly used in health care applications, they may develop a reputation for being secure. If they do not, their role in health care will be limited. If they do, their role in health care will be limited only by the imagination.

References

1. Hoffman J.A, Schneider SJ, Koman JJ, Flynn PM, Luckey JW, Cooley PC, Wish ED, Diesenhaus HI. The centralized intake model for drug abuse treatment: The role of computerized data management. *Comput Human Behav.* 1995; 11:215–222.

2. Potterat JJ, Spencer NE, Woodhouse DE, Muth JB. Partner notification in the control of human immunodeficiency virus infection. *Am J Public Health.* 1989; 79:874–876.

3. Wyckoff RF, Jones JL, Longshore ST, Hollis SL, Quiller CB, Dowda H, Gamble WB. Notification of the sex and needle-sharing partners of individuals with human immunodeficiency virus in rural South Carolina: 30-month experience. *Sexually Transmitted Dis.* 1991; 18:217–222.

4. Landis SE, Schoenbach VJ, Weber DJ, Mittal M, Krishan B, Lewis K, Koch GG. Results of a randomized trial of partner notification in cases of HIV infection in North Carolina. *N Eng J Med.* 1992; 326:101–106.

5. Rutherford GW, Woo JM. Contact tracing and the control of human immunodeficiency virus infection. *JAMA.* 1988; 259:3609–3610.

6. Wyckoff RF, Jones JL. Letter. *N Eng J Med.* 1992; 327:436.

7. Osborn JE. AIDS: Politics and science. *N Eng J Med.* 1988; 318:444–447.

8. American Public Health Association. Contact Tracing and Partner Notification. Washington, DC: Author; 1988.

9. Cates W, Toomey KE, Havlak GR, Bowen GS, Hinman AR. Partner notification and confidentiality of the index patient: Its role in preventing HIV. *Sexually Transmitted Dis.* 1990; 17:113–114.
10. O'Reilly J, Hubbard M, Lessler J, Biemer P. Audio computer assisted self-interviewing: New technology for data collection on sensitive issues and special populations. Presented to the American Statistical Association, Boston; 1992.

Section III

Information Networks and the Delivery of Care

The five chapters in Section III describe network-based health promotion services that are still in an experimental stage and not yet widely available. Some of these applications have been developed with financial support from the National Institutes of Health, the Alberta Cancer Board, and other agencies that nurture new approaches to health care; some are services on the Internet, where almost everything is new and experimental. Although not all of the network applications described in this section may develop beyond their present experimental stage, some may break ground leading to frequently used, effective public health interventions.

The section raises many questions about network-based health promotion services: Who will offer preventive services on information networks? What will be the principal goals of these services? Will network-mediated health promotion services be effective in changing behavior? Will these services be targeted to the individuals who most need them? What should be the demeanor or "personality" conveyed in computer-mediated services?

Who Will Offer Services Through CHINs?

Employers, preferred provider organizations (PPOs), health maintenance organizations (HMOs), and managed care organizations might wish to offer network-mediated services that reduce the number of times patients make non-essential face-to-face visits to providers. Physicians and hospitals might offer network-mediated services to publicize themselves and improve communication with their patients.

Users of network-based services like CHESS (Chapter 9), "Cancer Me?" (Chapter 11), the network for caregivers of Alzheimer's Disease patients (Chapter 10), or the telephone network for drug abusers (Chapter 13) might rely on these network-based services in place of some face-to-face services. When network-mediated services are available, users might be less in need of face-to-face visits with providers to obtain information and reassurance. Boberg and his colleagues (Chapter 9) found that HIV-positive CHESS users tended to have shorter hospital stays than HIV-positive patients who did not have access to CHESS. Boberg's group conjectured that CHESS users might be better informed about discharge planning, making them better able to live independently of the hospital. If network-based services can reliably bring about reductions in non-essential use of face to face services, managed care organizations will be eager to offer them.

Also, if these network-mediated services work — that is, if they bring about more healthful behaviors in large numbers of people — they potentially can reduce the overall need for health care services. For example, Alemi's telephone network (Chapter 13) could easily justify its cost if it improved prenatal care among crack-abusing pregnant women; Smyth's network for caregivers (Chapter 10) could justify its cost if it shifted some of the care of Alzheimer's patients to caregivers at home. Managed care organizations might see in these network-based services a way to improve the efficiency of face-to-face health services.

Of all the network-based services discussed in this section, only CHESS is presently being offered by a managed care organization. Its level of success in the managed care environment will help to determine whether many other network-based services will be offered in the future.

Physicians and hospitals may view network-based services as tools to generate referrals and to increase patient loyalty. Networks provide an avenue of communication with patients without requiring much staff time. For example, Schwartz (unpublished data) developed a computer system that periodically telephoned patients who were receiving treatment for hypertension and played prerecorded, personalized information about their treatment. He found that the patients who received the calls gained better understanding of their treatment, although the effects upon their compliance with treatment and their blood pressure itself were less clear. Schwartz did not attempt to assess the patients' satisfaction with their medical care. If further research shows that network-based services increase patient satisfaction with treatment, these services may be offered more widely as an adjunct to treatment.

In sum, network-based services must first show what they can accomplish before they will be routinely offered. While managed care organizations and HMOs might be most interested in network-based systems that reduce non-essential face-to-face visits to providers, physicians and hospitals might be more interested in systems that lead to patient referrals and enhance communication with patients.

What Should the Goals of Network-Mediated Services Be?

The principal goal of the systems described in this section is to promote healthful behavior among large numbers of people, using a minimum amount of professional staff time. For the most part, the systems use a behavioral approach in which the focus is upon central, problem behaviors, not upon the feelings or emotions that might surround the behaviors. This behavioral approach is relatively easy to adapt to computer-mediated interventions. For example, Schneider, Walter, and O'Donnell[1] offered a behaviorally oriented smoking cessation program on the CompuServe network. At the start of each session, the users answered a series of questions about their smoking and their progress in the program. The system chose its communications with the users on the basis of the users' responses. The "expertise" of the computer system was its ability to pick message segments and assemble them into complete messages and interactions with the users.

Network-mediated services can in principle reach an almost unlimited number of people, at any time of the day or night. Users can access the system when they are most willing to participate. Face-to-face interventions, by contrast, are usually available only at a scheduled time. Face-to-face interventions usually attract only the most motivated people, while network-based services are easily available to anyone willing to take part, even those who participate out of idle curiosity without real commitment. Health promotion programs such as smoking cessation and weight-loss programs are usually not covered by health insurance plans. When they are offered over a computer network — particularly when access is free of charge — they can reach the maximum number of people, particularly those not yet ready to change their behavior.

More research is needed to assess the ability of network-based services to reach people who are missed by face-to-face services and to determine which particular health risk behaviors are most easily modified through network-based services. More research is especially needed to determine which network-based approaches are most effective.

For example, some face-to-face health promotion services are based on a "health belief" model,[2] which holds that people change a health risk behavior when they believe that they are vulnerable to the ill effects of their behavior, that changing the behavior would reduce their vulnerability, and that they are capable of changing their behavior. The systems described by Boberg (Chapter 9) and Smyth (Chapter 10) include discussion groups, which provide a means for participants to continually model health-promoting behavior to one another. In the discussions, participants convey the idea that behavior change is feasible and effective. The discussion groups are nonjudgmental, so that participants may feel safe raising personal issues.

The smoking cessation program on CompuServe[1] was offered both with and without a discussion group. Comparisons showed that participants who had access to the discussion group were more likely to report that they had quit smoking at the 1- and 3-month postenrollment follow-up assessments.

The easy accessibility of network-based services allows them to reach people who can benefit from health-promotion services, including those who would not otherwise seek them. Network-based communications can be tailored to each participants' level of motivation; for example, some persons may be guided to make the decision to change their behavior, while others who have already made the decision to change receive suggestions on how to effect the change they seek.[3]

Are Network-Based Health Promotion Programs Effective?

The evaluations of network-based services such as CHESS and Alemi's telephone-based program suggest that network-based services can be an effective public health approach. However, most of the existing network-based services, like the dozens on the Internet listed in Chapter 12, have never been evaluated.

Evaluations of network-based health promotion programs should attempt to identify the components that make for effective programs. For example, Schneider, Schwartz and Fast[4] tested four versions of a computerized telephone-based stress management program. In some versions, the system gave callers assignments to practice specific stress management techniques. In some versions, the stress management messages were personalized to the individuals callers' responses to a questionnaire about stress. Participants stayed in the program longer, made more calls, and expressed more satisfaction with the program when the messages were personalized and contained homework assignments. Also, they were more likely to practice the stress management techniques when the messages were personalized. When the messages were not personalized, the participants were more likely to leave messages for the staff of the program; perhaps they were attempting to compensate for the lack of personalization this way. Thus, computer-mediated programs might be most effective when they personalize their communications to each individual user. Users might even regard the personalization of the messages as evidence that a computer-based program is credible and trustworthy.

Should Network-Based Programs Be Targeted to Those Who Most Need Them?

CHINs contain patient databases. If patients become participants in CHINs, it is possible that the information in those databases will be employed to direct information to specific users. For example, the databases on a CHIN could easily identify all smokers, or all known alcohol users among the patients in the database. It will be straightforward to identify all patients with certain characteristics on the network, and offer them network-based services. For example, it might be possible in the future to contact all Alzheimer's Disease patients' family members who log on to a network and ask them to participate in a network-based system like the one described by Smyth (Chapter 10). If the CompuServe network had kept data about which users were smokers—the way a CHIN would—the smoking cessation program could have contacted all CompuServe users who were smokers rather than waiting for smokers to learn about the program and join voluntarily.

What "Personality" Should Network-Based Services Convey?

The network-based services described in this section were designed so that personalized messages were sent to each participant. When Taenzer and his colleagues (Chapter 11) developed their program, they first had to decide upon the tone of these messages. They eventually agreed that the messages should be conversational in tone and contain a good deal of humor. Their decision appears to have been a good one, judging from the popularity of their service on the Alex network. However, Taenzer's group was taking a risk; users could have found humor and conversation by a computer to be disingenuous or artificial, like a machine that says "We appreciate your patience" to telephone callers waiting on hold.

The staff of the telephone-based stress management program[4] has run focus groups with some of the users of the program. Several users said that they strove to be polite in their interactions with the computer, as if the computer had feelings. Some said that they never interrupted computer-generated messages until the computer was finished presenting them. Some said that they had feelings of gratitude toward the computerized program, and felt as though they had established an ongoing relationship with the computer during the course of the interactions.

As computer technology improves, human-computer interactions will gain greater similarity to person-to-person interactions. Developers of network-based systems will have to determine what "personality" their programs will portray.

Information networks will take on new roles as patients gain access to them, and as the means for access evolves to interactive television and other technologies. Networks will increasingly provide information to patients, especially patients who have limited access to information. Networks will also become the medium for social support. Smyth's program for the caregivers of homebound patients and the CHESS program appear to be satisfactory ways to bring social support to hard-to-reach populations. Those programs also suggest that many patients will trust software that offers to help them make decisions about their medical care. Network-based health promotion programs that are both easy to use and consonant with users' expectations may become an important component of community-based health care.

References

1. Schneider SJ, Walter R, O'Donnell R. Computerized communication as a medium for behavioral smoking cessation treatment: Controlled evaluation. *Comput Human Behav.* 1990; 6:141–151.
2. Hornik R. Alternative models of behavior change. In: Wasserheit JN, Aral SO, Holmes KK, Hitchcock PJ (eds.). *Research Issues in Human Behavior and Sexually Transmitted Diseases in the AIDS Era.* Washington, DC: American Society for Microbiology; 1991.
3. Prochaska JO, DiClemente CC. Common processes of self-change in smoking, weight control, and psychological distress. In: Shiffman S, Wills TA (eds.). *Coping and Substance Use.* Orlando: Academic; 1985.
4. Schneider SJ, Schwartz MD, Fast J. Computerized, telephone-based health promotion: II. Stress management program. *Comput Human Behav.* 1995; 11:205–214.

9

CHESS: The Comprehensive Health Enhancement Support System

ERIC W. BOBERG, DAVID H. GUSTAFSON, ROBERT P. HAWKINS,
EARL BRICKER, SUZANNE PINGREE, FIONA MCTAVISH,
MEG WISE, BETTA OWENS, and RENEE BOTTA

The Comprehensive Health Enhancement Support System (CHESS) is a computer-based support system designed to empower people facing major illnesses and other health concerns to become partners in their own health care. Designed for in-home use, CHESS can also be installed in health care settings and community sites. CHESS provides users with a wide range of services for information, social support, decision support, skills training, and referrals.

The conceptualization of CHESS is based on change[1-3] and crisis[4,5] theories. The foundation of CHESS is the recognition that both the barriers to and strategies for successful patient empowerment are multifactorial. Barriers include limited access to information, due to financial, geographical, or educational constraints,[6] as well as the failure of formerly successful coping strategies.[4,5] To help people overcome these barriers, a variety of tools are needed, and different tools will be needed by different types of patients. Some patients will focus on information-gathering; others on social support, others will need support in making and implementing difficult decisions. The key feature of CHESS is that it accommodates these various needs by offering a wide range of services in an easy-to-use format that allows users to choose the type and order of services, and the rate of use that best meets their needs and situation.

CHESS

Design and Services

CHESS operates on IBM-compatible personal computers (PCs). The minimum individual work station requirements are a 286 microprocessor, 640 KB RAM, 40 MB hard disk drive, color VGA monitor, and a 2400-baud modem. Communications are transmitted via modem to a "host" computer (a 386 or 486 PC, based on size of the network) with multiple modem connections. To date, CHESS has been maintained as a DOS-based system to allow the widest possible compatibility with existing hardware. However, with the rapidly decreasing cost and speed of PCs and with advances in multimedia technology, a Windows™-based version of CHESS is being developed and is currently nearing completion.

Extensive experimentation and development have made the user interface attractive and easy to use, even for people with low educational levels and no prior computer experience. A graphical user interface provides easy-to-understand prompts. The information needed to navigate through CHESS is displayed on the screen at all times. Color and pictures are used to highlight key information.

CHESS is organized into "modules" that provide information on specific health-related crises or concerns (see Topics and Content section). Within each module, CHESS offers these services:

Questions & Answers offers answers to a wide range of questions people may face when dealing with a health crisis. Most of the questions are derived from an extensive needs assessment process described below. The one- to five-screen answers provide a brief introduction and overview of each specific issue and may refer users to sources of more detailed information. Anywhere from 100 to 500 questions and answers are provided, depending on the scope of the module. Experts and patients in each field have reviewed answers for accuracy and readability.

Instant Library stores and indexes publications, newsletter articles, abstracts of scientific articles, brochures, and other materials. While the material in Questions & Answers is designed to be brief, the Instant Library either provides more depth and detail or integrates several questions and answers. Each article contains information about the source of the article, often including an address and phone number in case users wish to get on a mailing list. Articles are anywhere from a few screens to nearly 100 screens long. Longer articles are broken up into chapters accessible through an additional menu. The number of articles on each topic varies, from about 50 to over 300.

Getting Help/Support is a tutorial that helps empower consumers of health, mental health, support, and other community services. The service was developed based on an assessment of consumer-perceived barriers to seeking and receiving satisfactory service, as well as providers' frustrations with service delivery to people facing health-related crises. Getting Help/Support describes hundreds of services, including specific medical specialists, financial services, and community psychosocial support. Descriptions include an overview of the service, what to expect, how to prepare for an appointment, how to find a compatible practitioner, and how to develop a partnership with a provider. In most cases a list of specific questions is supplied to help users overcome the problem of not knowing what to say.

Referral Directory is a comprehensive list of national services and providers. A local directory may also be included depending upon the availability and willingness of a partner (hospital, community-based organization, etc.) to research the necessary information, organize it using the keywords and enter it into a database created by CHESS programming staff. Entries contain all or most of the following pieces of information: agency name, hours of operation, phone number(s), availability of TDD phone service, and a brief description of the services provided.

Personal Stories are first-person accounts written by professional journalists from in-depth interviews of people facing the crises addressed by CHESS. The original idea of providing Personal Stories was to dissolve the perception of computers as a "cold" technological delivery system. However, it soon became clear that the stories also provide a wealth of practical information, insights, models of behavior, support, and a sense that CHESS is in touch with real people's lives. Structurally, Personal Stories are designed to be "created" by the user, according to his or her information or support needs. Each story has a three- to five-screen core, covering how the illness affects the person's life, and how he or she deals with issues on a day-to-day basis. At several points within each story, readers are asked if they would like to know more of the person's story on that topic. These "expansions" range from 1 to 10 screens and address topics of interest to specific users. By selecting some expansions, but not others, the user is able to construct the story that is most relevant and useful.

Dictionary assists users by providing easy-to-understand definitions of confusing medical, legal, and financial terminology. Definitions are between one and three sentences long. Care is taken to maintain a simple language level, although this is often difficult with medical terms. The Dictionary is available both as a menu choice and through a "hotkey" that allows the user to call up the dictionary from anywhere in CHESS, merely by pressing a specific key.

Assessment includes a number of different types of programs, depending on the topic (Table 9.1). The programs are similar in that they all help users identify behaviors or symptoms that can place them (or those around them) at increased risk of injury or illness. For example, persons with HIV may be more likely to change their behavior if they understand how their lifestyle affects their risk of transmitting the infection to others. To develop this particular assessment, a panel of experts in HIV transmission identified factors they felt would strongly predict a person's risk of transmitting the infection, suggested a way to assess these factors, and estimated the amount of prediction. A subjective Bayesian statistical model, designed so the predictive factors were conditionally independent,[7] yielded a posterior odds estimate for and against transmission.

The user is asked a series of questions about behaviors that might lead to transmission (e.g., frequency of unprotected anal intercourse) and health status (e.g., symptoms of HIV infection that might facilitate transmission to others). Graphics portray the relative risks of transmission and the extent to which different aspects of the person's lifestyle contribute to the risk. Then users are shown why those lifestyles have that effect on risk and how

TABLE 9.1. Topic-specific content in CHESS.

Topic	Questions and answers	Instant library	Getting help/support	Referral directory	Personal stories	Dictionary	Decisions and conflicts	Assessments
AIDS/HIV infection	451	372	177	340	29	856	1. Who to tell about HIV/AIDS for support 2. When to tell a potential new sex partner about being HIV-positive 3. Clinical trials	1. Risk of HIV transmission 2. Health charts 3. What uplifts you? 4. Handling your stress
Breast cancer	364	134	221	243	38	535	1. Breast surgery 2. Chemotherapy 3. Tamoxifen 4. Clinical trials 5. Oopherectomy	1. Health charts
Sexual assault	157	102	97	205	11	129	1. Who can you talk to about a sexual assault? 2. What kind of formal report can you make?	1. Road blocks to healing
Stress management	139	177	167	490	7	0	1. Who to talk to about a stressful situation 2. What professional help to seek	1. What uplifts you? 2. Handling your stress
Making in school	129	73	4	0	5	0		1. Academic problems
Adult children of alcoholics	45	14	54	184	8	0	1. Who to talk to	1. Family patterns

to change those lifestyles. Users may opt to see how changes in lifestyles will affect their risk. If they want more information on a risk behavior, they are taken directly to an article in the Instant Library for details.

Health Charts is really a specific type of assessment, but deserves additional explanation. Health Charts allows users to answer questions about their symptoms, emotional status, and quality of life, and track their responses over time; they can also access the responses of other system users (who agree to make their files available) for comparison. The program also offers feedback on the symptoms reported, providing appropriate courses of action based on severity and duration. This program allows users to track their own physical and mental health and compare their situation to that of other users.

Decisions & Conflicts is designed to guide people through difficult decision-making. Two different types of programs are available. One helps users through specific decisions related to a particular topic (Table 9.1); the other helps users with any decision. The underlying model for these decision programs is an additive multiattribute utility model.[8] It has four basic elements: options, decision criteria, weights, and utility functions. A panel of experts and patients identify the primary options the user is likely to face, suggest decision criteria that others have used to make the choice, and suggest how to measure each criterion. Users select the decision problem of interest and are guided through a seven-step process that helps them:

1. understand the available options (they can read descriptions of each option or a personal story of someone who chose that option);
2. understand possible decision criteria (by reading descriptions of what those criteria are, how they are related to the options, and why someone might choose each as a criterion to be considered in making a choice;
3. select criteria they will use and assign weights of relative importance to them;
4. reduce the set of available options to a manageable size (they may also add their own options if the expert-generated list does not contain them);
5. rate how well each criterion satisfies each option;
6. choose the option they are leaning toward and see which option CHESS predicted they would lean toward (CHESS won't tell users which option to choose, but will tell them which option the model predicted they would choose); and
7. understand how the computer arrived at that prediction.

The interface uses a combination of text and graphics to help users through the task. Users weigh decision criteria by creating a bar graph displaying the relative importance of all criteria. Another graphic combines a Likert scale on which users assign a utility score to each criterion-option pair with a summary of what is known about how well each option satisfies each criterion.

The second form of Decisions & Conflicts is more general in focus. It allows users to examine *any* decision by entering the options and decision criteria they wish to use. Then they weigh the decision criteria and rate how well each option satisfies each decision criterion. The model then predicts the decision they will make. This model can also be used as a conflict analysis aid. For instance, three different people can weigh the decision criteria and rate how well each option satisfies each decision criterion. Then, CHESS will compare the weights and utilities of the different people to help them understand how their views of the decision differ and why that might be a source of conflict. CHESS then identifies areas in which compromise might be possible.

Action Plan helps people plan how to implement their decisions and also offers a way to examine the plan and identify ways to improve it. Hence, Action Plan has two subservices. One helps users design an implementation strategy. Users are asked to: (1) specify the goal; (2) examine the level of social support and opposition they have; (3) identify the resources they will need to bring about the change; (4) list the major barriers they will face; (5) identify the rewards that can be obtained from success; and (6) develop a specific set of action steps they will follow. A summary plan is then presented to the user, who can go back and change items as desired. The second subservice (which can be used independently of or following plan development) asks users to assess factors predictive of success in their change plan, including the user's personal commitment level, self-efficacy, social support, information and skills, environment, resources, goals, and monitoring strategy. A subjective Bayesian statistical model[7] predicts the chances of successful implementation. The user is not given a numerical estimate of success, but is shown a traffic signal with either a green, yellow, or red light showing. The strengths and weaknesses of the plan are summarized and the mechanisms by which the weaknesses have their effects are shown. Finally, a steepest ascent operations research algorithm is used to identify the smallest set of improvements needed to move into a green light (success) prediction.

Ask an Expert provides users with a source of accurate, up-to-date information on health-related questions, which they can obtain anonymously. Questions can be written and sent to the expert at any hour of the day or night, and the user will get a response within 24 to 48 hours. Users type messages to the expert on their individual computers. The messages are then sent to the central "host" computer via modem. A CHESS staff expert logs into the host computer once or twice a day to read and respond to questions. Users retrieve the expert's responses by dialing in to the host computer and downloading the responses to their own computers, where they can read them at their convenience. Only the expert and the sender have access to the questions and the responses; others cannot read these interactions. Responses are written by a trained health care provider, usually a nurse or other professional with experience in patient education, not a physician. CHESS experts have a broad range of knowledge specific to the module topic and the ability to translate complex terms into clear, easily understandable English. Experts do not give medical advice. Complex or obscure questions may require the expert to consult the scientific literature or a panel of specialists who are available to the project. If the research or consultation will take longer than 48 hours, the expert lets the user know and gives a time frame for the final response.

New features of this service allow CHESS experts to provide even more personalized and detailed responses. User profiles (demographics, diagnoses, treatments, and social support), can be input by users, and made available to the experts for review. Experts also have access to databases of all previously asked questions and answers related to the current question, and all other related material in CHESS. From these databases, the expert will be able to select additional material from CHESS to attach to the answer and thus provide additional detail or explanation.

Discussion Group acts as an online support group that is available 24 hours a day, 7 days a week. Its objective is to provide users with a safe space to give and receive support in regard to health-related issues. Users exchange information and experiences, ask questions, offer insights, and generally do all of the things found at in-person support groups. Discussion Group is generally the most heavily used service when CHESS is placed in the user's home. Users type messages on their individual computers. The messages are then sent to the central host computer via modem. All messages are posted in common lists in each Discussion Group; there is no private, one-to-one mail between subjects. When a user selects the "receive new messages" option in Discussion Group, the host computer sends all unread messages from the host to the user's computer, where they are stored and can be read at any time. Messages in each group are listed in menus in chronological order, showing date, time, sender, and a topic. Messages are composed and written offline; that is, without using the telephone lines. Telephone lines are used only to send and receive messages. Because of the relatively small number of people who have the system at any one time, interactions generally do not take place in real time. That is, users will write a message and then come back several hours later or the next day to read responses. Fortuitously, this means that users often read of experiences and topics beyond their initial interests. Each Discussion Group is monitored by a trained facilitator. The facilitator reads all messages each day, prods discussion as needed, provides expert information when requested, reminds users of appropriate behavior in the group (only rarely necessary), and generally keeps the discussions on track.

Users have reported several advantages to this type of computer-based support. They were able to write messages 24 hours a day, 7 days a week, not just when the group met. They could remain anonymous if they wanted to. Those who were healthy did not have to be faced with the sight of people with more advanced disease. They could relate to other people based solely on what they wrote, without the influence of automatic prejudices based on race, dress, sex, or other factors. Users have reported a few disadvantages to this format also: the lag time in getting responses to messages (from a few minutes to a few days), difficulty in conveying certain emotions through written comments (especially sarcasm), and having to read many messages the user was not interested in (although the individual message selection was entirely in the user's control).

For convenience, CHESS services are often grouped into information services (Questions & Answers, Instant Library, Getting Help/Support, Referral Directory, Personal Stories, Dictionary), communication services (Ask an Expert, Discussion Group), and analysis services (Assessment, Decisions & Conflicts, Action Plan). These groupings are quite artificial, however, and depend on the biases of the user (or researcher). For example, Ask an Expert and, to some extent, Discussion Group are also used for information gathering and exchange. Someone interested in the social support aspects of CHESS might focus on Discussion Group and Personal Stories. However, Ask an Expert and many Instant Library articles also provide significant social support. The key point here is that by providing users with an array of services, CHESS can address a wide variety of needs and styles of support. Indeed, CHESS services address virtually all aspects of the change and crisis models upon which CHESS is based.

Topics and Content

The structure of CHESS is designed to accommodate content on virtually any health-related topic. Current CHESS topics include AIDS/HIV Infection, Breast Cancer, Sexual Assault, Stress Management, Academic Crisis, Adult Children of Alcoholics, modules for Parents and Partners of Alcohol Abusers. Heart Disease and Alzheimer's Disease are under development and many other topics are planned.

The content developed for a CHESS module (topic) is determined by a needs assessment,[9] because thorough understanding of the needs of potential users is critical to the success of the program. The needs assessment process used to develop CHESS content includes surveys of potential users as well as focus groups, literature reviews, and interviews with health care providers. The key is to focus on what patients ("customers") want, not what providers or others think they need. Addressing patients' needs ensures that patients will become engaged in the program and respond positively to it.

With the variety of CHESS services available, content in different topic areas can be tailored to the particular needs and desires of a given population. For example, in the AIDS/HIV module, a broad spectrum of information is a key element, because of the varied nature of complications and lack of consensus on optimal treatment patterns. Therefore, the Instant Library contains multiple articles on topics whenever possible and is thus larger in this module than in any other. The smaller range of complications and more standard treatments for breast cancer resulted in a somewhat smaller Instant Library in that module, because a single article from a definitive source meets the needs of most users. In the proposed diabetes module, the needs assessment identified tailored Action Plans (for diet modification and blood-sugar monitoring) as perhaps the key element for a successful CHESS module. The content of each module is constantly changing as new material becomes available and as technology is advanced. Table 9.1 outlines the current content of completed modules.

Navigating Through CHESS

To provide as much flexibility and tailoring as possible, users can access CHESS services in three ways:

- "All CHESS Services" (the whole topic);
- "Table of Contents" (groups of ideas related to the topic); and
- "Keyword Index" (particular subjects related to the topic).

All CHESS Services brings up a menu of all the services available to users. Many of the information services (Questions & Answers, Instant Library, Getting Help/Support, Referral Directory, Personal Stories) are also organized into a "Table of Contents" with a hierarchical structure of broad categories, and by "Keyword Index." Thus, a user can quickly select the content of interest or browse generally.

The *Table of Contents* helps users browse through a broad category such as social support or finances. After choosing this option at the beginning of CHESS, users select from a menu of broad topic areas. Choosing one of these broad topics leads to a number of additional menus, each more specific and designed to guide the user to where he or she wants or needs to be. For example, in the AIDS/HIV module, selecting the topic of Medical Issues leads to other menus containing more specific topics, where one might select "Symptoms and Specific Illnesses," and then, perhaps, "AIDS Dementia Complex." Choosing AIDS Dementia Complex provides the user with a menu of the available CHESS services on that topic: Questions & Answers, Instant Library, Getting Help/Support, and Dictionary.

Users with very directed information needs can quickly choose a specific key word from a *Keyword Index* offering hundreds of specific topics from which to choose. The Keyword Index is analogous to a book index. When a particular keyword is chosen, the user is given a menu of services that contain relevant material. To use the previous example, the term AIDS Dementia Complex is an option in the Keyword Index. Choosing that will lead to the menu of services described above. The Keyword Index functions globally within the module and is accessible from any part of CHESS simply by pressing the [F9] key.

Several of the problem-solving and communication services (Discussion Group, Ask an Expert, Decisions & Conflicts, and Action Plan) are process-oriented rather than content-oriented. Therefore, these services are accessible via all three navigational paths, and they can be useful for almost any specific issue. For example, in the case of AIDS Dementia Complex, a user could: (1) ask others about experiencing loss of mental acuity in Discussion Group; (2) get expert advice on Power of Attorney in Ask an Expert; (3) use Decisions & Conflicts to decide in whom to invest Power of Attorney should loss of mental competence occur; and (4) use Action Plan to implement their Power of Attorney decision.

Data Collection

A data collection program within CHESS can, if activated, collect data on nearly every keystroke a user makes while using CHESS. The data can be used in many ways. Analysis of what keywords are most often selected, what Instant Library articles or Questions & Answers are most frequently read, and what topics are discussed in Ask an Expert and Discussion Group can help us keep abreast of users' interests and priorities. Analysis of Decisions & Conflicts data provides an opportunity to analyze the values and perceptions of people in crisis. Data on the frequency and sequence of service uses can be used to examine the styles and patterns by which people seek help. The opportunities are virtually endless.

Pilot-Testing and Evaluation

AIDS/HIV Module

The AIDS/HIV module of CHESS has been extensively tested, with a 3-year, controlled evaluation funded by the Agency for Health Care Policy and Research. In this study, over 200 men and women at all stages of HIV infection were randomly assigned to either receive CHESS (experimentals) for 3-6 months, or receive no intervention (controls). All subjects were given pre- and posttests to study the effects of CHESS on quality of life, risk behaviors for HIV transmission, and health service utilization.[10-13]

Subjects who had access to CHESS used it extensively, on average 138 times for a total of 39 hours over 17 weeks, an average of over once per day throughout the study. Communication Services, particularly Discussion Group, were used most frequently (Table 9.2); in fact, Discussion Group accounted for 76 percent of all uses. Women and minorities used CHESS at least as frequently as their male and Caucasian counterparts; younger people and people living alone tended to use CHESS more, but level of education did not predict CHESS use.[10,13]

Differences between pre- and posttest scores ("change scores") of subjects

TABLE 9.2. Use patterns of CHESS services in various studies.

	\% of Total Uses of CHESS In Each Type of Service				
	HIV/AIDS	Breast cancer	Sexual assault	Campus	Workplace
Site(s)	Home	Home	Dorms/sororities	Various	LAN/kiosk
Length of use	3–6 months	3 months	4 months	6 weeks	6 months
Information	14.8	24.2	32.3	48.1	57.8
Communication	81.6	72.0	59.3	32.5	26.3
Analysis	3.6	3.7	8.4	19.4	15.9

who had access to CHESS were better, compared to the change scores in controls, on measures of cognitive functioning, social support, leading an active life, participation in health care, and negative emotions. No significant differences in change scores between the groups were seen on measures of depression, physical functioning, or reported level of energy. In subjects who had CHESS for 6 months, some of these effects (greater social support and participation in health care) remained even 3 months after CHESS was removed.[11,12]

Differences between control and experimental subjects in utilization of ambulatory care services were generally small and not statistically significant. Experimental subjects, however, spent significantly less time during ambulatory visits than control subjects. This suggests that experimental subjects became more efficient in the use of provider time during their visits.[11,12]

The most noticeable effect of CHESS on health service utilization was that hospitalization costs for experimental subjects were significantly lower than for controls, during and after use of CHESS (Table 9.3). Little difference was seen between controls and experimentals in the probability

TABLE 9.3. Hospitalizations per month in AIDS/HIV study.

	Time period	Control	Experimental
Probability of admission[1]	Before CHESS	0.108	0.131
	During	0.154	0.152
	After	0.181	0.149
Average length of stay (days)[2]	Before CHESS	4.90	8.38
	During	7.89	5.95
	After	6.60	6.24
Estimated hospital costs per person per month[3]	Before CHESS	$438	$816
	During	$906	$668
	After	$891	$713

[1]Probability of admission to the hospital during the 2 months prior to each survey.
[2]Average length of stay per hospitalization (for only those subjects hospitalized).
[3]Average length of stay per subject (for all subjects, regardless of whether they were hospitalized) times average cost per day of stay for AIDS care in the Madison area, $1485.

of admission to hospital. However, average length of stay rose for the control subjects during the study, while it fell for the experimentals. Because of an unexpected pretest difference between groups in length of stay (the only significant difference between the groups at pretest), a conservative approach was taken to the cost analysis. That is, the differences at pretest were considered to be unrepresentative, and a pretest average of all subjects was used as a baseline for comparison of study effects. Using this approach, the pretest average hospital costs (for all subjects) of $633 per person per day rose to $906 in controls, but only to $668 in subjects who had CHESS, a difference of 36 percent. This difference was maintained, at a slightly lower level of 27 percent, even after CHESS was removed.[11,12]

At least two possible explanations may account for this effect of CHESS in reducing length of hospitalization. It is possible that people using CHESS, through increased education and social support, were more aware of symptoms of opportunistic infections and had these infections diagnosed and treated more rapidly, before they became serious or life-threatening. Another explanation, offered by a physician at the University of Wisconsin Hospital HIV clinic, is that patients with CHESS may have taken a more active role in discharge planning, ensuring that they were released as soon as medically appropriate. A follow-up study, also funded by the Agency for Health Care Policy and Research and currently underway, will analyze this question in detail. Subjects given CHESS for 1 year will be compared to controls, and data from medical and billing records will be compared to determine in greater detail how CHESS affects health status and use of health services.

Breast Cancer

The Breast Cancer module of CHESS has been extensively pilot-tested with women recruited from the breast clinic at the University of Wisconsin Hospital and Clinics and from Cook County Hospital in Chicago. In all of these tests, CHESS has been very well received and extensively used, with more positive emotions and fewer negative emotions experienced as a result of using the system. Use data from two of the pilot tests is shown in Table 9.4. In these two studies, women with Stage I or II breast cancer (20 recruited from UW-Madison and 8 from Cook County) had CHESS for approximately 10 weeks.

The difference in use between the women recruited from UW-Madison and from Cook County Hospital is noteworthy. The women from Cook County (all African-American) used the system on average twice as frequently, and for four times as many total minutes as women from UW-Madison (all Caucasian).[14,15] The women from both studies were similar in age (average of 52 years for Cook County, 54 years for UW-Madison) and prior computer experience (38 percent Cook County, 40

TABLE **9.4.** Use of CHESS services in breast cancer module pilot tests.

	UW Madison		Cook County	
	Average total number of uses	Average total minutes of use	Average total number of uses	Average total minutes of use
Discussion group	35.9	178.4	49.1	560.1
Ask an expert	5.8	26.0	25.2	165.2
Questions and answers	5.6	13.3	9.2	68.6
Instant library	4.6	26.6	5.3	37.9
Personal stories	1.6	17.1	4.8	56.1
Getting help/support	1.4	1.0	2.0	8.8
Decisions and conflicts	0.5	2.0	2.2	22.3
Action plan	0.6	4.8	0.6	5.3

percent UW-Madison), but only 50 percent of the Cook County women had completed high school, while all of the UW-Madison women had. Thus, education was not at all correlated with use.

Use also did not correlate with perceived ease of use. While average scores for ease of use were high in both studies, UW-Madison users rated CHESS easier to use (6.7 on a 7-point scale) than did women from Cook County (5.8 average). Women from Cook County, however, rated the value of CHESS (6.9 average on a 7-point scale) higher than women from UW-Madison (6.1 average), although both scores were very high. Women in both studies reported feeling high levels of acceptance, motivation, understanding, and relief when using CHESS, and experiencing low levels of stress, boredom, fear, sadness, indifference, helplessness, and anger.[15]

A study funded by the National Institute on Child Health and Human Development is currently underway to evaluate the effects of CHESS on quality of life, functional performance, and level of disability of women under age 50 with breast cancer at Stages I to IV. A total of 300 women (100 women of color) will participate from Cook County Hospital and Rush-Presbyterian-St. Luke's Medical Center in Chicago and the University of Wisconsin-Madison Hospital in Madison.

Sexual Assault

The Sexual Assault module of CHESS was pilot-tested for a 4-month period in 13 dormitories and sororities on the campus of the University of Wisconsin-Madison. CHESS was used by 371 of the 700 women who had access to it at these sites, a substantial proportion for a single-purpose service not immediately relevant to all women. CHESS services were used a total of 1264 times. As shown in Table 9.2, Communication Services (primarily Discussion Group) were used most frequently (59 percent of all uses), followed by Information Services and Analysis Services (32 and 8 percent of all uses, respectively).

Thirty users voluntarily completed both pre- and post-use questionnaires; 16 of these users were survivors of a sexual assault. CHESS was used most by women who felt the least comfortable talking about and disclosing acquaintance rape, and by those who had less exposure to, and felt more of a need for, information about acquaintance rape. Among women who had been assaulted, CHESS was used more by women who blamed themselves, who had less support, and who were uncertain about whether their experience was rape. CHESS was also used heavily by two women who were assaulted during the 4-month implementation period. In other words, use of CHESS was self-selected by those most in need of its information and services; lack of comfort with the subject in interpersonal situations was no bar to exploring it with the computer. A typical user comment on CHESS was, "I was getting very hopeless and depressed and CHESS aided in helping me out of a path that could have led to suicide. I also did not allow anyone to pressure me into sex."

Workplace Implementation

A 6-month pilot test of CHESS was carried out at a large local employer, CUNA Mutual Insurance. CHESS was installed on the company's local area networks (LANs), giving over 2000 employees access to CHESS at their own workstations. In addition, free-standing kiosks were available for those employees without access to the LANs or who wanted more privacy. All CHESS topic modules were available in this study. Extensive promotional campaigns made employees aware of CHESS through electronic memos, posters, brochures, table tents, and so forth. Video orientations were also offered.

CHESS was well-received and accepted in this setting. Fully 25 percent of the work force made use of CHESS one time or more. Regardless of whether or not it was used, an overwhelming 76 percent of employees responding to a postimplementation survey felt that a service like CHESS had potential value for people in a workplace setting. Survey responses and use patterns suggest that a combination of life management and health issues will maximize workplace utilization. Time constraints and a perceived lack of privacy were the main barriers to use.

In this study, use patterns differed significantly from those seen in other tests of CHESS. Here, Information Services were the most frequently used, accounting for 58 prcent of all uses (Table 9.2). Analysis Services were also more frequently used than in other studies (16 percent of uses), and Communication Services were used correspondingly less frequently (only 26 prcent of all uses). This different use pattern may be explained in at least two ways. The perceived lack of privacy, as well as less frequent overall use, may have made workplace users feel less comfortable than in-home users about opening up their feelings and using the Discussion Groups as support groups. Also, because multiple topics were made available to a general population, rather than a single topic to a group specifically affected by it, there may not have been enough people with strong interest in any one topic to generate sustained, widespread interest in ongoing conversations.

This same type of use was seen in an early pilot test of CHESS at 14 locations on the University of Wisconsin-Madison campus, including residence halls, libraries, health clinics, athletic facilities, and campus-based social organizations. In a 6-week test, almost 1500 uses were registered, with the greatest amount of use at a Computer Resource Center and in dormitories. Academic Crisis, AIDS and Sexual Assault were the most frequently used programs, accounting for 22, 17, and 16 percent of system uses, respectively. As in the workplace implementation, Information Service use was most frequent, followed by Communication and Analysis (Table 9.2).

Conclusions and Future Directions

The controlled evaluations and pilot tests have demonstrated that CHESS is widely accepted, heavily used, and can have a significant impact on quality of life and health service utilization. Many issues remain to be explored, however.

Dissemination of CHESS is the key to ensuring that it does not become another demonstration project that never makes it in the real world. Two methods of dissemination are currently being pursued. The CHESS Health Education Consortium, consisting of health care providers around the United States, has been established to continue to develop CHESS and research on its effects and the best ways of implementing CHESS through health care settings. The first member of the consortium, HealthPartners (a large Minneapolis-based HMO), has completed controlled studies using the breast cancer and AIDS/HIV modules. Data from that study is still being analyzed and no results are yet available. Group Health Cooperative – Puget Sound began a study with their HIV population in the spring of 1996. The University of Wisconsin has also licensed the copyright for CHESS to a private company, Health Companion Systems, which has begun marketing CHESS to both individuals and organizations.

Expanding the number of topics covered by CHESS is also a key to its ultimate success. Plans call for development of up to 30 new modules over the next few years. Potential topics include depression, diabetes, heart disease, spinal cord injury, various cancers, endstage renal disease, and so forth. Funding for new module development will probably come from a variety of sources, including the Research Consortium, public and private grants, and revenues from Health Companion Systems.

A variety of questions remain to be addressed; for example: (1) comparison of CHESS versus nontechnology-based interventions of similar cost; (2) impact and utility of the various CHESS services; (3) ways of making

CHESS more accessible to disadvantaged populations; (4) impact of CHESS in areas other than HIV/AIDS and breast cancer; and, (5) the most cost-effective means of widespread dissemination. The rich potential for collecting data on CHESS will also allow research into such important questions as: (1) the dynamics of computer-mediated discussion; (2) values and perceptions of people in crisis; (3) the effects of these values and perceptions on decision-making in crisis; and (4) styles and patterns by which people seek help.

Finally, the rapid pace of technological advance means that CHESS and programs like it need to be able to grow and change rapidly. While in-home PC workstations are the most viable delivery option today, alternatives are not far off. The rapidly expanding capability to transfer graphics via the Internet will make an on line version of CHESS a relatively easy modification. The anticipated widespread introduction of interactive television systems may allow greater access to low-income populations, as well as expanded opportunities for full-motion video and sound capabilities. Other options will exist in the near future.

The challenge is to maintain a focus on the end user. The questions to ask as we continue to develop and enhance CHESS and systems like it are these: (1) Will this better satisfy the user's need for information, social support and help in decision-making?; (2) Will this be more effective in meeting those needs?; and (3) Will this get the system into the hands of more people who need/want it? The extent to which the answer to these questions is "yes" is the extent to which systems like CHESS will be successful.

The final word on CHESS should always come from users. This message was posted in Discussion Group one day by a man in the AIDS/HIV study:

Hello all,

I'm such a compulsive reader that it never fails to surprise me how much I want to WRITE when I have this keyboard in my lap. I thought I HATED writing, hmm . . . I am constantly learning from this system. Learning how people relate, learning how people think of themselves, and learning how much people like to help others. What a wonderful education I'm getting! I have watched each of us:

Give thoughtful, well thought out advice;
Gripe about the lousy day we had;
Laugh;
Lash out;
Try to comfort another in pain;
Cry;
Apologize;
Be UNBELIEVABLY irreverent;
And, just BE THERE for each other.

We have done this with the simple goals of helping ourselves, and helping each other. And its working! Every one of us is growing and gathering strength from these contraptions, I am dealing with this disease better than I ever thought I would, and we're helping each other in the process! What a concept! Call the papers, I think it's working!

These are my thoughts,
Alec

Acknowledgments. Major funding for development of CHESS was provided by the W.K. Kellogg Foundation. Funding for evaluation of CHESS was provided by the Agency for Health Care Policy and Research (for the AIDS/HIV module) and the National Institute for Child Health and Human Development (for the breast cancer module). Funding for the development of the Parents and Partners of Alcohol Abusers module was provided by the Robert Wood Johnson Foundation.

References

1. Bandura A. Self-efficacy: Toward a unifying theory of behavioral change. *Psych Rev.* 1977;84:191–215.
2. Strecher VJ, McEvoy-Devellis B, Becker MH, et al. The role of self-efficacy in achieving behavior change. *Health Ed Quart.* 1986;13:73–91.
3. Bosworth K, Gustafson DH. CHESS: Providing decision support for reducing health risk behavior and improving access to health services. *Interfaces.* 1991; 21(3):93–104.
4. Moos RH, Schaffer J. The crisis of physical illness: An overview and conceptual approach. In: Moos RH (ed.). *Coping With Physical Illness II: New Perspectives.* New York: Plenum Medical Book Company; 1984:3–25.
5. Aquilera D. *Crisis Intervention: Theory and Methodology.* St. Louis: CV Mosby Company; 1990.
6. Slovic P, Fischoff B, Lichtenstein S. Behavioral decision theory. *Ann Rev Psych.* 1977;28(1):1–39.
7. Gustafson DH. Health risk appraisal: Its role in health services research. *Health Serv Res.* 1987;22(4):453–465.
8. Sainfort FC, Gustafson DH, Bosworth K, et al. Decision support systems effectiveness: Conceptual framework and empirical evaluation. *Org Behav Human Decision Processes.* 1990;45:232–252.
9. Gustafson DH, Taylor JO, Thompson S, et al. Assessing the needs of breast cancer patients and their families. *Qual Manage Healthcare.* 1993;2(1):6–17.
10. Boberg EW, Gustafson DH, Hawkins RP, et al. Development, acceptance and use patterns of a computer-based education and social support system for people living with AIDS/HIV infection. *Comput Hum Behav.* 1995;11(2)289–311.
11. Gustafson DH, Hawkins RP, Boberg EW, et al. Quality of life and hospitalization cost benefits of a computerized health support system for HIV-positive patients. *Ann Int Med.* Submitted for publication.
12. Gustafson DH, Hawkins RP, Boberg EW, et al. The use and impact of a computer-based support system for people living with AIDS and HIV infection. In: Ozbolt JG (ed.) *Transforming Information, Changing Health Care. Proceedings of the Eighteenth Annual Symposium on Computer Applications in Medical Care;* 1994; Nov 5–9, Washington, DC. Philadelphia: Hanley & Belfus, 1994:604–608.
13. Pingree S, Hawkins RP, Gustafson DH, et al. Will HIV-positive people use an interactive computer system for information and support? A study of CHESS

in two communities. In: Safran C (ed.) *Patient-Centered Computing. Proceedings of the Seventeenth Annual Symposium on Computer Applications in Medical Care;* 1993; Oct 30–Nov 3, Washington, DC. New York: McGraw-Hill, 1993:22–26.

14. Gustafson DH, Wise M, McTavish F, et al. Development and pilot evaluation of a computer-based support system for women with breast cancer. *J Psychosoc Oncol.* 1993;11(4):69–93.

15. McTavish FM, Gustafson DH, Owens BH, et al. CHESS: An interactive computer system for women with breast cancer piloted with an under-served population. In: Ozbolt JG (ed.) *Transforming Information, Changing Health Care. Proceedings of the Eighteenth Annual Symposium on Computer Applications in Medical Care;* 1994; Nov 5–9, Washington, DC. Philadelphia: Hanley & Belfus; 1994:599–603.

10

The Alzheimer's Disease Support Center: Information and Support for Family Caregivers Through Computer-Mediated Communication

KATHLEEN A. SMYTH, STEVEN J. FEINSTEIN, and SUSAN KACEREK

The special information and support needs of caregivers of persons with Alzheimer's disease and related dementias have been well documented. Help lines, support groups, education programs and materials, and other services have been developed to address these needs, but many caregivers cannot or will not use them.[1,2] One reason is that dementia-related caregiving typically limits caregivers' time, energy, and other resources. Another is that the mechanics of connecting with services may be beyond caregivers' capacity when they are already facing significant competing demands and wide ranging and unpredictable responsibilities.[3,4] Further, only the most common problems and issues are typically addressed through printed materials and educational programs, and support groups meet only for limited time periods on a fixed schedule, usually no more than twice per month. As a result, the specific issues important to an individual caregiver may not be addressed in a timely way. Finally, not all caregivers feel comfortable seeking support from strangers and/or in public settings.

Computer-mediated communication (CMC) systems simultaneously function as a mass communication medium, because they can reach multiple users, and as an interpersonal communication medium, because they allow for interaction between the system and those who access it.[5] These functions make the use of CMC to meet caregivers' information and support needs feasible. CMC systems have the potential to address the problems of accessibility and specificity inherent in many current information and support efforts because they are characterized by asynchronicity (exchange of messages need not be concurrent); demassification (capacity to exchange a special message with each individual in an audience); and multiple levels of anonymity. These features put control of the education and support process into the hands of users.[5-8]

By exploiting the potential of CMC, the Alzheimer's Disease Support Center (ADSC), a joint project of the University Hospitals of Cleveland/ Case Western Reserve University (CWRU) Alzheimer Center and the Cleveland Area Alzheimer's Association, is designed to complement existing services for caregivers by making education and support more accessible and more responsive to specific needs.[9] ADSC modules have been developed as analogs to more traditional health and social service information and social support activities. They provide for both private and shared communication among caregivers (analogous to self-help groups) and between caregivers and professionals (analogous to counseling and health education), and for the dissemination of current information on research, treatment, and care in Alzheimer's disease (analogous to information and referral services).

The ADSC, begun in 1989, is a part of the Cleveland Free-Net community telecomputing system, located on the campus of CWRU. Anyone with a microcomputer (or terminal) and a modem can connect to the system via telephone and access a variety of electronic services and features 24 hours a day, paying only for the cost of the telephone call. Individuals become registered users of the Free-Net by completing a short form on line and signing and mailing in a release form. Users are assigned a user name and choose their own password. It takes about 2 weeks to complete the registration process. Registered users have access to the ADSC as well as all other areas of the Free-Net. They move through the system by selecting options from menus.

ADSC modules use standard telecomputing features: electronic bulletin boards (posting of public messages by identified individuals to which (multiple) individuals can respond); Q & A (posting of anonymous questions by system users that are answered by persons designated to do so; once questions and answers are posted to the Q & A module, they can be read by all system users); and static information files (reading and/or copying of files of information selected by the user from a menu of options). Electronic mail (e-mail) (sending and receiving of private messages between individuals) also is available. The ADSC is comprised of seven modules, four of which focus on family caregivers' needs: About the Support Center; Alzheimer's Disease Q & A; Alzheimer's Disease Information Rack; and Caregiver Forum. The other modules are targeted to health care and social service professionals.

Once "inside" the ADSC, a user types in the number of the desired module and module feature. The Free-Net limits each session to 60 minutes, but caregivers can access the system as many times a day as they wish. Six incoming modem lines are dedicated to the ADSC, with access controlled by screening user IDs. Table 10.1 provides a summary of the menu structure and content of the ADSC modules targeted to family caregivers. The left-hand column details the main menu of the ADSC and the middle column indicates the submenus, if any, that are displayed when each main menu option is chosen. The right-hand column describes the material presented to users at each main menu or sub-menu choice.

This chapter describes how the ADSC meets the adoption and diffusion requirements of innovations generally and CMC systems specifically, and summarizes what we have learned about the role of CMC in the provision

TABLE 10.1. Summary of ADSC menu structure and content for family caregiver modules.

Main menu	Submenu	Material presented
1. About the Support Center	None	Description of the ADSC
2. Alzheimer's Disease Questions and Answers	1. About the Q & A	Description of the Q & A Module
	2. Comon Q & A's about Alzheimer's Disease	Text of common questions and answers
	3. When Can I Expect a Response to my Question?	Information about when the answer to a question will be posted
	4. Questions and Answers	Numbered list of questions posted by users and answered by Alzheimer Center professionals; when number of question is typed in, text of question and answer is displayed
3. Alzheimer's Disease Information Rack	1. About the Information Rack	Description of the Information Rack Module
	2. Calendar of Upcoming Events	Location, time, date and other details about events of interest to family caregivers
	3. Caregiver Support Group Meetings	Location, time, date and contact person for meetings
	4. Books for Caregivers and the General Public	Annotated bibliography
	5. Books for Professionals	Annotated bibliography
	6. Videos	Annotated listing
	7. Brochures and Handouts	Text of brochures and handouts
	8. Electronic Brochure Rack	Text of Alzheimer's Association brochures
5. Alzheimer's Disease Caregiver Forum	1. About the Forum	Description of the Caregiver Forum Module
	2. Helpful Hints for Caregivers	Suggestions for handling common problems in dementia care
	3. The Caregiver Dialogue	Numbered list of topics posted by caregivers; when number of item is typed in, text of item is displayed
	4. User Histories	Brief biographical sketches posted by users including a description of the user's caregiving situation

of health and social service information and social support to persons caring for a family member with Alzheimer's disease or a related dementia. We concentrate here on interactive aspects of the system: the Caregiver Dialogue (a bulletin board for public postings by caregivers emphasizing peer-to-peer support and monitored by a professional from the Alzheimer's Association), and the Q & A module through which anonymous user questions are answered by clinical experts from the University Alzheimer Center.

Interaction plays a pivotal role in the delivery of effective health and social service information and social support. A CMC system designed for this purpose must be able to demonstrate that the quality of interaction on the system is sufficient for the service delivery envisioned. The ADSC seeks to create an electronic version of caregiver support groups, professional/caregiver consultation, and information and referral services.

The ADSC is an ongoing information and support intervention; it is not an experimental system embedded in a formal research project. Consequently, observations about its use and impacts must be descriptive, rather than analytic. Further, access to the system is not strictly controlled. Although most of the known users were recruited and trained by staff of the sponsoring organizations, anyone who has Cleveland Free-Net access, including Internet and World Wide Web users, can access the ADSC. Finally, we are able to track system use only at the aggregate level.

Adoption and Diffusion of New Technology

General Issues in Innovation Adoption and Diffusion

Drawing on Roger's theory of innovation diffusion, Brennan and colleagues[10] have noted that to be adopted, new technology developed to meet specific needs (such as the ADSC) must be: (1) perceived as an advantage over currently used technology; (2) compatible with other aspects of the potential user's life; and (3) accessible to and observable by potential users.

Unsolicited ADSC evaluations posted by system users in the Caregiver Dialogue, reported in Table 10.2, indicate that some users perceive the ADSC to offer tangible advantages, and have incorporated it into their day-to-day lives. We cannot assume, however, that these comments reflect all users' views. Volume of use (discussed in more detail below) suggests that some caregivers who have been trained use the system infrequently. These caregivers may not see an advantage to using the ADSC but we have not determined whether this is the case. As Table 10.3 shows, ADSC users are not confined to those fitting the typical computer user profile (young, male, highly educated, affluent). This evidence of compatibility is important. It is well documented that care of persons with dementia is provided primarily by women; that dementia is not a respecter of race, ethnicity, or socioeconomic status; and that many caregivers are spouses in their seventies and eighties. The need for accessibility and observability has been dealt with in a variety of ways. System use is free, except for the cost of telephone calls;

TABLE **10.2.** Unsolicited user evaluations of ADSC advantages and compatibility with other aspects of life.

Advantages:

"The computer family is the best source for help and sharing. . . ."

"My husband wants to know if I'm getting any information out of this thing or if it's just interesting. I can't really explain the kind of help you get just being able to 'talk' with someone who has the same problems."

"What makes this board so great is that it relates 'real life' experiences and not a text-book dissertation of some untested ideas."

Compatibility:

"Whenever I get frustrated and need to talk to someone, I come to this forum. It has never let me down. Although I am only typing my feelings, it is the same as talking, and this starts the process of relieving my tension."

"This computer has also become an important part of my day."

---

computer terminals, (hot keyed to perform login functions), modems, and user manuals are provided on long-term loan for use in caregivers' own homes; and training is provided at a time and place convenient to caregivers. Given the volume of Free-Net use, dedicated phone lines were purchased for ADSC users to ensure accessibility at a level compatible with their needs. Observability is facilitated both by system demonstration during training, and by the ability of new users to access the system without being detected by other users. Observability may be particularly important for CMC systems like the ADSC, targeted to groups who may have little previous familiarity with computers.

TABLE **10.3.** Profile of known ADSC users as of December 31, 1995 (numbers in parentheses).[1]

Age (138)		
	Range:	10–84
	Mean:	51
Gender (189)		
	Female:	71% (134)
	Male:	29% (55)
Race (119)		
	African American	17% (33)
	White	83% (156)
Relationship to diagnosed (168)		
	Spouses	25% (46)
	Children/children-in-law	56% (101)
	Other	15% (33)
Residence of Person with Dementia (138)		
	Home	52% (72)
	Nursing home	17% (23)
	With other family	11% (15)
	Deceased	12% (16)
	Alone	9% (12)

[1]Not all information is available on all users. Some percentages do not add to 100 percent due to rounding error.

Issues in Adoption and Diffusion of CMC Systems

In his later work, Rogers[5] identified special considerations for the adoption of communication technologies: (1) critical mass, (2) reinvention, and (3) degree of use.

Critical Mass

Rogers maintains that a critical mass of users is essential to a successful communication innovation and that the value of the technology to those who have already adopted it increases each time a new person does so. By and large, our experience is congruent with this observation. Activity on the ADSC was very sparse when only a few caregivers had agreed to adopt the technology. Some ADSC users knew one another prior to joining the ADSC and that may have influenced system message volume. As a result, we are unable to trace the independent effect of number of users on volume of system use.

We know of 189 caregivers who have used the ADSC; the majority of them were recruited and trained by us. Our most recent available usage statistics show that in 1995, there were an average of 41 different system users per week. A group of this size would be considered too large for a face-to-face support group. Whether the group of active users can continue to grow without adversely affecting system use or satisfaction with use is not known. We have yet to receive any complaints from users about the number of caregivers with access to the system. However, users have observed from time to time that it is a challenge to keep up with the volume of messages on the system, especially if one does not log on each day. Rice[11] cited evidence that CMC system users develop login schedules such that they can keep the number of asynchronous messages to be dealt with in a session to about six. If most users consider most messages of personal relevance (as ours appear to), the challenge of keeping up may increase. Hence, it is likely that at some point there will be a decrease, rather than an increase, in the value associated with adding each new user, unless attrition keeps pace.

Reinvention

Adoption of communication technologies is an active process, and because these technologies are "tools," they are amenable to reinvention or modification by the user. Users have modified the ADSC in two primary ways. The first is philosophical: they have significantly broadened the use of the Caregiver Dialogue. When the ADSC was designed, the Dialogue was conceptualized as a place where caregivers would discuss common concerns related to caregiving and receive empathy and concrete advice from others who had had similar experiences. Messages reflecting this goal are prevalent on the ADSC. However, user communication themes are much broader and include a wide range of events, such as pregnancies, births, weddings, anniversaries, and deaths involving children, siblings, parents, and other relatives; reports of leisure activities such as bike rides, movies, and vacations; and commentaries on day-to-day events or special topics like the weather and cooking, selling a house, and buying a car. Jokes, poetry, and prayers are common. These themes reflect the degree of "social presence" on the system, discussed in more detail below. The point here is that CMC system content can depart substantially from that envisioned by system developers. In the case of the ADSC, the departure appears to foster one of the system's goals, but this may not be true for all CMC systems.

Users also have been directly involved in the modification of system modules. Several users are recruited to the system each month. Over time, existing users began to observe that part of welcoming new users involved introducing themselves and summarizing their own caregiving stories. One user proposed a biography module, where new users could become quickly acquainted with current users. Other users supported the idea, and an optional "user history" section was added to the system. Users post their own biographies, and can modify or delete them at will. To date, 55 users have posted biographies.

Through a questionnaire, we have determined that some users desire other system changes, such as removing personal identification from Dialogue postings, deleting old Dialogue postings, or limiting access to the Dialogue to caregivers. These changes have not been implemented because they would not be optional and are not endorsed by all users. They illustrate, however, the fact that user involvement in reinvention should be anticipated by interactive CMC system developers; anecdotally, we know that usage is affected by users' satisfaction with specific system characteristics.

System designers might overtly identify a moderator whose role would be to influence the way in which a CMC is used, but moderators also can emerge from among users. Several ADSC users have taken on such a role. We monitor the Q & A and Forum modules daily. We make it a policy to respond to Q & A postings within 2 working days, and also have instituted a component in the Q & A where we can let questioners know if it will take longer to respond to their questions. We read Dialogue postings daily, but rarely post messages to it, and do not attempt to influence Dialogue topics or the course of discussions. Clearly, ADSC-like systems could vary widely in this regard. The extent to which the nature and amount of CMC can be influenced by a group leader, either a professional designated to monitor the system or a system user who emerges as an opinion leader, warrants careful study.

Berge[12] notes that moderators can play many roles, including facilitator (e.g., keeping things on track); manager (e.g., archiving, deleting/adding subscribers, removing inappropriate messages); expert (e.g., answering substantive questions); editor (e.g., editing, summarizing, or formatting postings); promoter (e.g., stimulating discussion); marketer (e.g., recruiting or orienting new users); or helper (e.g., responding to general needs not appropriate for experts). Danowski[13] asserts that user postings to a system can be manipulated to conform to specific purposes and objectives if moderators periodically post "optimal messages." Danowski indicates that optimal messages can be identified by using mathematical formulas, but does not provide examples.[13] The effects of various levels of monitoring on CMC systems have yet to be studied.

Degree of Use

Degree of use, not mere adoption or implementation, is a crucial variable in the success of CMC systems. With over 180 known users and an average of 41 unique logins per week, it is clear that degree of ADSC use varies by individual. We know little about the causes for this variation but have observed that some users log in daily or more often, while others do so only when they have a specific need for information or support. We have anecdotal evidence that caregivers are sometimes uncertain as to whether they should continue to use the ADSC when their situation changes (e.g., care recipient is placed in a nursing home or dies). Whenever a user poses such a question publicly, responses are uniformly in favor of the user continuing to use the system. However, some decide privately to discontinue or reduce use in response to changed circumstances, or they may be unconvinced by the views of other users. We also know from message content that travel, competing demands on time from family or community activities, and illness of the caregiver or care recipient cause usage fluctuations. In most cases, however, it appears that each ADSC user establishes and maintains a fairly consistent level of use.

ADSC usage also varies by module. The number of items posted in the Q & A module has doubled in each of the last 2 years; a total of 266 items had been posted there by the end of 1995. In 1995, 66 questions were posted. Through a content analysis of the first 225 questions posted, we have identified several common themes that represent the majority of the questions. Table 10.4 gives these themes and the number of questions in which they appear. (Note that more than one theme can be represented in a single question.) The topics show a clear interest in symptoms, treatments, and daily care, and in research. We are in the process of grouping the questions into these 12 categories on the system itself to facilitate access.

Nearly 6700 messages had been posted on the Caregiver Dialogue module by the end of 1995. Message volume per year has grown substantially (e.g., from 474 in 1992 to 2145 in 1995). Users also communicate by private e-mail, but we do not monitor the number or content of these messages. Table 10.5 shows average weekly system usage for selected portions of the ADSC during 1995. Clearly, users prefer caregiver-to-caregiver interaction (Caregiver Dialogue) over other system offerings.

TABLE 10.4. Themes represented in questions posted to the Q & A module.

Category	Number of questions
Caregiver support and respite services; support groups; public policy; finances	45
Behavioral symptoms management	45
Dementia medications (uses and side effects)	41
Research in Alzheimer's disease (causes and treatment)	40
Basic information (definitions, risk factors, epidemiology)	35
Dementias related to Alzheimer's disease	33
Nursing home (transition to and care)	28
Age of onset, initial symptoms, and diagnosis	23
Physical problems of persons with AD (causes and responses to)	23
Autopsy and other late stage issues	20
Talking to/communicating with persons with dementia	15
Genetics	9

Social Presence and Individuation/Deindividuation in CMC

Social scientists continue to debate the meaning of social support. One widely accepted conceptualization characterizes social support as interpersonal transactions that demonstrate positive affect, affirmation of actions or ideas, or direct aid.[14] In CMC, capacity to provide social support is most closely linked to two concepts, social presence and deindividuation.

Social Presence in CMC

The extent to which CMC allows for "social presence" is a key factor in determining its usefulness as a source of social support, and it is the subject of much scholarly debate. There is no single agreed upon definition of or operationalization of social presence.[15] Typically, the term refers to the extent to which a communication medium conveys person-oriented elements such as sociability, sensitivity, warmth, and personal interest.[16,17] Analyzing the influence of social presence and other interactive media

TABLE 10.5. Average weekly system use overall and by most frequently accessed modules or module components, 1995.

Module/component	Mean accesses per week
Caregiver Forum	
Caregiver Dialogue	287
User Histories	26
Information Rack	11
Q & A	21
Overall (unique users)	41

theories on thinking about CMCs, Walther[16] notes the strong influence of Short and colleagues' assertion that social presence is inherent in the medium itself.[18] Most of the social meaning of face-to-face communication is thought to come from nonverbal cues. Because it lacks nonverbal elements and other types of cues, CMC has been considered a priori to be low in social presence in comparison to face-to-face communication. Walther's[16] critical evaluation of this perspective and the experimental research growing from it, however, challenges this view. Citing evidence from field studies rather than experiments, Walther argues convincingly that given sufficient time, "as goes face-to-face goes CMC, given the opportunity for message exchange and accompanying relational development" (Ref. 16, p. 75).

Social Presence on the ADSC

Taking a social information processing perspective, Walther makes several observations about strategies for social interaction in CMC that are congruent with ADSC usage, illustrated in Table 10.6 below. These include "relational icons" (forming faces from combinations of punctuation marks), and electronic "paralanguage" (intentional misspelling, lexical surrogates, spatial arrays, grammatical markers, absence of corrections, and capitalization). Users also have developed a shared set of abbreviations for terms they frequently use (e.g., NH [nursing home]; AD [Alzheimer's disease]; CF [computer family]; and CFL [computer family luncheon]).

TABLE 10.6. Examples of relational strategies employed by ADSC users.

Relational icons:	:-) :)ing :-o :-(:-| [faces]
	( )s [to indicate hugs]
Electronic paralanguage:	
intentional misspelling:	soooooooo
	toooooooo
	reeeeeeal
lexical surrogates:	HA HA HA
	. . .and in a forceful way, I said: "let's go."
	Yeah Browns!
spatial arrays:	. . .this is one way I have to think not to go way
	D
	O
	W
	N
	o/⌒ o/⌒ o/⌒ [accompanying song lyrics]
manipulated graphical display:	GOOD MORNING FAMILY
	ZZZZzzzz
	* I *
	* cold *

Although communication on the ADSC system is asynchronous, the tone of many Dialogue messages suggests that when posting messages, users envision others as actually present. In some cases, they log on at times when they know certain other users also are likely to be on the system, and they post messages that approximate real-time conversations with those other users.

Rice and Love[19] cite evidence to suggest that users' experience with the system, group norms, and the nature of the communication task all influence the proportion of socio-emotional content in CMC systems. ADSC Dialogue messages are replete with examples of social support in the form of affect, affirmation, and aid. Users themselves cite the centrality of social support to the system when welcoming new users. The following excerpts are taken from recent postings:

"You will find this 'family' closer in many ways than 'blood' family. Certainly you won't experience a lack of understanding from this family. They are eager to lend a hand in any way they can."

"You'll find this to be a wonderfully supportive group and amazingly upbeat."

" . . ., I would like to welcome you to the best family around."

"Feel free to 'jump' in on this board at any time. I am sure you will always get a response and the computer family will warmly welcome you."

"I hope that you will become a part of our computer family. It has been my most important support from the day I signed on."

Note the reference to "computer family," a name system users adopted for themselves.

User development of a biography module was clearly motivated not only by a desire to streamline system function, but also by a desire to foster interpersonal linkages between old and new users. In the biographies, users tell their age, gender, family composition, and details about their caregiving situations. Generally, Dialogue messages are clearly targeted to individual receivers, and reflect prior knowledge of the intended recipient. Users also respond quickly to the first posting by a new user. It is not uncommon for a new user to receive three or more welcoming messages within a few hours of posting an initial message.

Several key thinkers in the field of CMC have observed that social presence is not inherent in the medium, but is a function of the willingness of users to develop strategies to overcome the barriers presented by the medium.[15,16,20] Two key steps in this process, which are borne out by our experience with the ADSC, are establishing expectations for the type of communication desired and allowing time for interpersonal communication to develop.

Individuation and Deindividuation in CMC

A number of communication theorists have warned that CMC may result in deindividuation, or the loss of private and/or public self-awareness.[21,22]

Private self-awareness refers to personal feelings, attitudes, values, and beliefs. Public self-awareness refers to aspects of self that can be seen and evaluated by others, such as physical characteristics.[23] Reduction in public self-awareness is generally thought to be positive, because it reduces interpersonal barriers often related to physical characteristics that may be less socially desirable, and it allows users to control the creation of their identities. Loss of private self-awareness, however, is generally considered negative.[21,23]

Individuation and Deindividuation on the ADSC

The potential for public self-awareness on ADSC-like systems varies considerably. Many of our users are trained in groups. Further, users who may not have been trained together have met, either fortuitously at other caregiver-oriented events, or by design at "Computer Family Luncheons," monthly face-to-face meetings at Cleveland area restaurants organized online by system users. Even without these meetings, however, users convey public characteristics such as age, gender, and socioeconomic status as they share their caregiving situations and other happenings in their lives. Hence, the potential benefit of deemphasizing personal characteristics in CMC may be mitigated over time both on and off the system.

The ADSC enables users to at least partially control public self-awareness through the Q & A module, where questions are posted anonymously. By careful message construction and avoidance of face-to-face events, ADSC users could control what is known about their personal characteristics. However, this is likely to reduce the information and support they can obtain from the system.

With regard to private self-awareness, we have found no evidence in the Dialogue or Q & A postings of impersonality. The extent to which this is due to use of real names instead of pseudonyms on the Dialogue is not known. We have had reports of system use for journaling rather than interpersonal communication: Users have described occasionally typing a lengthy message into the Dialogue to "get something off my chest," and then deleting it instead of posting it.

There is clear evidence that time is needed for some individuals to become comfortable with participation in the Dialogue. It is not unusual to find that a first posting to the Dialogue acknowledges that the user has been reading the postings of others for weeks before gaining the confidence to "say" something to other users. Rather than being a weakness, however, we view this as an advantage of the ADSC over face-to-face groups, where the pressure for interpersonal interaction is great.

CMC System Life Cycle Issues

This analysis points out the dynamic nature of interactive CMC systems. Because the use of CMC in health and social services is in its infancy, the life cycle of such systems is not known. Further, the health problems such systems might address are not static. In Alzheimer's disease, for example, the last 10 years have witnessed a dramatic increase in professional and lay awareness of the disease. The first drug treatment has received FDA approval. Dementia-specific services are becoming more widely available. These and other changes in the way the wider community responds to the disease have implications for the role of ADSC-like systems in the lives of affected families. There are numerous life cycle issues of importance. We select only a few for comment here.

The Past as Part of the Present

The memory capacity of CMC systems sets them apart from other modes of communication. Whether to retain all messages or periodically delete them is a key question. As noted earlier, some users are not in favor of retaining messages. Our system is designed so users can delete messages they have posted at any time. However, this option is not frequently exercised. The current challenge is to organize past messages in a way that maximizes their value to users. We have obtained content analysis software to assist us in grouping messages in such a way that they can be accessed by keyword and/or menu options. We anticipate introducing a message archive organized by topic in 1996.

Maintaining a Future

Local funding (from the Cleveland Foundation and University Hospitals of Cleveland) and national funding (from The National Institute on Aging and the Gerontological Society of America) have supported the development and implementation of the ADSC, and Case Western Reserve University has provided it a "home" on the Cleveland Free-Net. Recognizing the contribution the project makes, the Alzheimer Center and the Cleveland Area Alzheimer's Association have incorporated the ADSC into their ongoing programs of service and are committed to sustaining it. Individuals and organizations have donated time and equipment to the project. This unique package of funding and organizational backing is not necessary to develop and maintain an ADSC-like system. But the need for ongoing staffing for recruitment and training, and sufficient hardware and software to maintain a user base representative of the target population, should not be underestimated. Level of technology also is important. We have created a World Wide Web home page (http://www.cwru.edu/orgs/adsc/intro.html) to facilitate sharing ADSC resources with a broader community of users. However, access to the ADSC will move beyond the reach of some potential users as more cutting-edge CMC technologies are employed. Our ability to attract users who do not fit the typical computer user profile has depended in large part on our ability to keep the interface simple and minimize costs.

Conclusions

The ADSC is a new service delivery mechanism that complements existing approaches. Like other approaches, it is not appropriate for all caregivers, nor will it meet all the needs of those who use it. However, it provides a new service option that can reduce barriers to care. We have demonstrated that a CMC system to deliver information and support to family caregivers can be designed and implemented and that it will be adopted and used. Some of the ADSC's effects (e.g., Computer Family Lunches, range of topics covered in the postings) were not anticipated. They show that CMC systems are not static and that their characteristics and effects are determined over time by both system developers and system users. Our experience has been encouraging, but continued work is needed to refine this approach to care. Replication and rigorous longitudinal evaluation are essential.

Acknowledgments. This project was supported in part by the Cleveland Foundation, the Gerontological Society of America, the National Institute on Aging (Grant #AG08012), and University Hospitals of Cleveland. We wish to thank Karen Bensing, Nancy Catalani, Rory Dick, Linda Rechlin, and Stephanie Schach for assistance in preparation of this manuscript.

References

1. Smyth KS, Eckert S, Bass D. Information and referral processes in provision of dementia-oriented care: Provider and consumer perspectives. *Presented at the 41st Annual Scientific Meeting of the Gerontological Society of America.* San Francisco, CA. November 20; 1988.
2. U.S. Congress Office of Technology Assessment. *Losing a Million Minds: Confronting the Tragedy of Alzheimer's Disease and Other Dementias.* OTA-BA-323. Washington, DC: U.S. Government Printing Office; 1987.
3. Schmall VL. It doesn't just happen: What makes a support group good? *Generations.* 1984;9:64–67.
4. Wright SD, Lund DA, Pett MA, Caserta MS. The assessment of support group experience by caregivers of dementia patients. *Clin Gerontol.* 1987;6:35–59.
5. Rogers EM. *Communication Technology: The New Media in Society.* New York: The Free Press; 1986.
6. Dutton WH, Rogers EM, Jun S-H. Diffusion and social impacts of personal computers. *Commun Res.* 1987;14:219–250.
7. Grundner TM, Garrett RE. Interactive medical telecomputing as an alternative approach to community health education. *N Eng J Med.* 1986;314:982–985.
8. Kerr E, Hiltz R. *Computer Mediated Communication Systems.* New York: Academic Press; 1982.
9. Smyth KA, Harris PB. Using telecomputing to provide information and support to caregivers of persons with dementia. *Gerontologist.* 1993;33:123–127.
10. Brennan PF, Moore SM, Smyth KA. ComputerLink: Electronic support for the home caregiver. *Adv Nursing Sci.* 1991;13:14–27.
11. Rice RE. Mediated group communication. In: Rice RE et al. (eds.). *The New*

Media Communication, Research and Technology. Beverly Hills: Sage Publications; 1984:129–154.

12. Berge ZL. Electronic discussion groups. *Commun Ed. 1994;43:102–111.*

13. Danowski JA. Computer-mediated communication: A network-based content analysis using a CBBS conference. *Commun Yearbook* 1982;6:905–924.

14. Antonucci TC, Jackson JS. The role of reciprocity in social support. In: Sarason BR, Sarason GR, Pierce GR (eds.). *Social Support: An Interactionist View.* New York: Wiley; 1990:173–198.

15. Rice RE, Williams F. Theories old and new: The study of new media. In: Rice RE et al. (eds.). *The New Media Communication, Research and Technology.* Beverly Hills: Sage Publications; 1984:55–80.

16. Walther JB. Interpersonal effects in computer-mediated interaction: A relational perspective. *Commun Res.* 1992;19:52–90.

17. Walther JB, Anderson JF, Park DW. Interpersonal effects in computer-mediated interaction: A meta-analysis of social and antisocial communication. *Commun Res.* 1994;21:460–487.

18. Short J, Williams E, Christie B. *The Social Psychology of Telecommunications.* London: Wiley; 1976.

19. Rice RE, Love G. Electronic emotion: Socioemotional content in a computer-mediated communication network. *Commun Res. 1987;14:85–108.*

20. Myers D. "Anonymity is part of the magic": Individual manipulation of computer-mediated communication contexts. *Qual Sociol. 1987;10:251–266.*

21. Kiesler S, Siegel J, McGuire TW. Social psychological aspects of computer-mediated communication. *Am Psychol.* 1984;39:1123–1134.

22. Jessup LM, Connolly T, Tansik DA. Toward a theory of automated group work: The deindividuating effects of anonymity. *Small Group Res.* 1990;21:333–348.

23. Matheson K, Zanna MP. Computer-mediated communications: The focus is on me. *Social Sci Comput Rev.* 1990;8:1–12.

11

Cancer, Me??: Health Care Advice Goes Online

PAUL TAENZER, IVAN ZENDEL, JUDY M. BIRDSELL, S. ELIZABETH McGREGOR, and SIMON FREIWALD

The long-heralded information age has become a reality with the arrival of the Internet in North American homes. The exponential growth of Internet activity is a sign of the public's thirst for adventure in the form of information and interaction. The challenge before us now is to provide information services that both sustain public interest and provide a public benefit.

Several years ago our research group had the opportunity to explore a new concept in online health services. Using expert system technology, we piloted a software program that provided personalized advice rather than information. We then implemented this program on Bell Canada's public access telecommunication network. This chapter describes the development and preliminary evaluation of Cancer, Me??, a computer-network delivered health promotion and advice intervention to reduce cancer risk. The chapter describes program goals, interface design and implementation, building of the knowledge base, and a field evaluation conducted in 1991 in the city of Montreal.

The Origins of Cancer, Me??

The Role of Prevention in Reducing the Burden of Cancer

Cancer is a major health problem for industrialized countries. In Canada, cancer is the second most common cause of death, following cardiovascular diseases; it accounted for 26 percent of all deaths in 1988.[1] Cancer is the leading cause of lost years of potential life in Canada, accounting for 29 percent of premature mortality from all causes in 1992.[2] Even with massive research efforts, progress in effectively treating cancer has been disappointing.[3] The United States National Cancer Institute has noted that to diminish the impact of cancer on society, more attention must be placed on prevention.[4] Lifestyle-related causes of cancer include use of tobacco products and alcohol, unhealthy diet, risky reproductive and sexual behavior, occupational exposure to carcinogens, and sun exposure. Using the analytical method of Doll and Peto,[5] the proportion of cancer deaths in Alberta which are attributable to lifestyle and to environmental exposure is estimated at 74–77 percent.[6] Miller[7] has estimated that if current knowledge were effectively used in practice, at least 50 percent of cancer deaths would be prevented.

The Steve Fonyo Cancer Prevention Project

The Alberta Cancer Board's Epidemiology and Cancer Prevention Division initiated an ambitious multi-site cancer prevention project in 1986. Known as the Steve Fonyo Cancer Prevention Program, this project involved the evaluation of three programs of community-based cancer prevention delivered in medium-sized cities across the province of Alberta.[6] As part of the project, a comprehensive cancer prevention questionnaire was developed and delivered to households in two of the four test cities. Responses to the questionnaires were coded and entered into a database that produced a personalized cancer prevention letter for individual respondents. The database selected appropriate cancer prevention advice that matched the personal and family medical histories and lifestyles of individual respondents. The knowledge base for the program was developed on the basis of a review of the epidemiological literature in 1986/1987 and the views of a consensus panel of prevention experts convened by the project staff. We used this information to produce the basic "rules" for Cancer, Me??

The Cancer, Me?? project was developed to test three questions: whether computer-illiterate domain experts could transfer their expertise to a computer program with minimal training in computer programming; whether this program could be delivered on a public access videotex network; and finally, whether users would be attracted to an automated advice service and how they would react to this type of service. We chose to use a proprietary expert system shell (described later) because of our positive experience in developing other advice systems. The authors of Cancer, Me?? were specialists in cancer risk factors and behavioral medicine.

Design of Cancer, Me??

Interview Style

In designing Cancer, Me?? we departed from the established tradition of converting paper and pencil questionnaires to computer-based electronic questionnaires. We decided instead to use the facilities of rule-based expert system technology to have Cancer, Me?? simulate an interview with a cancer prevention specialist. Our intent was to provide the program with a "personality" by using an "interview style" based on our understanding of a therapeutic conversation. We even tried to capture the wording and pace of an experienced psychotherapist. We believed that providing a "personality" to the program would increase engagement and "trust" in the information and advice provided.

The program opens by introducing itself and explaining its intended purpose and limitations. As with any interviewer, it asks an opening question: "Have you ever used an advice program before?"

Unlike a questionnaire, however, Cancer, Me?? responds with a light-hearted reply: either "Then this will be a new experience for you" or "Then this should be very familiar." Cancer, Me?? next asks users to introduce themselves with their first name and teaches users about the keyboard interface, again using interactive encouragement. At this point, 1 or 2 minutes into the interaction, Cancer, Me?? continues the interviewer style by exploring users' motivation. Users are presented with the menu displayed in Fig. 11.1.

The response to the query about motivation leads to an exploration of users' interests in cancer prevention and attempts to shape their under-standing of the prevention material that will be presented during the interaction. Each response to the menu generates a unique pathway through

---

Oh you're 33 years old. I would have never guessed.

Although most of my advice can apply to people of any age, I was designed specifically for people your age.

People are interested in learning about cancer prevention for a variety of reasons.

Which of the following best describes why you are interested?

------------------------(Choose one answer only.)----------------------------

I am curious about cancer and would like to know more about it
Even though I don't have symptoms, I worry about getting cancer
A friend or relative has had cancer
I have symptoms which are concerning me
I have had cancer
Another reason

FIGURE 11.1. Screen prompting users about their motivation for consulting Cancer, Me??

the interaction. For example, people who indicate that they have symptoms that they fear are related to cancer are encouraged to discuss these with their doctor and are also told that cancers that are detected early are most likely to be curable. Users who indicate that they have previously had cancer are queried about their current well-being and, further, about their motivation for using Cancer, Me?? If they wish to understand why they themselves got cancer or wish to prevent recurrences, they are directed to a discussion with their physician.

These aspects of Cancer, Me?? mimic the initial phase of a skilled interview. The interaction not only provides valuable information about the interviewee that serves to clarify the role and purpose of the interview, but it also assists in the establishment of "clinical rapport." In designing the program, we believed that this would be important because traversing the program as a whole can take 20 to 40 minutes. If users were not engaged in the process, we reasoned that it would be unlikely that they would maintain interest throughout the interaction.

Another way in which we tried to mimic an interview with a human health provider was by having the software use the first person. That is, Cancer, Me?? uses the personal pronoun "I" in responding to the user's input. It also employs appropriate emotional language such as "I'm glad to hear that you . . ." or "I'm sorry that. . . ." The software also responds with emotionally supportive comments when appropriate. For example, when the program learns that a user has a relative with a cancer diagnosis, it responds by indicating that "This must be a difficult time for you" and goes on to ask about the person's state of health. In this way, we attempted to provide Cancer, Me?? with an "electronic persona"; that is, a consistent style of interaction that acknowledges emotional issues, provides support and gives feedback to the user in a timely conversational style.

Another method of engaging users was to ask them which aspects of cancer and cancer prevention they were most interested (e.g., tobacco, diet, sun exposure, and early detection). This information was used to customize the interaction so that the person's primary cancer prevention interests were explored early on. Areas of lesser interest were explored later. The program returned each time to a menu to allow people to choose their next preference or end the interaction. This menu is displayed in Fig. 11.2.

Each domain of cancer prevention information took advantage of information acquired earlier in the interaction and asked the questions necessary for selecting appropriate advice. Advice on each domain was delivered as soon as adequate information was collected from the user.

Cancer, Me?? Development Tool

Rule-based shells have a proven track record in the implementation of expert systems,[8,9] but the role of dialogue in such systems is secondary. To support the dialogue needs of Cancer, Me??, we used a rule-based shell

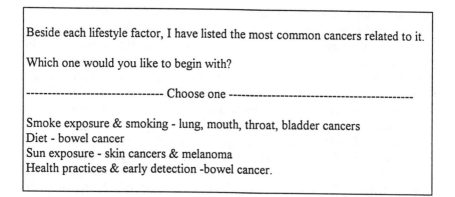

Beside each lifestyle factor, I have listed the most common cancers related to it.

Which one would you like to begin with?

------------------------------ Choose one --

Smoke exposure & smoking - lung, mouth, throat, bladder cancers
Diet - bowel cancer
Sun exposure - skin cancers & melanoma
Health practices & early detection -bowel cancer.

FIGURE 11.2. Screen offering users options for which aspect of cancer prevention to explore first.

enhanced with unique text handling capabilities (EXP is available from Paradigm Solutions, #420 910-7th Avenue, SW Calgary AB, Canada T2P 3N8). This approach proved effective in earlier cases in which professionals with no programming background authored applications in their domains (arthritis patient interview, diabetes adviser, organ transplant coordinator).

The simple and consistent syntax elements—rules and parameters— constitute a high-level declarative language, hiding low-level programming details like execution control or the user interface. The inference engine semantics are more abstract, but within the grasp of a person who is capable of the conceptual design of the application.

The portability of the development/delivery environment has proven vital. Not only can applications be developed on most common personal computers (PCs), but also, the knowledge bases—standard ASCII files— can be shared between co-developers, and ported easily to a variety of target systems. Portability is largely due to the separation of the user interface, which makes ported applications immediately usable. The author is concerned only with the content of textual entities like prompts, responses, checklists, help, or hypertext entries. Their presentation to and manipulation by the user are handled automatically by interchangeable user interface drivers, communicating with the inference engine through a formal protocol. The ALEX driver conforms to general and ALEX-specific user interface guidelines, relieving the author of this responsibility.

Implementation of Cancer, Me?? on the ALEX Network

ALEX was Bell Canada's experimental public access videotex network. Patterned after the successful Minitel network in France, ALEX used Bell

Canada's telephone network to connect telephone subscribers to digital service providers. Customers used either a PC and modem or specially designed ALEX terminals to access the network through their telephone line (see Fig. 11.3).

At the time of this trial in the winter of 1990/1991, there were approximately 440 service providers on the network. Service providers used either their own computers or a service bureau to present services to network users. Typical services included entertainment guides, restaurant listings, want ads, descriptions of telephone services, and horoscopes, as well as chat lines of various sorts. All ALEX-based services were required to adhere to a uniform interface standard. This allowed users to use the different services without specific training. Cancer, Me?? was implemented on ALEX to assess user response to advice services. The project involved a cooperative arrangement between Bell Northern Research (S.F.), the Alberta Cancer Board (P.T., J.B., and E.M.) and the Foothills Hospital (I.Z.). The expert system-based adaptation of the Steve Fonyo knowledge base was designed and developed in Calgary. The technical implementation of the system on a UNIX-based PC server was done in Montreal.[10] During the trial the system was accessed by up to five simultaneous users.

ALEX users were made aware of the availability of the Cancer, Me?? project by means of a catalogue of services provided monthly to ALEX users in Montreal. Because Montreal is a predominantly French-speaking (80 percent) city, the catalogue of services listed Cancer, Me?? in both the French and English indexes, but indicated that Cancer, Me?? was available only in English. Cancer, Me?? was offered at no cost to users during this trial.

The data analyzed for this project included connection information, which included the number of connections, the length of each connection, the number of users, and the number of connections per user. Cancer, Me?? produced a log of each user selection, which provided information on the user's motivation, medical history, family history, and lifestyle. In addition, users were invited to complete an online evaluation at the end of each Cancer, Me?? session.

Results

Contacts with Cancer, Me??

During the analysis period, which was the first 7 weeks that Cancer, Me?? was available, there were 948 connections with the service. During its initial month of operation, Cancer, Me?? was the sixth most popular service available on the network. This is particularly meaningful given the predominance of unilingual French speakers in the service area. The most popular

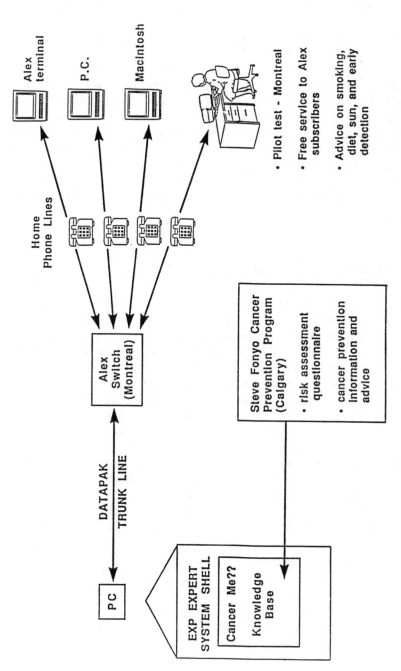

FIGURE 11.3. Schematic of the Methodology of the Cancer, Me?? trial on ALEX.

service was the electronic yellow pages, followed by four gay digital chat lines.

During the study period, 66.4 percent of users signed on once, 25.7 percent two or three times, and 7.8 percent four or more times. Repeaters signed on to complete previously started sessions, review the advice given, or change their answers. When more than one complete session was available for a particular user, the first complete session was used in the analysis. Forty-eight percent of the session logs involved responses to fewer than three questions. We presumed that the majority of these signons were francophone subscribers who were unable to complete the English-only interaction. An additional 18.1 percent of sessions were repeat sessions by the same user and 4.1 percent were test sessions conducted by the project staff (these were dropped from further analyses). A total of 308 complete sessions were included in our analysis.

User Demographics and Motivation

Table 11.1 displays the demographic profile of the Cancer, Me?? users. They were predominantly male, young, and well-educated, not a surprising profile of early adopters of a computer telecommunication system.

Users spent an average of 32 minutes interacting with the system. Table 11.2 displays users' responses to the initial question on motivation for learning about cancer. One half were curious about cancer and one quarter expressed concern about getting cancer. This is intriguing because this demographic segment does not typically seek out health promotion services or programs. Users who contacted the system more than once were asked why they had called back. Thirty-nine percent were completing a previous session. Twenty-two percent, however, wanted to go through the program again and try different answers. Ten percent wanted to see if a change they made would change the advice they received.

Twenty-six percent of the Cancer, Me?? users were regular smokers. The tobacco section of the program was the most popular. It was traversed by

TABLE 11.1. Demographic characteristics of Cancer, Me??: users.

Gender	
Males	75.6%
Female	24.4%
Mean age	31.7 (SD = 11.9)
Education	
University	34.1%
Post Secondary	33.8%
High School or less	32.1%

TABLE 11.2. Motivation for using Cancer, Me??

Curious about cancer	49.8%
Concerned about getting cancer	25.7%
A friend or relative has cancer	14.9%
Has symptoms that are concerning them	7.3%
Have had cancer themselves	2.3%

65.3 percent of the program users ($n = 201$). The other sections were engaged by approximately 50 percent of the users. One third of the users went through all four cancer prevention advice segments.

Users' Evaluation of Cancer, Me??

At the completion of the advice section of Cancer, Me??, users were offered the opportunity to respond to an online evaluation survey. Of the 308 users, 138 (44.8 percent) completed the evaluation. There were no significant differences in the demographic characteristics of the evaluation sample and the total sample. Table 11.3 presents the results of the survey. Users were presented with a series of evaluation questions using a 4-point response format. For example, they were asked, "Did you find the questions to be clearly stated?" and were offered the response options "perfectly clear, clear, somewhat unclear, and very unclear." The percentages listed in Table 11.3 are for respondents to the first two categories.

In addition to these rating scale items, users were also asked a series of yes/no questions. Seventy-nine percent indicated that they would not have sought this information from another source if they had not received it on ALEX. Eighty-eight percent indicated that they would use Cancer, Me?? or a similar health advice program in the future. Users were also asked if they would access programs similar to Cancer, Me?? if there were a charge for this service. Twenty-five percent indicated that they would. Finally, 72 percent of users indicated that they intended to take action as a result of their interaction with Cancer, Me?? The most frequently indicated action was changing their diet (50 percent), followed by losing weight and exercising (10 percent) and changing in their smoking habits (12 percent).

FIGURE 11.3. Evaluation of Cancer, Me??

Questions were clearly stated	97.1%
Information was understandable	98.5%
Information was interesting	82.4%
Like the way the program took on a "personality"	85.9%
Would use Cancer, Me?? or a similar program again	88.3%
Were not frustrated at any point during the program	76.9%

Implications of the ALEX Trial

The results of the trial are a strong endorsement of the popularity and acceptance of online health advice among ALEX subscribers. The style of the program, which mimics a "live interview," was also well-received. The intriguing suggestion that respondents may use the health advice to initiate behavior change is the subject of a randomized community trial currently being conducted. The ALEX trial in Montreal was conducted during the winter of 1990/1991 when public access online services were a novelty in North America. The profile of users of Cancer, Me?? is what one would expect of early adopters of a computer-based service. The degree of acceptance of the health advice system by this predominantly young and male population suggests that health promotion/disease prevention advice may be accessed by this population if packaged in a technically innovative manner. If online health advisory services are attractive to a typically resistant demographic group such as young males, [11] they should be even more attractive to population segments who traditionally seek health information.

Automated health advice has both advantages and limitations. Expert advice is a scarce commodity. The automation of such advice creates the potential for wide dissemination. This has broad implications for community health. Individuals who may not have convenient access to personally relevant health promotion advice through a health professional can obtain quality advice without requiring face-to-face contact. It is conceivable therefore that the dissemination of personally tailored health advice can be far more cost effective if done through computer networks.

Another advantage of automated advice is its consistent quality. Unlike human experts who may be distracted, fatigued, rushed, or misinformed, a computer advisor will methodically ask the same questions and provide consistent advice to patient after patient, day after day. It is conceivable therefore that in some health care domains, a computer advisor may provide higher quality, more accurate advice than a human advisor. In a similar vein, computer advisors do not require users to travel to their offices, make appointments, or pay for parking. Computer advisors could be available in communities where trained professional health advisors are unavailable.

Health knowledge is constantly advancing. Research results reshape our understanding of disease processes and affect the advice we give patients. Research over the past 30 years on the process of diffusion of innovations has made clear the difficulties of moving from a research innovation to adoption of the innovation by the health care community. [12] However, a panel of experts can periodically review and update computer advisors, which will thereafter provide consistent up-to-date advice. Thus, the use of computer advisors makes it possible for a much broader population to have access to the expertise.

Our discussion has highlighted the potential benefits of automated advice. We have not, however, considered whether there are advantages to having this advice available online rather than distributed on storage media such as diskettes. It might be argued, for example, that at this point in time there are many more people with access to stand alone PCs than with access to computer networks. Therefore, relying on online services may limit access. However, there are several potential advantages to providing online advice. We noted earlier that one advantage of automated advisors is that they can be periodically updated to reflect advances in medical knowledge. If the advisor is distributed on diskette, the problem of diffusion becomes a matter of upgrading outdated software. In contrast, if advisors are primarily provided online, updating the network servers completes the upgrade cycle.

Another way in which online health advice may be preferable to stand alone PC delivery is by making users' data available to their health providers. That is, it is conceivable that an advisory service could generate a report for the user's physician or community health clinic. Such a report would be a useful addition to the medical record and could be followed up on subsequent clinic visits. Network delivery could also promote the use of messaging services between the user and human provider around issues raised in the automated health advice session. In addition, health service providers could conduct research using advisory systems delivered on community networks. This research could be directed toward improving service delivery based on increased understanding of users' information needs and how they have used the advice they have already received.

A number of limitations related to automated advisory services are also worthy of consideration. Foremost is the problem of making an automated advisor sufficiently comprehensive to recognize when its limits have been surpassed. For example, in the Cancer, Me?? project, advice was given to women to reduce dietary fat in order to reduce the risk of breast cancer. If this advice were given without awareness of other illnesses, such as kidney disease or diabetes, the user would be at risk for receiving naive and possibly dangerous advice. The panel of experts that established the knowledge base for Cancer, Me?? included questions about other diseases that would affect the nature of dietary advice. Expertise is critical for reducing the number of instances of naive and inappropriate advice.

This raises the issue of legal liability for the advice given. A human health professional who provides substandard advice is vulnerable to legal action. However, the author of a book that includes speculative information as the basis of inappropriate advice will not be the object of a suit. Where do advice programs fall on this continuum? They purport to provide personalized, individually specific and relevant health advice. Who is responsible—the author, the publisher, the service provider, or the user? At this point we are unaware of a legal precedent in this regard.

The information generated by online advisory systems raises further ethical and possibly legal issues. Who owns the electronic record of the advice session that includes the user's personal health information? Should these data be treated as a medical record? Who should have access to it? Are network service providers subject to the confidentiality standards that health service professionals endorse? What level of security is appropriate to protect this electronic record from tampering?

This is a new field with enthusiastic adventurers eager to explore the benefits of reaching out to others in a novel way. In our enthusiasm we would be wise to pause and reflect on the potential for violation of fundamental principles of human rights. The history of public adoption of new technologies has much to teach us about the subtle and unexpected negative effects that new technologies have brought.[13]

Although Cancer, Me?? continued to be available to Alex users for a number of months following the analysis period, the question of financial support for ongoing use was not resolved and the program was removed from the network. Initially Bell Canada indicated interest in maintaining and expanding these types of services, but regulatory issues regarding service provision ultimately prevented this from happening. Who will pay for the development and delivery of this type of service remains an important question.

Conclusions

Our experience with the Cancer, Me?? ALEX trial provides a strong endorsement of public acceptance of online health promotion advice. The potential benefits of online advice include extending access to health advice to populations who are not well served by our current system due to either limited access or limited motivation. The development of such systems requires expert attention to the accuracy of the decision rules that determine which advice to give and also to issues relevant to the interaction between the user and the "advisor." We use the concept of the persona to describe a programming style that attends to the manner of interaction and seeks to engage the user in the advice delivery session by simulating the style of an experienced human interviewer. As public access to online services becomes broader, further development of these concepts seems warranted.

References

1. *Canadian Cancer Statistics 1990*. Toronto: National Cancer Institute of Canada; 1990.
2. *Canadian Cancer Statistics 1995*. Toronto: National Cancer Institute of Canada; 1995.
3. Bailar J, Smith E. Progress against cancer? *N Eng J Med*. 1986;314:1226–1232.
4. Greenwald P, Cullen JW, McKenna J. Cancer prevention and control: From research through applications. *JNCI* 1987;79(2):389–407.

 5. Doll R, Peto R. The causes of cancer: Quantitative estimates of avoidable risks of cancer in the United States today. *JNCI* 1981;66(6):1191–1308.
 6. Birdsell JM, Campbell S, McGregor SE, Hill GB. Steve Fonyo Cancer Prevention Program: Description of an innovative program. *Can J Public Health*. 1992;83(3):237–239.
 7. Miller AB. Planning cancer control strategies. *Chronic Dis Canada*. 1992;13(1):S1–S40.
 8. Buchanan BG, Shortliffe EH. *Rule-based expert systems: The Mycin experiments of the Stanford Heuristic Programming Project*. Reading, MA: Addison-Wesley; 1984.
 9. Harmon P, King D. *Artificial Intelligence in Business*. New York: John Wiley; 1985.
10. Freiwald S, Zendel IH, Benjamin D, Rubinov E. Health expert goes on-line. In: *Operational Expert System Applications in Canada*. Suen CY, Shinghal R (eds.). New York: Pergamon Press; 1992, pp 45–55.
11. Finnegan JR, Rooney B, Viswanath K, et al. Process evaluation of a home based program to reduce diet related cancer risk: The "WINN" at home series. *Health Ed Quarterly*. 1992;19(2):233–248.
12. Rogers EM. *Diffusion of Innovation*. 3rd ed. New York: The Free Press; 1983.
13. Franklin, U. *The Real World of Technology*. Concord, Ont: House of Anansi Press Ltd.; 1990.

12

Improving Health Through Computer Self-Help Programs: Theory and Practice

Thomas L. Patterson, William S. Shaw, and Daniel R. Masys

In this chapter, we examine the use of computer self-help programs, a logical but controversial extension of community health intervention networks. We will use the term "computer health care services" to refer broadly to interactive, self-help computer programs or computer networks that can be accessed directly by patients for information or advice about their health or to obtain emotional support. Although many ethical concerns remain unresolved, a surprising number of prototypes have been developed and researched, driven by the high cost of conventional medical care. In the following paragraphs, we provide a partial listing of these programs, the primary dilemmas associated with their use, and factors that are likely to affect their utilization and effectiveness. Our goal is to provide a behavioral framework for analyzing the pros and cons of computer self-help health care services from our existing knowledge of health care utilization, health behavior, and social support. These considerations are critical in setting realistic goals for the implementation of computer health care services.

The concept of self-help in health care is not new. A perusal of any bookstore will provide evidence of the continuing demand for books and videotapes on physical and mental health. Mechanization of educational programs is also not new. In 1926, S.L. Pressey[1] invented a "teaching machine" that presented educational materials in a didactic, but mechanized fashion to ensure uniformity of stimulus exposure in experimental psychology studies. Later, B.F. Skinner[2] extended this concept so that the machine could make simple judgments about correct and incorrect responses, providing individuals with corrective feedback. Today, personal computer (PC) technology provides a rich and interactive educational medium. However, little is known about how this technology might be used to influence health behavior and complement conventional health care services.

Computer health care services can be grouped into two principal categories: *computer-mediated* services and *computer-directed* services. Charac-

TABLE **12.1.** Characteristics and examples of computer health care services.

Computer-mediated services	Computer-directed services
Characteristics:	Characteristics:
Computer as communication device.	Computer as instructor/trainer.
Requires MODEM/network.	Modem/network requirement optional.
Time flexibility variable.	Time flexibility high.
Requires personnel time.	No personnel time.
Highly interactive.	Moderately interactive.
Highly customized.	Moderately customized.
Moderate to high degree of medical oversight.	Low to moderate degree of medical oversight.
Affordability variable.	Affordability variable.
Examples:	Examples:
Electronic patient support groups.	Take-home educational software.
Online communication with health care provider.	Interactive illness monitoring programs.
"Talk to the Experts" internet services.	Motivational/health change programs.
Symptom, diet, or exercise diaries.	Computer psychotherapy.
Caregiver communication links.	Electronic health encyclopedia.
Public electronic bulletin boards.	Health decision support systems.

teristics and examples of these services are provided in Table 12.1. *Computer-mediated* services are those in which a computer link is the principal mode of communication, whether between patients and their health care providers, or among patients themselves in an electronic discussion group. For example, a new mother might be able to communicate with a nurse practitioner about neonatal care via an interactive computer network established by an HMO for its members. Or, a family caregiver of an Alzheimer's Disease patient might receive assistance from other caregivers on general care guidelines through the network. In contrast to *computer-mediated* services, *computer-directed* services are instructional software packages that operate without the explicit participation of another individual. These programs may pertain to specific illnesses or provide general information about diet, exercise, and other health habits. Despite mounting ethical concerns about how they are used or disseminated, these software applications represent a logical next step in medical technology, with a vast potential for reducing health care costs.

Computers and the Health Care Crisis

In the current health care crisis in the United States, the three issues are: affordability, accessibility, and accountability[3]. Spiraling health care costs are the driving force behind the advancement of computer health care services. While technological advances in most industries have reduced costs to the consumer, this has not been the case in medicine. Though generally improving the quality of care in the United States, advances in medicine have had the unfortunate side effect of disproportionately increasing costs relative to benefits. As shown in Fig. 12.1, health care costs in the United States have spiraled upward from $4.0 billion in 1940 to an estimated $662.0 billion in 1990. Making up nearly 14 percent of the gross national product, these health care costs have jeopardized U.S. industries' competition for international markets. Therefore, any proposed technological advances in health care delivery that reduce rather than inflate health care costs should not go unstudied.

Despite the exorbitant cost of health care in the United States, between 32 and 38 million Americans have no health insurance.[4] Therefore, access to health care is severely limited. For example, it has been estimated that nearly 7 million people with emotional disorders do not receive any type of care.[5] The use of computers may be a part of the solution to the accessibility problem (Fig. 12.2). The unequal geographical distribution of medical expertise between urban and rural areas might be offset by allowing patients to access self-help information and medical advice by computer. Other media, including interactive video conferencing, have already proven viable links to health care services in rural areas.[6] Computer health care services may also provide health information to individuals who might not otherwise seek the advice of health care providers. These include patients who are geographically or socially isolated, patients who fear the embarrassment of

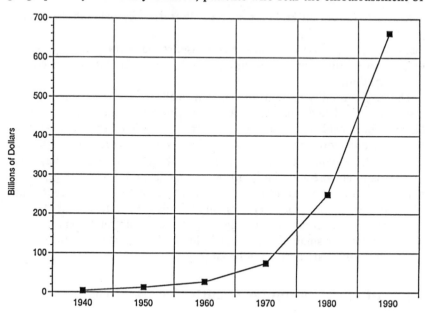

FIGURE 12.1. The escalation of U.S. health care costs.

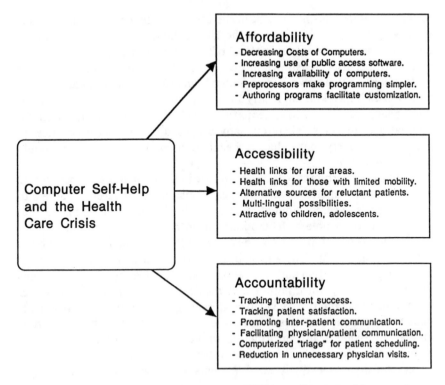

Affordability
- Decreasing Costs of Computers.
- Increasing use of public access software.
- Increasing availability of computers.
- Preprocessors make programming simpler.
- Authoring programs facilitate customization.

Accessibility
- Health links for rural areas.
- Health links for those with limited mobility.
- Alternative sources for reluctant patients.
- Multi-lingual possibilities.
- Attractive to children, adolescents.

Computer Self-Help and the Health Care Crisis

Accountability
- Tracking treatment success.
- Tracking patient satisfaction.
- Promoting inter-patient communication.
- Facilitating physician/patient communication.
- Computerized "triage" for patient scheduling.
- Reduction in unnecessary physician visits.

FIGURE 12.2. The potential role of computer self-help services in health care reform.

disclosure (e.g., those with substance abuse, sexually-transmitted diseases, or psychiatric disorders), and patients with limited mobility or access to transportation.

The accountability issue in the current health care crisis focuses on the way in which advances in treatments are evaluated. In the past, treatments have not been held accountable to produce their desired benefits in terms of long-term and global well-being. With a limited health care budget, the cost of heroic life-saving attempts for a single patient with an extremely poor prognosis might preclude basic preventive medicine measures (e.g., vaccinations) for thousands of others. Like any other health care policy, the use of computer health care services should also be put to the test of accountability. Preliminary findings suggest that computer services may produce relatively small effects at the individual level; however, the savings in system health care costs may be large.

Utilization of Computer Health Care Services

As with other voluntary self-help programs, computer health care services are likely to be used only by a subset of the population, although future advances in technology may change this dramatically. A number of factors will be critical in determining which individuals will be likely to use this new service. A widely accepted framework for analyzing individual differences in use of conventional health care services has been developed by Anderson and Newman,[7] who divide variables into three categories: *predisposing* factors, *enabling* factors, and *need* factors. *Predisposing* factors are demographic characteristics and basic beliefs that provide a backdrop for specific patterns of health behavior. *Enabling* factors are those family or community variables that act to facilitate or obstruct the use of services in the presence of a health care need. *Need* factors are both individual traits and self-perceptions of illness that give rise to the desire for service use. We will use this three-factor framework for examining variables related to the use of computer health care services (see Table 12.2).

The primary predisposing factor for use of computer health care services is accessibility to computer equipment and the necessary communication linkages. An estimated 15 million homes in the United States (17 percent of all households) had a home computer in 1994, and many of these were

TABLE 12.2. Characteristics and examples of computer health care services.

Health care utilization factor	Potential impacts associated with computer self-help
Predisposing factors	
Age	More computer familiarity among younger patients.
Sex	More positive computer attitudes among males.
Marital status	Unknown patients.
Past illness	Computer self-care might prevent relapse.
Education	More computers among high education households.
Occupation	Employers could provide computer self-help links.
Family size	Unknown impacts.
Ethnicity	Fewer computers among disadvantages groups.
Religion	Unknown impacts.
Residential mobility	Provide homebound patients with health information.
Enabling factors	
Income	Cost of computer hardware may be prohibitive.
Health insurance	Self-help health care information for the uninsured.
Type of regular source	Computer self-help might help to standardize care.
Access to regular source	Links to primary physician may be more flexible.
Ratio of health personnel to patients	Computer self-help might aid in allocation of resources.
Price of health services	Computer self-help extremely affordable.
Region of country	Health information customized to address local needs.
Urban-rural character	Computers may link rural areas to health care information.
Illness factors	
Disability	Computer-directed cognitive or physical rehabilitation.
Symptoms	Programs to encourage early detection of symptoms.
Perceived diagnoses	Programs may help to differentiate serious symptoms.
Perceived general state	Programs may address coping skills, provide support.
Evaluated symptoms	Computers may provide link for monitoring symptoms.
Evaluated diagnoses	Computers may promote physician/patient exchanges.

tailored for telecommunications.[8] In households with a family annual income in excess of $35,000, nearly 30 percent are equipped with a home computer. In the past 10 years, elementary and secondary schools in the United States have increased their computer availability substantially, from 63 students per computer to 12 students per computer.[8] Despite these gains in computer accessibility, use of computers remains largely divided along lines of race, gender, age, education, and income. Middle- and high-income households are four times more likely to own a computer than households with an annual income of less than $15,000.[8] Because health is generally compromised among lower income groups, computer health care services may be ineffective in reaching those with the greatest needs. In the future, however, advances in technology are likely to make computers more accessible to disadvantaged groups by making them more affordable. Also, future home computers may interface with other more popular devices in the home, like radio and television,[9] to increase their mass appeal.

Computer attitudes may pose a hurdle to computer health care services. Many individuals with available resources choose not to use computers when given a choice of media. One explanation is that software packages have not properly addressed the human factors of computer use and decliners perceive computers to be taxing, tedious, and unfriendly. Another explanation is that some individuals experience computer anxiety, an aversive response to computers (and often technology in general) that is marked by a strong physiological stress response to computer interactions. A third explanation is that computers are simply unable to capture the interest of people in the same way that personal interactions do, an issue that is addressed later in this chapter.

Several aspects of computer health care services represent enabling factors. For patient populations with either limited mobility or disability, a home computer may provide access to health care information or advice. Examples include deaf individuals, people for whom transportation is difficult or unavailable, and individuals who are bound to their homes for other reasons (e.g., family caregivers, social phobics). In an experimental intervention for Alzheimer's Disease caregivers,[10] 68 percent of caregivers took advantage of a supportive computer link at home and caregivers used the service an average of nearly five times per week. Computers also may provide opportunities for individuals to receive health care information when they otherwise would not.[11] For example, patients may be more likely to request information about sexually transmitted diseases by computer than in person because of the fear of embarrassment. Training in breast self-examination provides another good example of preventive medicine that might be more acceptable to patients when delivered through a computer medium. Minor ailments that frequently go untreated because individuals fear expensive, painful, or inconvenient health care services might also be targeted for patient education using computer networks.

One population that may be especially receptive to computer health care services is children and adolescents. For reasons not well studied (perhaps merely a cohort effect of technological advancement), younger people are more engaged with computers than older people. Among adolescents, this interest in computers is often coupled with a general distrust of authority figures (who, incidentally, are well represented in the health care field). Therefore, computers may provide a feasible substitute for classroom health educators, especially because some subjects have been given poor coverage by educators in the past (e.g., sex education, drug abuse). For both adolescents and younger children, computers may be more efficient than conventional instruction, because they possess fewer social nuances to digest and interpret along with technical information. Children prefer colorful, animated, and competitive formats for computer instruction to maintain their interest. Based on age-related differences in computer attitudes, computer health care services should be differentially designed for children and adults.

Need factors are the last ingredient in the Anderson and Newman[9] model of health care utilization. Computer health care services may play an important role in the way in which patients assess their need for medical assistance by guiding their decisions to make physician appointments. Group interventions aimed at educating patients about when to seek services have demonstrated long-term cost savings and improved well-being among patients.[12] Similar interventions could be designed using computer-directed instructions. Based on a series of questions related to the nature and severity of symptoms and background characteristics, patients could be prompted to seek a physician, obtain home treatment, or merely monitor symptoms for changes. This information could be electronically relayed to the health care provider to keep abreast of the patient's condition. This "computer triage" system is particularly attractive given the affordability and accessibility issues of the current health care crisis.

Computers and Health Education

For those who find computer health care services both accessible and desirable, three health outcomes need to be considered: (1) the ability of computers to educate patients about health-related subjects, (2) the ability of computers to bring about changes in health behavior, and (3) the ability of computers to provide social support or assist in obtaining social support. We will address each of these three issues separately, although we recognize that they are highly interactive. The educational value of computers in health care settings has received the most study. The ability of computer services to change health behavior and the ability to provide social support are much more recent.

As noted earlier, the mechanization of educational materials is not new. Several recent improvements in software, however, have made the computer a more attractive medium for the delivery of patient education. Research into the human factors of computing and intuition suggest that users prefer instructional systems that are customized, interactive, illustrative, and nonrepeating. A meta-analysis comparing various forms of computer-assisted instruction in 47 studies[13] found that interactive videos and computer-enriched instruction that included realistic computer simulations were most effective in providing health instruction. The meta-analysis also found that computer-based instruction was more effective (*effect size* = 0.41) than traditional instruction.

The initial applications of computer instruction have been in preventive medicine, where programs have educated patients about substance abuse,[14-17] sexually transmitted diseases,[18] sexual dysfunction,[19] and diet control in diabetes.[20,21] Interestingly, these are some of the health care topics least comfortable for physicians in face-to-face encounters with patients. Despite the availability of these programs, a 1983 survey revealed that only 4 percent of family physicians in the United States used computers for patient education.[22] Several studies,[23] including Skinner, Siegfried, Kegler, and Strecher,[24] suggest that physicians' negative attitudes toward computers may be one of the primary hurdles to computer patient education.

Computers can be used in many ways to guide or complement patient education, with a full spectrum of complexity and interaction. The most passive use might involve the positioning of computer stations, preprogrammed with pertinent disease information, in the waiting rooms of specialized clinics. These types of computer services appear to garner support from passers-by who use the computer,[25,26] although little is known about the sustained value of such programs. More deliberate uses of computers in health education have shown remarkable instructional value. Table 12.3 gives a partial list of research results on computer patient education including applications for cystic fibrosis,[27] cardiovascular disease,[25] adolescent health,[28] diabetes,[29] and prenatal care.[30] These programs appear to match or exceed the effectiveness of both written and live presentations of educational materials.

Computers and Health Behavior Change

Health psychology studies have demonstrated that many health behaviors are resistant to change, and merely educating patients about their condition may not produce positive change. Therefore, computer health care services that target changes in health behavior should be interactive and motivationally based, and they should guide patients through incremental changes in behavior while providing positive feedback, encouragement, and (possibly) tangible rewards. Several theoretical models have been proposed to explain the process of health behavior change. Three well-recognized

TABLE 12.3. A partial listing of studies incorporating computers in patient education.

Authors	Target population	Health topic	Results
Petzel, Ellis, Budd, and Johnson[27]	Parents of children with cystic fibrosis	Behavior management	Parents reported that computer instruction was more helpful, more informative, and more likely to change behavior than lessons in a written format.
Chen, Houston, Burson, and Comer[25]	Waiting room patients	CVD risk factors	97% of patients favored use of computer services and 90% reported easy to use.
Bosworth et al[28]	Adolescents	General health information	70% of ninth-grade students chose to use computer health services.
Wheeler and Wheeler[29]	Diabetic patients	Nutrition education	Education was effective and more efficient than dietician services.
Kinzie, Schorling, and Siegel[30]	Low-income, rural women	Prenatal care	97% enjoyed the program, 75% learned important information, 81% preferred computer to other educational media.

theories of behavioral change are: the *social cognitive theory*, which emphasizes the role of external influences; the *health belief model,* which emphasizes internal influences; and the *communication-behavior change model*, which is especially valid for examining media effects. While other more complex models for health behavior have been proposed, these three capture many of the issues related to changing health behavior.

Social cognitive theory, first advanced by Albert Bandura,[31,32] involves reciprocal determinism between a *person*, the *environment*, and the person's *behavior*, as shown in Fig. 12.3a. This model recognizes that a person not only responds to the environment, but also shapes the environment. Similar feedback systems exist between a person's internal thoughts and emotions and the person's overt behavior (the person/behavior reciprocity concept). Social cognitive theory also stresses the importance of *outcome expectations* and *self-efficacy expectations*, beliefs of the person in his or her ability to control both behavior and the environment. In terms of health behavior, "environment" is considered to include the "bodily environment," or physical health and symptomatology. Social cognitive theory predicts that those with strong beliefs in their abilities are more likely to succeed in changing their behavior.

The computer now plays a role in reinforcing both outcome expectations and self-efficacy expectations. We will propose two changes to the basic model to understand the potential role of the computer. First, we will add the clinician/support source as a fourth element that may also have reciprocal effects with persons and their environment (Fig. 12.3b). A patient has expectations about the ability of health care providers to improve her health (the bodily "environment") directly or to guide her through behavioral changes which may improve her health. In conventional health care, the clinician serves a primary function as "healer" and a secondary function as "motivator" of improved health behavior. With computer health care services, the motivational relationship between a person and the clinician is enhanced by the computer (in the case of computer-mediated services), or the computer acts as a surrogate provider (in the case of computer-directed services). This model (Fig. 12.3c) suggests that both confidence in the computer and confidence in the physician are important in increasing an individual's self-efficacy for behavioral change.

If a patient has high confidence in her physician, then computer health care services should be introduced as a "prescription" of the attending physician, and should be customized to include repeated "messages" from the patient's physician. For example, communication links might be provided to allow physicians a glimpse at a patient's progress in completing an instructional program for managing chronic illness. Based on this report, the physician might respond electronically with words of encouragement and recognition of accomplishments, acting as the primary reinforcer in continuing the use of computer services. Also, confidence in computers to

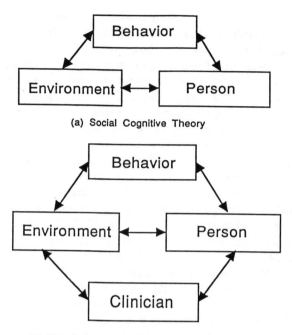

(a) Social Cognitive Theory

(b) The Role of the Physician in Health Behavior

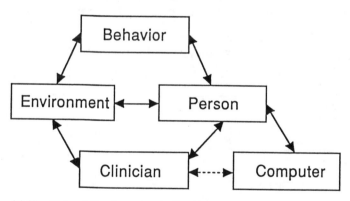

(c) The Role of the Computer in Health Behavior Change

FIGURE 12.3. Social cognitive theory and computers in health behavior change.

provide accurate and beneficial information is critical to the efficacy of computer health care services. Early attempts at installing computer health care services for patients should be carefully planned and monitored, so that negative public attitudes do not develop as a result of haphazard attempts to use computers in patient care.

A second widely accepted model for understanding changes in health behavior is the health belief model[33]; this model is particularly useful in explaining preventive health behavior. The model (Fig. 12.4) suggests that decisions about health behavior are made based on the perceived threat of illness. This threat is made up of two components: perceived *susceptibility* to the illness and perceived *severity* of the illness. In addition, the *benefits of action* or *barriers to action* affect the decision to act. The health belief model suggests that software applications that increase perceived susceptibility to, severity of, or benefits of a particular health behavior will be successful in promoting the behavior.

A third theoretical model for understanding health behavior, the communication-behavior change model, was developed to understand the role of large-scale media campaigns in promoting positive health behavior.[34] The model includes a 12-step sequence of events that occur to link media exposure to behavior change (see Fig. 12.5). Like billboards, television ads, and radio announcements are today, computers may become a medium for large-scale public health campaigns. Brief announcements about safe sex and smoking cessation might be added to the start-up programming of popular software packages or computer bulletin boards. As with other media, however, public health announcements must compete with better-funded commercial advertising interests.

The communication-behavior change model might also be applied to lengthier software applications developed to promote changes in health behavior. To this end, the model works nicely within the information-

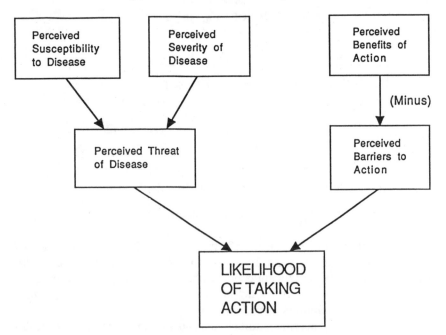

FIGURE 12.4. The health belief model.

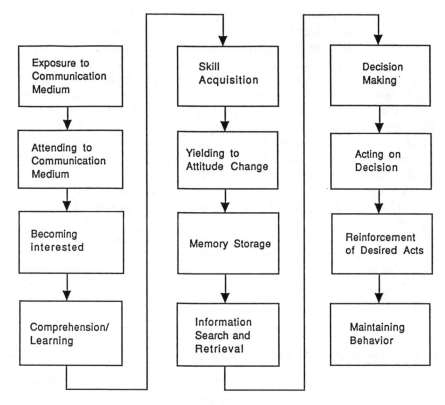

FIGURE 12.5. The communication-behavior change model.

processing framework that we customarily associate with computers. For example, the model applies terminology like "search and retrieval" or "memory storage" to describe cognitive processes associated with behavior change. Health information software might be designed to take advantage of these theoretical similarities between mental and computer processing.

Ecological validity is a primary concern in the use of computers to improve health behavior. Does information presented in a computer medium have less relevance to people in their day-to-day lives than material presented through live presentation? If we look historically at the advent of other technological advances (e.g., radio, telephone, television), we see a familiar pattern of reluctance, resistance, and, finally, acceptance for each of these media in a variety of settings. Today, no one would deny the influence (and hence, ecological validity) that these media enjoy in shaping the behavior of millions. Interestingly, television and radio have become important instruments for encouraging negative, rather than positive health behaviors through commercial advertising of unhealthy foods and beverages.

The ecological validity of computers in health behavior change can be increased by incorporating realistic images, scenarios, and problem-solving elements in health education software. For example, cognitive rehabilitation software has been developed that includes video scenarios for testing and strengthening memory and decision-making processes.[35] In such software, the patient in treatment for alcohol abuse may be asked to imagine situations at a party or restaurant where they are tempted to drink. Choices that the patient indicates lead to feedback and presentation of further dilemmas requiring additional decisions and appropriate feedback. The efficacy of computers in shaping behavior change has not been clearly documented by controlled experiments and, thus, the debate over ecological validity continues. Nevertheless, several studies suggest that behavior change may be a byproduct of computer instruction (see partial listing in Table 12.4). These include behaviors as specific as the proper collection of urine specimens,[36] or more general health behaviors including the reduction of interpersonal conflict among psychiatric patients,[37] dietary intervention to reduce cardiovascular disease[11] and obesity,[38] and depression.[39] More controlled experimental research is needed to demonstrate whether computers, when used in realistic settings and with ecologically valid software, can produce changes in health behavior.

Social Support and the Computer

How important is human contact in relaying messages about health behavior? The importance of social support in maintaining good physical and mental health is well documented. Individuals who become socially isolated tend to experience more symptoms of poor health. Social support has also been shown to buffer the health impacts of negative life events and improve health habits and medical compliance. Social support, however, is a broad construct. The three components of social support that have been associated with health decrements are small network size and restricted access to helping resources, and thus insufficient emotional intimacy.[40] Computer health care services can help to increase network size and increase access to helping resources, and thus may provide at least some forms of emotional support to those experiencing difficulties.

Event-centered support groups probably represent the most common form of social support intervention in health care settings, and support groups usually consist of patients or families of patients who are coping with a common illness. Other support groups may be formed to motivate changes in health behavior (e.g., smoking or diet groups) or provide help with common forms of life adversity (e.g., U.S. veterans groups or single-parent groups). Initial contact with support groups is most often through referrals from friends, family members, or health care professionals, with nonprofit social service agencies or patient associations playing a lesser role. Groups typically meet weekly with a loosely formatted agenda

TABLE 12.4. Partial listing of studies incorporating computers in patient behavior change.

Authors	Target population	Health behavior	Results
Fisher, Johnson, Porter, Bleich, and Slack[36]	Women patients	Collection of clean-catch urine specimens	Computer instruction was more effective in instructing collection of urine specimens than written or oral instructions.
Ellis, Raines, and Hakansan[11]	Waiting room patients	CVD high-risk behavior	35% of patients self-reported that they would probably or definitely change their behavior.
Colby, Gould, and Aronson[37]	Psychotherapy patients	Relieving inhibition in stressful interpersonal conflict	80% effective in motivating action to relieve interpersonal conflict.
Burnett, Taylor, and Agras[38]	Obese, middle-aged females	Dietary change	Ambulatory microcompters providing dietary guidance produced larger weight loss than controls.
Selmi, Klein, Greist, Sorrell, and Erdman[39]	Depressed outpatients	Mood elevation	Computer-administered cognitive-behavioral treatment showed mood improvements equal to therapist-administered therapy. Both groups improved more than controls.

that allows for the free exchange of information and supportive reinforcement. While the general premises of electronic support groups are identical to those of conventional support groups, the computer as the facilitator and mediator of the support group introduces some unique qualities to patient interactions.

The most exciting opportunity of electronic patient support groups is the possibility of providing access to thousands of patients with common health concerns in the privacy of their own homes. Unlike the conventional support group, whose membership may be limited by geography, accessibility, group membership, health insurance coverage, and serendipity, an electronic link has none of these obstacles. Therefore, patients in need of information may draw upon the experience of thousands. Another advantage is that patients with rare disorders for whom conventional support groups are impractical may now correspond with others who are similarly affected. This potential benefit is enormous, given that patients with rare disorders often feel stigmatized by, and isolated from, their normal sources of social support. The large number of patients potentially accessible by computer link is likely to increase the patient's perceptions of available network size and, in turn, result in positive outcomes. A number of social theories, including social comparison theory,[41] and social learning theory,[32] have described feasible mechanisms by which increased network size may lead to reduced helplessness and improved health practices.

Another advantage of computer support groups (as well as other types of computer health care services) is the ability to guide patients to other forms of community and medical resources. This information may be dispatched through patient-to-patient interactions or through a separate software component of the computer link, which provides an index of community resources. Another possibility is a medical referral service that lists health care professionals with disease-specific expertise by geographical region. Providing guidance to patients in accessing community services is critical in resolving the accessibility issue of the current health care crisis. This "access to resources" function of computer links is perhaps more in line with popular notions about computers and their applicability as merely a data source. This direct use of computers by patients is highly feasible and has undisputed benefits. The primary obstacles to its adoption are the unavailability of computers and the lack of comprehensive lists of available patient resources.

The most obvious argument against the use of computer-mediated patient support groups is the loss of face-to-face contact among individuals. Facial expressions, speech inflections, physical gestures, and physical contact are important ingredients in the experience of social support. While it seems unwise to dispute this point, we might point out, however, that social psychology has only begun to investigate the role that technological media play in social interactions.[42,43] We might expect computer interactions among individuals to be briefer, more focused, and less likely to lead to long-term relationships. One interesting aspect of electronic patient support groups is the relative anonymity with which patients can converse. Given this high level of anonymity, patients may interact more honestly and less guardedly, potentially resulting in greater therapeutic value than conventional forms of interaction. The electronic patient support group also offers more selectivity and control of specific interactions. From a large pool of online patients, one might identify several individuals with backgrounds or interests like one's own in an "electronic room" consisting of a self-selected support group. The role of computers in mediating social relationships is an interesting direction for research, given the rapidly rising rates of computer-assisted communication. If we assume that computer support groups are less beneficial than conventional face-to-face groups, this disadvantage may be offset by the advantages of accessibility, volume, and ease of use.

Another question with regard to computer-directed programs for promoting positive changes in health behavior, is whether face-to-face contact with a health care provider is necessary to effect changes in patient behavior (e.g., diet, exercise, high-risk behavior). Although early research suggests that face-to-face contact may not be necessary, the power of the physician (or other providers) in instilling motivation and compliance is not to be underestimated. In fact, in terms of health care satisfaction, patients rate sympathy and understanding of health care providers as important as technical quality of care and expertise.[44,45] Nevertheless, health interventions using creative forms of technology seem to show results comparable to other, more social forms of education and training. As mentioned earlier in this chapter, the success of behavioral change computer programs may depend in part upon personalized endorsements from attending physicians.

The Special Case of Computer Psychotherapy

Unlike most health care services, psychotherapy does not require invasive medical procedures. Therefore, psychotherapy represents an interesting platform for testing the limits of the computer in health care services. These services may be computer-mediated (involving a computer link between a client and therapist) or computer-directed (in which therapy is actually guided by the computer). Until recently, software was the limiting factor in the ability to produce a computer-directed therapy session. However, several experimental software packages are currently undergoing the scrutiny of the clinical research community (not to mention therapists everywhere), and preliminary results suggest that in at least some situations, the computer therapist can produce therapeutic benefit equal to that of a human therapist, although the ethical implications of circumventing clinical judgment and face-to-face therapeutic interaction may be insurmountable in real clinical practice.[46]

One requisite for performing psychotherapy (whether human or machine) is a relatively sophisticated knowledge and use of language. Natural language processors may provide a means for computer "comprehension" and production of English language with substantial allowances for colloquialisms and idiosyncratic verbalisms. This Herculean task has been attempted in several recent programming efforts. GURU, a computer program designed to simulate natural human conversation in a therapeutic milieu,[47] produces some common-sense therapist prompts in response to client statements about an interpersonal relationship. The program searches client responses for semantic information that it recognizes, pieces together these ideas with a set of interpretive functions, then responds from a list of preprogrammed therapeutic messages that can be customized to match incoming information. Computer modeling of lexical units is a science unto itself, and programmers admit that natural language processors have some severe limitations. Nevertheless, these programs are limited more by operating capacity and input sets than by programming complexity. The perseverance of programmers may over time produce some very natural-sounding computer conversations.

The Growing Popularity of Electronic Patient Support Groups

Computer-mediated and computer-directed self-help services available via networks are growing in scope and in number of users. The commercial online services designed for consumers, such as those provided by America Online® CompuServe® and Prodigy,® are converging rapidly upon access to the information services and discussion groups of the Internet, which is the world's largest network of computer networks, public and private. The growth has been fueled by intensive media exposure about information available on the Internet, commitments by the federal government to promote the "Information Superhighway," and the development and widespread deployment of easy-to-use graphic software for creating electronic mail and reading network-based discussion groups and "bulletin boards." The newest and fastest growing type of information access to Internet sources is that provided by browsing programs such as Gopher and the World Wide Web clients "Mosaic" and "Netscape."

Table 12.5 gives a sample of Internet computer-mediated discussion groups (called "newsgroups" by common convention) that have formed on a wide variety of medical topics; these topics represent a tiny fraction of the more than 10,000 current newsgroups, to which individuals add approximately 100 million characters of new text daily.[48] By the naming conventions of the Internet, most of these groups are "alternative" topics (noted by the naming prefix of "alt.", i.e., controversial or unusual topics; not carried by all computer host sites). Newsgroups are created by a populist process

TABLE 12.5. Sample computer-mediated health discussion groups (newsgroups) of the Internet.

Internet Addresses	
alt.adoption	alt.support.cerebral-palsy
alt.health.cfids-action	alt.support.crohns-colitis
alt.infertility	alt.support.depression
alt.med.allergy	alt.support.diet
alt.med.cfs (chronic fatigue syndrome)	alt.support.dissociation
alt.med.fibromyalgia	alt.support.divorce
bit.listserv.autism	alt.support.eating-disord
misc.health.aids	alt.support.epilepsy
misc.health.alternative	alt.support.grief
misc.health.arthritis	alt.support.learning-disab
misc.health.diabetes	alt.support.loneliness
misc.kids.health	alt.support.multi-sclerosis
misc.kids.pregnancy	alt.support.non-smokers
alt.abuse.recovery	alt.support.obesity
alt.sexual.abuse.recovery	alt.support.post-polio
alt.support	alt.support.shyness
alt.suport.abuse-partners	alt.support.sleep-disorder
alt.support.anxiety-panic	alt.support.stop-smoking
alt.support.arthritis	alt.support.stuttering
alt.support.asthma	alt.support.tall
alt.support.attn-deficit	alt.support.tinnitus
alt.support.big-folks	alt.support.tourette
alt.support.cancer	misc.handicap
alt.support.cancer.prostate	soc.support.fat-acceptance

that allows any individual to propose a name and topic for a discussion group, which is then posted to existing newsgroups for voluntary voting by interested readers; current procedures require that a newly created group have 100 more "yes" votes than "no" votes, and two thirds of all counted votes must be "yes." With tens of millions of potential readers around the world, new special interest discussion groups can be quite easily created on medical topics (in theory, requiring only 100 persons to vote "yes" if there are no dissenters). The actual number of readers of any particular newsgroup is difficult to determine, because unlike paper publications, where the number of physical objects produced is an approximate surrogate for usage, there are no widely applied monitoring methods for determining who only reads (as opposed to submits messages to) a given newsgroup; even the most popular of newsgroups are read by less than 1 percent of the global online community.

The character of interactions on the newsgroups has been likened to "an electronic cocktail party" where anyone can say anything about anything. The commonest start of a new "thread" of discussion (a related group of messages posted to a newsgroup) in a medical self-help newsgroup is a question of the form, "I have a friend who has just been diagnosed with [*name of disease*]. What are good sources of information about this problem?" Almost invariably, one or more other readers of the newsgroup will respond with a synopsis of information sources. Such responses are so common that they are often incorporated into a "Frequently Asked Questions" (FAQ) message, edited by the self-help group's informal "leader," often the individual who cared sufficiently about the topic to initiate the newsgroup. The FAQ is posted at regular intervals to the newsgroup, because most computer hosts that store and provide access to newsgroup messages use archiving methods to delete messages more than a few days or weeks old.

Other messages posted to self-help newsgroups often take the form of a specific technical question (e.g., "I know of someone who has diabetes and is now having difficulty with hair loss; is this a complication of diabetes, and if so, what can be done about it?"). It is here that the real strength of an international electronic community is evident, for among the hundreds or even tens of thousands of subscribers to a newsgroup there is a broad base of experience, and even uncommon events will have happened with sufficient frequency that a personal, firsthand reply is promptly posted for all to read.

Though the potential for misinformation is an oft-cited concern of self-help groups, online discussion groups are, in one sense, self-correcting in a fashion unprecedented in the history of human communications. An assertion made in a message posted to the discussion group may be true, may be doubtful, or may be provably incorrect, but it will almost invariably be followed (often within hours) by a set of responses that either validate it by others' descriptions of similar experiences and beliefs, or quickly call its accuracy into question. Though the "truth" may not be evident from the to-and-fro controversy that follows a provocative statement posted to a discussion group, the fact that there is controversy is not lost on even the most naive of readers. Contributors who post useful and compassionate answers to questions submitted to medical newsgroups win the compliments and respect of other participants, but in general, no participant in the electronic community is granted "tenure"; reputations made over months or years of sustained contributions to a particular newsgroup can be dashed by an eccentric or ill-worded observation about a single topic. In this sense, online self-help groups are a fragile meritocracy of written fact and opinion, in which each reader must decide what is true and what is merely unsubstantiated belief.

The growing numbers of computer network users and the power of recently developed information access tools to represent multimedia documents composed of images and sound, as well as text, have led to the creation of an increasing number of consumer health information sources. Though such electronic databases and documents existed before on numerous small, proprietary electronic bulletin boards and commercial sources, the convergence of information providers and online users on the Internet is the dominant theme in current developments. Table 12.6 lists

TABLE 12.6. Examples of current computer-directed self-help and consumer health information.

Source	Content	Access information
Government		
U.S. National Institutes of Health	Consumer health information for specific diseases, such as cancer and AIDS	http://www.nih.gov
U.S. Centers for Disease Control and Prevention (CDC)	Immunization and infectious diseases	http://www.cdc.gov
World Health Organization	Travelers health alerts and recommendations	http://www/who.ch/
Academic		
Emory University	Directory of online consumer health information sources	http://www.cc.emory.edu/ WHSCL/medweb. consumer.html
University of Washington, Seattle	"HealthBeat" consumer health articles	http://www.hslib.washington. edu:80/your__health/
University of Pennsylvania	OncoLink Cancer Information	http://cancer.med.upenn. edu:80/
Professional Societies		
American Medical Informatics Association	"Medical Matrix" guide to health information on the Internet	http://kuhttp.cc.ukans. edu/cwis/units/medcntr/ lee/homepage.html
Charitable Organizations		
American Cancer Society	Online versions of consumer health pamphlets	http://nysernet.org/bcic/ac2/ pat.fam/index.html
Amerian Heart Association	Consumer health articles	gopher://amhrt.amhrt.org: 70/11/about.aha
Individuals		
Dr. Jeanine Wade, clinical psychologist	"Specifica" list of self-help medical information sources	http://www.realtime.net:80/ ~mmjw/

examples of Internet consumer health publications available electronically from sources that include government, universities, societies, and even individuals. Most of these sources provide multimedia online documents composed of text with associated graphics, in an electronic form that parallels closely the appearance of printed materials made available by the same organization. Use of the sources varies widely and is not systematically monitored; however, use is substantial and growing. For example, the University of Pennsylvania's OncoLink cancer information service reported over 36,000 online inquiries per month in its first year of operation.[49]

The growth of interconnected public and private computer networks is expected to continue for the foreseeable future. Currently the Internet is estimated to provide online access to 30 million users in over 120 countries, and users have been doubling approximately every 18 months since 1989;

over 110 million connected computers in the United States are projected alone by the year 2000.[50] The current era of public domain, freely accessible information sources will be supplemented by growing numbers of "electronic bookstores" offering multimedia self-help information on a subscription or fee-for-service basis as technologies are developed to permit secure electronic commerce over public networks. A predictable result will be redefinition of the notion of "community" in the term community health information networks, for communities of interest will develop in a fashion independent of geography: defined by language, electronic connectivity, and the seemingly boundless energy and interest of our species in communicating and seeking new knowledge.

The Ethics of Computer Health Care Services

Little has been written on the ethical and legal issues related to the use of computer programs in clinical practice. We have summarized several areas of ethical concern for the use of computers in direct patient care in Table 12.7. The most salient topics are confidentiality, responsibility, competence, and public welfare. While computer interactions may be partly anonymous, all computer transactions are ultimately stored on an electronic tape somewhere, and access to this information is not well policed. Concerns about the exchange of electronic patient medical records and information are also applicable to records of direct computer use by patients. When patients log on to bulletin board support groups, for example, no confidentiality warnings are issued and patients have little knowledge about the privacy of their interactions. New technologies may be necessary to encode all information with obscured personal identifiers.

Professional responsibility and competence are special problems for

TABLE 12.7. General ethical guidelines and their significance to computer health care services.

APA ethnical guideline	Level of concern	Comments
Confidentiality	High	Does anonymity compensate for lack of confidentiality?
Responsibility	High	Who is responsible for liability associated with computer use?
Competence	High	Should state agencies or professional organizations accept watchdog/licensing responsibility?
Pubic welfare	High	Do potential benefits outweigh potential risks?
Legal standards	Moderate	Do mandatory reporting requirements apply?
Moral standards	Moderate	Are computers dehumanizing?
Professional relationships	Moderate	Is there less control over the therapeutic milieu?
Research	Moderate	Is "informed consent" necessary?
Pubic statements	Low	How should services be promoted/advertised?

computer health care services because conventional professional organizations have been slow to recognize computers as a domain requiring ethical oversight. Users, therefore, are provided with no means of judging the validity and efficacy of various programs. Until disputes related to computer use emerge among ethics boards or within the legal system, software programs are unlikely to be licensed or undergo peer evaluation. The question of who is ultimately responsible for the health effects of computer software is critical for understanding the potential liability of hospitals and health care professionals who provide computer services. Also, responsibility for meeting mandatory reporting requirements (in the case of a homicidal patient, for example) has not been established.

In a standard text on psychology ethics, Keith-Spiegel and Koocher[51] make relatively brief mention of computers. While they define computer applications more narrowly than we do, they did note the universal temptation of users to adopt computer-generated results simply because they "look good." Although not well studied, there seems to be a propensity among users to attribute high levels of precision and accuracy to the computer, at times in spite of good judgment and common sense. One of the challenges to software designers has been to promote computer use while stressing infallibility and educating users about their vital role in interpreting computer results ("garbage in, garbage out"). Ironically, however, the mistaken notion of computer infallibility may represent a powerful tool in shaping health behavior change (if the computer said it, it must be true!).

Public welfare is another area of ethical concern. Some would argue that the use of computers is an unhealthy behavior. In a study of physiological measures during typical computer use, Emurian[52] observed that data clerks and college students showed autonomic changes similar to the "anger" component of Type A behavior. From this research, he concluded that repeated use of computers may lead to blood pressure elevations that pose a risk for coronary heart disease. His research, however, did not include control groups of students and clerks using other media to do their work; therefore, the apparent negative impact of computers may have been simply a negative impact of desk work. There have been earnest efforts among computer manufacturers to improve ergonomic designs and educate people about proper use of computers to avoid carpal tunnel syndrome, vision problems, headaches, and muscle tension. Nevertheless, if not unhealthy, computer use certainly is sedentary. In comparison to television and radio, however, computers are a less sedentary activity (at least mentally so), because programs can be interactive and require constant user input.

Colby[53] emphasized that the computer is simply a mechanical device and software is the medium needing study of ethical soundness. Indeed, the breadth of possible computer applications prevents any ethical analysis of computers in a general sense. The most popular concern about computers is their potential to "dehumanize" the frequent computer user. However, the complexity and interactive qualities of computer programs make them highly dependent on human input and decision-making. Therefore, it seems unlikely that computers will be capable of "dehumanizing" a person, at least in any measurable or direct way. Nevertheless, this remains a sticking point among computer nay-sayers. Although we might concede that technology is generally "nonhuman" and does not share human capacities, we see no reason to vilify the computer more than other forms of electronic gadgetry.

We might suggest that the use of computers in health care is only a small step in a century-long pattern of increased efficiency, mechanization, and changes in styles of professional communication. For example, in the early part of this century most contacts with physicians were made at home. This idealized physician, immortalized by Norman Rockwell, has now been replaced by a system that is less personalized and more specialized, and encourages rapid and efficient treatments. These changes in health care have been driven by population growth, limited resources, and a rapid growth in medical knowledge. Computer health services may well become a tool for customizing services to the individual needs of the consumer at relatively low cost . Whatever the future prevalence of computer health care services, it is unlikely that health care providers will ever be "replaced" by computers regardless of the nature of futuristic innovations. To illustrate, one might note that in "Star Trek," Gene Roddenberry's popular television epic describing his vision of the 25th century, a physician was cast as one of four principal characters.

Early investigations of computer attitudes found that individuals who opposed computer technology attributed their opposition to the fear of being dehumanized by the computer.[54,55] More recent work suggests that attitudes may be changing.[56] However, this work also suggests that attitudes may be improving more rapidly among males than among females. In addition, most work on computer attitudes has been conducted with younger populations of students, where improvement would be most likely. Nevertheless, work with Alzheimer's disease caregivers[10] with a mean age of 68 years supports the notion that there can be acceptance and use of computer support networks by those who are not typical computer users. Indeed, the successful diffusion of computer technology in many settings in recent years suggests that the threat of dehumanizing features is easily overcome simply by the overwhelming utility of the computer. While it is beyond the scope of this chapter, it will be important for future researchers to focus on how efficiently and effectively computerized interventions are accepted by various populations. Theories such as Rogers' diffusion of innovation theory[57] may provide a framework for such research. In such models, it will be important to consider attitudes such as dehumanization.

Summary and Conclusions

We are no longer experiencing a computer "revolution" — computers have already won the "war" and have revolutionized how we access and use information. We have now entered an evolutionary phase of human–computer interactions in which computers have begun to affect the way in which the public gains access to professional guidance and support. While computers in the past were instrumental in guiding and facilitating medical research, computers now have a great potential for directly influencing our health and health behavior. One of the ultimate challenges of computers may be to help us with our own psychological problems, as in the case of computer psychotherapy. As this chapter has demonstrated, many forms of computer technology are already in place and in use. As both an educational device and a communications link, the computer has many advantages. However, the critical question still remains relatively unstudied: *What is the efficacy of the computer in providing direct health benefits?*

In this chapter, we have provided the reader with some empirical evidence that computerized self-help programs are efficacious in educating patients. However, the computer's ability to change health behavior and provide a means of social support is not as clearly documented. The majority of the studies have been conducted with small samples of special patient groups. In addition, most of the studies involved a serious selection bias because investigators used nonrepresentative convenience samples or polled only those expressing an a priori interest in computers. There is a great need for randomized empirical studies of computer health interventions for diverse and representative populations. In the meantime, we can draw conclusions only about the *efficacy* of computer interventions among those who participate; studies of *effectiveness* must consider both effect size and participation rates.

As we noted earlier, discussion/support groups have become very popular with computer network users. These groups may be particularly helpful for bedridden patients, patients with relatively rare disorders, and individuals living in isolated locations. Currently, computerized support groups exist without professional/trained group leaders. This lack of clinical leadership in the computer environment could lead to abuses by ill-meaning individuals or to the proliferation of misinformation. The electronic support group for Alzheimer's disease caregivers described previously[10] was particularly successful in incorporating a professional oversight function into their network group software. Future computer groups should incorporate similar safeguards. The strongest leadership in safeguarding against computer abuses of this nature may come from the same nonprofit patient groups that currently sponsor face-to-face support groups.

Clinicians work with ill patients, not disease syndromes. While providing care, clinicians must consider a broad spectrum of biological, social, and psychological factors in diagnosis and treatment. Computer software, as an instrument of both clinicians and patients, must be written to consider the complex interplay of factors associated with health and health behavior. Implementation of computers in direct service to patients should be carefully planned, patient groups should be discriminately targeted, and patient attitudes closely monitored. In our zeal to apply new forms of technology, we should resist the temptation to install patient software systems without carefully studying the short-term and long-term effects of these changes in the health care system. Preliminary evidence suggests that direct use of computer software by patients may provide some elegant, effective, and cost-saving approaches to health care.

Acknowledgments. Support for this work was provided by the Medical Research Service of the Department of Veterans Affairs and a fellowship awarded to William S. Shaw from the Sam and Rose Stein Institute for Research on Aging. The authors are especially grateful to Ms. Patricia Whitney for her help in preparing the chapter manuscript.

References

1. Pressey SL. A simple apparatus which gives tests and score-and-teaches. *School and Society.* 1926:23.
2. Skinner BF. Teaching machines. *Sci Am.* 1960;205:90–102.
3. Kaplan RM. Quality of life, resource allocation, and the U.S. health-care crisis. In Dimsdale JE, Baum A (eds.). Quality of Life in Behavioral Medicine Research. Perspectives in Behavioral Medicine. Hillsdale, NJ: Lawrence Erlbaum; 1995.
4. Short PF. *National Medical Expenditure Survey: Estimates of the Uninsured Population, Calendar Year 1987: Data Summary 2.* Rockville: National Center for Health Services Research and Health Care Technology Assessment; 1990.
5. Regier DA, Goldberg ID, Taube CA. The de facto U.S. mental health services system. *Arch Gen Psychiatry.* 1978;35:685–693.
6. Tröster AI, Paolo AM, Glatt SL, Hubble JP, Koller WC. "Interactive video conferencing" in the provision of neuropsychological services to rural areas. *J Commun Psych* 1995;23:85–88.
7. Anderson R, Newman JF. Societal and individual determinants of medical care utilization in the United States. *Millbank Memorial Fund Quart/Health Society* 1973;51:94–124.
8. U.S. Department of Commerce, Economics and Statistics Administration, Bureau of the Census, Statistical Abstract of the United States; 1994.
9. Anderson B. Programming in the home of the future. *Int J Man-Machine Studies.* 1980;12:341–365.
10. Brennan P, Moore S, Smyth K. Computerlink: Electronic support for the home caregiver. *Adv Nurs Sci.* 1991;13:14–27.
11. Ellis LBM, Raines JR, Hakanson N. Health education using microcomputers: One year in the clinic. *Prev Med.* 1982;11:212–223.
12. Cronan TA, Shaw WS, Gallagher RA, Weisman M. Predicting health care use among older osteoarthritis patients in an HMO. *Arthritis Care and Research.* 1995;8:66–72.
13. Cohen PA. Computer-based instruction and health professions education: A meta-analysis of outcomes. *Evaluation & the Health Professions.* 1992;15:259–281.
14. Meier S, Scott T, Simpson JP. Use of computer-assisted instruction in the prevention of alcohol abuse. *J Drug Educ.* 1989;19:245–256.

15. Meier S. Alcohol education through computer-assisted instruction. *J Couns Dev.* 1984;66:141–144.
16. Reynolds N. *The Alcohol IQ Network (computer program).* Ithaca: Cornell University Health Services; 1988.
17. Thomas B. *Drinking and Not Drinking* (computer program). Santa Barbara: Kinko's Academic Courseware Exchange; 1987.
18. Alemi F, Cherry F, Meffert G. Rehearsing decisions may help teenagers: An evaluation of a simulation game. *Comput Biol Med.* 1989;19:283–290.
19. Binik YM, Servan-Schreiber D, Freiwald S, Hall KSK. Intelligent computer-based assessment and psychotherapy: An expert system for sexual dysfunction. *J Nervous Mental Disease* 1988;176:387–400.
20. Horan P, Yarborough M, Besigel G, Carlson D. Computer-assisted self-control of diabetes by adolescents. *Diabetes Educ.* 1989;16:205–211.
21. Mazzuca SA, Moorman NH, Wheeler ML, et al. The Diabetes Education Study: A controlled trial of the effect of diabetes patient education. *Diabetes Care* 1986;9:1–10.
22. Schmittling G. Computer use by family physicians in the United States. *J Family Prac.* 1984;19:93–97.
23. Peters R. Attitudes of community mental-health staff toward computers. *Can J Commun Mental Health.* 1990;9:155–162.
24. Skinner C, Siegfried JC, Kegler MC, Strecher VJ. The potential of computers in patient education. *Patient Ed. Counseling.* 1993;22:27–34.
25. Chen MS Jr, Houston TP, Burson JL, Comer RC. Microcomputer-based patient education programs for family practice. *J Family Practie.* 1984; 18:149–150.
26. Jones RB, Edgerton E, Baxter I, et al. Where should a public access health information system be sited? *Interac Comput.* 1993;5:413–421.
27. Petzel SV, Ellis LB, Budd JR, Johnson Y. Microcomputers for behavioral health education: Developing and evaluating patient education for the chronically ill. *Comput Human Services.* 1992;8:167–183.
28. Bosworth K, Gustafson DH, Hawkins RP, Chewing B, Day T. Adolescents, health education, and computers: The body awareness resource network (BARN). *Health Ed.* 1983;14:58–60.
29. Wheeler ML, Wheeler LA. Computer-planned menus for patients with diabetes mellitus. *Diabetes Care.* 1980;3:663–667.
30. Kinzie MB, Schorling JB, Siegel M. Prenatal alcohol education for low-income women with interactive multimedia. *Patient Ed Counsel.* 1993; 21:51–60.
31. Bandura A. *Social Foundations of Thought and Action. Englewood Cliffs: Prentice-Hall;* 1986.
32. Bandura A. *Social Learning Theory.* Englewood Cliffs: Prentice-Hall; 1977.
33. Becker MH. The health belief model and sick role behavior. *Health Edu Monographs.* 1974;2:409–419.
34. McGuire WJ. Public communication as a strategy for inducing health-promoting behavioral change. *Prev Med.* 1984;13:299–319.
35. Lynch WJ. Ecological validity of cognitive rehabilitation software. *J Head Trauma Rehabil.* 1992;7:36–45.
36. Fisher LA, Johnson TS, Porter D, Bleich HL, Slack WV. Collection of a clean voided urine specimen: A comparison among spoken, written and computer-based instructions. *Am J Public Health.* 1977;67:640–644.

37. Colby KM, Gould RL, Aronson G. Some pros and cons of computer-assisted psychotherapy. *J Nervous Mental Disease.* 1989;177:105–108.

38. Burnett KF, Taylor CB, Agras WS. Ambulatory computer-assisted therapy for obesity: A new frontier for behavior therapy. *J Consult Clin Psychol.* 1985; 53:698–703.

39. Selmi PM, Klein MH, Greist JH, Sorrell S, Erdman H. Computer-administered cognitive-behavioral therapy for depression. *Am J Psychiatry.* 1990;147:51–56.

40. Gottlieb BH. Social network strategies in prevention. *Psychiatric Epidemiol Prevention: Possibilities.* 1985:53–64.

41. Kulik JA, Mahler HI. Social support and recovery from surgery. *Health Psychol.* 1989;8:221–238.

42. Kiesler S, Siegel J, McQuire TW. Social psychological aspects of computer-mediated communication. *Am Psychologist.* 1984;39:1123–1134.

43. Turkle S. *The Second Self: Computers and the Human Spirit.* New York: Simon & Schuster; 1984.

44. Hall JA, Dornan MC. What patients like about their medical care and how often they are asked: A meta-analysis of the satisfaction literature. *Soc Sci Med.* 1988;27:935–939.

45. Kaplan SH, Greenfield S, Ware JE. Assessing the effects of physician-patient interactions on the outcomes of chronic disease. *Med Care* 1989;27:S220–S227.

46. Ghosh A, Greist JH. Computer treatment in psychiatry. *Psychiatr Ann.* 1988; 18:246–250.

47. Colby K, Colby P, Stoller R. Dialogues in natural language with GURU, a psychologic inference engine. *Philosophical Psychol.* 1990;3:171–186.

48. Gaffin A. *Electronic Frontier Foundation's Guide to the Internet.* Version 3.1 [online], Available at: http://www.eff.org/pub/net_Net_Guid/netguid.eff.; 1995.

49. Buhle EL, Goldwein JW, Benjamin I. OncoLink: A multimedia oncology information resource on the Internet. *Proc Annu Symp Comput Appl Med Care* 1994:103–107.

50. Internet Society. Internet Society Charts and Statistics [online]. Available at: ftp:/ftp.soc.org/isoc/charts/; 1995.

51. Keith-Spiegel P, Koocher GP. *Ethics in Psychology.* Hillsdale, New Jersey: Lawrence Erlbaum Associates; 1985.

52. Emurian HH. Human-computer interactions: Are there adverse health consequences? *Comput Human Behav.* 1989;5:265–275.

53. Colby K. Ethics of computer-assisted psychotherapy. *Psychiatr Ann.* 1986; 16:414–415.

54. Nickerson RS. Why interactive computer systems are sometimes not used by people who might benefit from them. *Int J Man-Machine Studies.* 1981; 15:469–483.

55. Wagman M. A factor analytic study of the psychological implications of the computer for the individual and society. *Behav Res Meth Instrumentation.* 1983;15:413–419.

56. Siguardsson JF. Computer experience, attitudes toward computers and personality characteristics in psychology undergraduates. *Person Individ Diff.* 1991; 12:617–624.

57. Rogers E. *Diffusion of Innovation Theory.* 3rd ed. New York: Free Press; 1983.

13

Electronic Communities of Patients: Computer Services Through Telephones

Farrokh Alemi and Richard C. Stephens

Numerous studies have shown that computers can reduce the cost of health care, improve quality of services, and increase access to care.[1] However, because computers have not been widely available, their demonstrated promise has not been realized. Recently, computer technology has changed. Computers can now play back recorded messages, and talking computers are accessible through any touchtone telephone. Computers used to talk to each other; now they can talk to human beings. These developments have created new opportunities for computers in health care delivery. Almost overnight, we have come to a new realization: every household can use a standard telephone to access a growing number of computer services (Fig. 13.1).

Most people are familiar with a telephone. Voice-interactive, or talking computers, enable one to call a computer, listen to a description of menu choices, and select an option by pressing numbers on the telephone pad. Not all interactions need be based on menu choices. Sometimes the computer questions are open ended, in which case, a caller's answers are recorded for later transcription. At other times, voice recognition is used.

When computer services are delivered through telephones, one computer can serve a large number of households. Patients do not need to buy a computer or set up new networking equipment. Computer services accessed through a standard touchtone telephone—without computers and without modems—may be referred to as telecommunications aids. The widespread availability of telecommunication aids, the low cost of creating distributed networks through existing telephone line connections, and the low cost of hardware (no need for a computer in every home) have made the technology

Disclosure. Cleveland State University has transferred the ownership of systems described here to TelePractice, and Farrokh Alemi, Ph.D. holds minority share of the company. This chapter is adapted from a similar article by Farrokh Alemi and Richard Stephens entitled "Computer services for patients: Description of systems and summary of findings," in *Medical Care;* 34(10), Supplement. Used by permission of Lippincott-Raven Publishers.

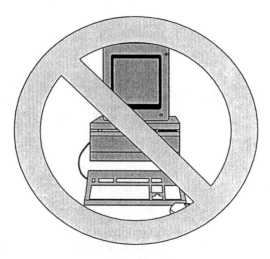

FIGURE **13.1.** Equipment needed by the patients.

not only possible but a viable mass medium. The question then is, "Who cares?" What can we do with this new medium that we couldn't do before and what benefit does it have beyond entertainment value?

In four major projects (Extended Case Management of Cocaine-Abusing Pregnant Patients, All Kids Count, CMHA Electronic Community, and AVIVA Health Risk Appraisal) and several other smaller projects, a team of researchers at Cleveland State University has developed a number of computer services through the telephone. This chapter reports the major findings of these researchers and speculates on how the new technology will require a different type of clinical practice pattern. The various computer systems described here constitute the building blocks of what some of us have come to call the "Telecommunication Practice Model": a practice pattern in which clinicians use computer services delivered through a standard telephone to address patients' medical, prevention, and self-care needs in the community and without a visit.

The technology seems simple—after all, most people are familiar with a telephone and to claim that this device will radically change practice patterns may seem farfetched. But the telephone itself has changed: it can now act as a window to computer services. Some may feel that technology can change without substantially influencing how health care is delivered. But first impressions may be deceiving. Changes in technology and in the organization of health care delivery go hand in hand; both the technology and the organization must change to provide quality services at the lowest cost. An analogy may illustrate this point. In the past, people walked to reach their destinations. When carts were designed, they were designed not with legs, but with wheels. The designers thought about transportation in a new way, and as a result, they not only solved an immediate transportation problem but also eventually changed our ideas about where and how far we wanted to go. Likewise, the computer systems described in this chapter abandon some existing health care practices (e.g., scheduling a follow-up visit, always requiring a visit to the doctor before laboratory tests are ordered for patients), emphasize other practices (active triage in the community), and introduce new practices (peer to peer education).

Still another example may highlight the point better: in one of our projects the computer reminded patients to keep their appointments. The system was so effective in bringing patients to the clinic that we were asked to stop the process! Too many patients were showing up. The entire scheduling system had to change because now when we scheduled 100 patients 82 showed instead of the few that used to show. Overscheduling of the patients was no longer a reasonable approach.

In this chapter, we will describe the telecommunication tools that we have used, review the empirical data on the impact of these tools, and discuss the implication of these tools for the organization of clinics. But before we discuss any of these topics, let's clear away the misconceptions that many have about patients' reactions to computer services.

Patients' Reactions to Computers

When discussing our work, the first reaction of clinicians, especially if they have not worked with computers, is that patients don't like interacting with computers. Critics describe a number of negative experiences with computers: "I hang up when computers call me to sell things." "Computerized telephone menus are frustrating, patients want to talk to people." Some critics argue that patients, especially those who turn to the health care system for care and not cure, will resist talking to computers.

Patients' reactions to computers are not simple. They may like some computers more than others. In addition, because clinicians often speak on behalf of patients, the issue of appropriateness of computer interviews may depend on the clinician's willingness to allow these innovations.

For the most part, the aids discussed in this chapter seem to patients more like interrelated answering machines than computers. Most of the proposed systems involve a short interaction with a computer followed by a free-form interaction with other people through the computer. Our data show that these aids are welcomed by most patients. When hard-to-reach individuals were asked to compare our computer calling them to an answering machine, or a computer sales call, they rated our services positively and similar to those of an answering machine, whereas they almost uniformly expressed a negative attitude toward computer sales calls.[2]

But some of the systems presented in this chapter (e.g., the patient assessment system) require that patients interact with the computer for a more extended period of time as they choose responses from fixed menus. Many fear that computerized assessment will anger and frustrate clients who have turned to the health care system in part because they needed human care and attention.

However, the data indicate that contrary to expectations, patients prefer computerized telephone assessments[3-6] and CRT-based computer assessments to assessments conducted by an interviewer.[7-16] This is especially true when patients must report on confidential matters (such as drug use, sexual preferences, suicidal thoughts, etc.).[17] Such preferences have been known since the late 1960s and have been demonstrated in far too many studies to be considered simply an artifact. One explanation for such preferences is that computer interviews are nonjudgmental, whereas clinicians, because of their status, may be perceived as judgmental. Another explanation is that patients prefer the self-paced, self-administered nature of computer interviews. Still another explanation is that patients prefer a nonverbal interaction because it helps them be more introspective. Whatever the reason, it is clear that computer interviews are liked by patients.

Our own experience is also telling.[18] We created AVIVA—a system for automatically interviewing patients about their health risks, advising them about what lifestyle they should change, and referring them elsewhere. Subjects' reactions to AVIVA were compared to reactions to receiving health information from magazines, television, or a health professional. Data were collected from a stratified random sample of 96 males and females who included faculty, professional, and non-professional staff from Cleveland State University. When subjects received a postcard and a letter announcing the availability of AVIVA, the majority (71 percent) used it. Those who did not use AVIVA gave various reasons for this (some did not use the system because they could not read the material mailed to them). Less than 4 percent did not participate in AVIVA because they objected to a computer giving advice on health risks. Those who used the system rated AVIVA as more accurate, easier to understand, more convenient, more affordable, easier to use, and more accessible than health education received from television, magazines, or health professionals. (See Table 13.1 for details.)

These data in Table 13.1 clearly show that subjects are open to and like computer interviews about their health risks, do not mind receiving advice from a computer, and prefer this to existing sources of health education. Our experiences confirm the finding that patients, once familiarized with the technology, accept and enjoy it.

Ironically, the most negative reactions to computers advising patients and triaging them to care come from patient advocates (some clinicians, newspaper journalists, and lawyers). An example can serve to illustrate this. At the beginning of our research, one local newspaper, *The Plain Dealer,* reported our funding on its first page and one of its editors wrote a very negative opinion claiming that we planned to reduce drug use by calling cocaine addicts and asking them to stop.[19] The writer went on to ridicule the

TABLE **13.1.** Average rating of source of health education (number of subjects are given in parentheses).

Dimensions	Control	AVIVA users
Accurate*	3.5(42)	4.2(35)
Current	4.0(43)	4.3(35)
Easy to understand*	3.9(43)	4.5(35)
Enjoyable	3.2(41)	3.7(35)
Convenient**	3.5(42)	4.3(34)
Affordable***	3.6(40)	5.0(35)
Easy to use	3.7(41)	4.4(35)
Interesting	3.7(42)	4.1(35)
Accessible*	4.0(42)	4.7(35)
Accomplishment	3.1(41)	3.6(35)
Involvement	3.1(40)	3.3(35)

All scales had a possible range of 1 to 6, with 6 being the best possible score. *, **, and ***, respectively, denote differences that were statistically significant for a one-sided test at the 0.025, 0.01, and 0.001 (alpha) levels.

project as an example of how Congress wastes tax payers' money on projects that are doomed. Now, there was some truth to their claim that we planned to call drug users, but that was the extent of their understanding of what we planned to do. We planned to call patients and provide them with information, but we also were going to provide drug treatment, prenatal care, pediatric care, home monitoring, home health education, and a host of other case management interventions. Shortly after the media attention, drug treatment groups organized a boycott of our work and refused to allow their patients to participate. Eventually the boycott broke and we were able to recruit patients and conduct our work. Contrary to the editor's claim, the data showed that patients liked our services, used our services, and these services improved their care. The self-appointed advocates of patients took a position different from the wishes and the best interests of these patients. So, do patients resist computer interviews? No, and certainly not as much as their advocates do.

Satisfaction with a computer system depends on how the system is organized. Most individuals are familiar with computer calls only through telephone marketing. Because these marketing calls are frustrating, most people think that if a computer calls, they will hang up on it. But consider the circumstances of marketing calls. Often they arrive at unwanted times, interrupting other activities, and furthermore, they are about topics of little interest to the receiver. Thus, it is not surprising that people hang up on these calls. Similarly, when a salesman shows up at the door, in the middle of dinner, and tries to sell you something that you do not need, you tell him to go away. If he were to come back every other day, you would naturally be frustrated. The point is that your frustration is not with the door-to-door salesman's existence, but with what he is selling and with his lack of judgment and timing. The same applies to computerized telephone calls. Computers that call when the patient has asked, deliver messages that the patient cares for, and do so in a reliable fashion are not frustrating.

When we asked drug-using pregnant patients if they were satisfied with computer services, the answer was a resounding "yes." They not only didn't mind that a computer called them and interacted with them, but they were angry when because of the unavailability of funds we had to discontinue our electronic job announcement system.

In the end, the most obvioius test of whether patients are satisfied with computer services over the telephone is their use patterns. In our studies, the systems (with some exceptions) were used heavily, as much as twice every week.

Description of Telecommunication Aids

We have designed and put in use telecommunication aids that affect different aspects of patient care. These include the following.

Community Health Rap

This system educates patients at home. Clients call the computer and record a question. The computer alerts experts who, at their convenience, record a response. The computer calls the client back with the response and keeps both the question and response in a public area, where other registered patients, who have not yet articulated their questions, can listen and benefit. Here is an example of an interaction that occurred in Community Health Rap:

Computer: "The public message forum is not for emergency use. Your question will be recorded in your own voice and be available on the system for others to listen. Cleveland State University does not guarantee that the answers or messages you receive in this forum are accurate and appropriate for your particular situation. To ask a question, press 1; to listen to questions and answers, press 2; to exit, press 3."

Caller: [Select asking a question by pressing 1].

Computer: "For pregnancy issues, press 1; for child care, press 2; for drug abuse issues, press 3, for other areas, press 4."

Caller: [Select asking a pregnancy-related question by pressing 1.]

Computer: "Record your question at the beep and press the pound key when finished."

Caller: "I came back from clinic and they told me I have cervical cancer. What is that?" [Caller presses the pound key.]

Computer: Thank you. We will call you back when an answer to your question has been recorded. [The computer alerts an expert that there is a question to be answered.]

Conference Calls

This system allows clients who cannot come to face-to-face meetings to participate in self-help and support group meetings through a telephone conference. Patients obtain a password valid at a particular time of a day from their provider. At the specified time, patients call a telephone switchboard, which then connects all patients calling with the same password to a telephone conference.

Talknet

This system enables patients to participate in self-help and support groups from the convenience of their home and without the need for coordinating schedules. Patients record a title for their group and thereafter record messages under that title for each other. Callers hear the last few recorded messages in a first-in first-out basis and can skip a message by pressing the pound key. Here is an example of an interaction that occurred after a client selected the Talknet system:

Computer: "For *what makes me feel good about myself* [italic is in the voice of a previous caller], press 1; for *dealing with the death of a loved one,* press 2; for *the Long Island killings,* press 3; for *abusive relationships,* press 4; for a new topic, press 5."

Caller: [Caller selects listening to the ongoing discussion about abusive relationships and presses 5.]

Computer: "[In the voice of another caller] . . . *Once you give that person that's abusing you the control and the right to violate you, it's over. You might as well reconsider abusing yourself. You are giving the person the right to beat you, that's not right. You have a choice, you have decisions. It's hard [pause] people have got to stop thinking about what they are going to lose and what they are going to have to do without. I mean, you might not have your life. . . .*" [Computer beeps to designate end of message.]

Computer: "[In the voice of still another caller]. *Yeah, hello. I want to comment on abusive relationships. Abusive relationships is wrong to me, but number one, you can't comment on it unless you've been in it [laughs, background voices and some more laughter].* [The computer beeps.]

Computer: "[In the voice of yet another caller]. *Hi, I am responding to abusive relationships, and I would like to comment on that — abusive relationships. I lived in an abusive relationship with my mother and my father because my father beat my mother all the time, you know. So, it was seven of us and all we could do was stand around and cry because my father had that much fear in us. So, when I got older, all we said that I would never get into an abusive relationship. Well, I've got an 11-year-old daughter. I found out with her father, he loved me, he loved me real hard and then things got to the point where, you know, he would get so [sighing] bent out of shape by the things that I would do that he would retaliate on me. But, you know, I went through that for maybe a little while and I got out of that relationship — well, in and out of the relationship and after that, I always made up my mind that I would never fall back into an abusive relationship, but you never really know, you know, until the things start happening. . ."*

Caller: [Caller presses pound (#) key to skip the rest of the comments.]
Computer: [The computer starts with the next message in the discussion. When all messages are played back the computer asks the following.] "To add a comment, press 1; to exit, press 2."

Announcements

One way of motivating patients to participate in self-care is to send them testimonials from other patients who have done so and have succeeded. We have developed a system to broadcast a message to all or a subset of patients.

Care Mail

One of the most important and easiest aids is to provide a voice mail box to every patient and every clinician caring for the patient. With such mail boxes, providers and clinicians can record messages for patients, but the computer takes over the difficult and frustrating task of locating the individual and delivering the message. Clinicians can use the voice mail system to query patients and monitor them at home. An example may illustrate how the system can be used to reach patients.

A provider records a message for the client asking her how she is feeling. The computer either calls or pages the client at the client's preferred calling times. Once a call is initiated, one of several situations may result. If the computer reaches a busy signal, it is programmed to call back in 5 minutes. If there is no answer, it will try to call again in 1 hour. If a person answers the telephone and then hangs up, the computer will call back in 24 hours. And if it reaches an answering machine, it will leave a message and then try to call back the next day. If a person answers the call and does not hang up, he or she will hear:

Computer: "This is the phone service at Cleveland State University. If you are [first name of client], press 1 now. If she will come to the phone shortly, press 2 now. If she is not there, press 3 now. If you don't know this person or need other assistance, press *0 now, or call us at [gives a staff telephone number]. To hear this message again, press *R."
Caller.   [The person who answers the telephone presses 1].
Computer: "Please enter your password and press the pound key."

When the identity of the caller has been established (a correct password has been entered), the computer will deliver the message. The caller will be able to keep, delete, immediately answer, verify who sent the message, or listen again to the message. If the caller decides to answer, she will record a message and the computer will deliver the message to the clinician.

Assessment

We have developed a system for assessing patients over the telephone at regular intervals. The computer calls the patient's home, verifies the identity of the respondent, and interviews the patient by playing recorded questions; the client answers by pressing keys on the telephone pad. An artificial intelligence package analyzes the responses and sends a facsimile to the patient's clinician. A sample interaction with the computer follows:

> Computer: "This is the assessment system. Your doctor has asked us to call you to collect information in anticipation of your upcoming visit. Please answer by pressing the keys on your telephone pad; if you do not have a touch tone telephone, please call us at [gives a staff telephone number]."
> "How old are you?"
> Caller: [Enters 3 and 7 for 37-year-old]
> Computer: [Continues questioning.]

Follow-Up

One way of monitoring patient conditions is to record a follow-up question every time one has had a contact with the patient. The follow-up system calls the patient, asks the recorded question, collects the response in a data base, and sends a recorded message to the case manager if the answer indicates a need for intervention.

Reminders

One way of improving patients' compliance is to remind them about their care. The computer calls the patient's home, verifies that the respondent is the patient, and reminds the patient to (1) make an appointment or (2) keep an appointment. If the patient cannot keep an appointment, the computer calls the person who set the appointment to cancel the appointment. The computer calls back in a few days with a reminder to make a new appointment. If the patient does not show up for an appointment, the computer contacts the patient with a reminder to make a new appointment.

Information and Referral

The computer records a description of the need, then either sequentially or simultaneously calls all numbers on a list of agencies to poll them to see if they can help. It maintains a waiting list for all the referrals to the agency until an admissions person from the agency calls in, listens to the referrals, and accepts or denies the referrals.

Key Findings

The fact that new technology exists is not a reason to use it. Progress in technology has raised questions about what role computers should play for patients, what are the patterns of use of the technology, and what benefits are associated with these new telecommunication systems.

Telecommunication Aids Brought Drug-Using Mothers to Treatment

In one of our first studies,[20] we examined the combined impact of Care Mail, Community Health Rap, Telephone Conferences/Talknet, Announcements, and Follow-up on the care of 179 drug-using pregnant patients. Patients were randomly assigned to control and experimental groups; only the experimental group had access to the telecommunication systems. Patients were enrolled during the prenatal period and followed for 6 months after the birth of a live child. Patients were interviewed at enrollment, at delivery, and at 6 months after delivery. Self-reported data were collected on subjects' participation in drug treatment programs, subjects' health status (using short form developed in the medical outcome study[21]) and subjects' addiction severity (using the Addiction Severity Index). The computer also collected data on the frequency of use of the telecommunication systems.

Systems were used regularly by patients, with one exception. The telephone conference system was not used despite repeated efforts to organize this type of group meeting. As a consequence of the failure of telephone conference system, we created Talknet and allowed patients to use Talknet to organize asynchronous discussion groups. Care mail, Announcement, and Follow-up were used on average 2.3 times per week per person by the patients. Community Health Rap was used 0.2 times per person per week to leave a question and 1.9 times to listen to questions.

Multiple and logistic regressions were used to identify the effects of the intervention after controlling for demographic and baseline variables. The dependent variables were participation in formal treatment during the course of the project and drug and alcohol use at exit interview. Variables were blocked so that variation was first explained by other variables and last by the intervention. The data showed that poor, drug-using pregnant, undereducated clients could use the services, and about 45 percent of the clients used the services more than three times a week. Mere access to the

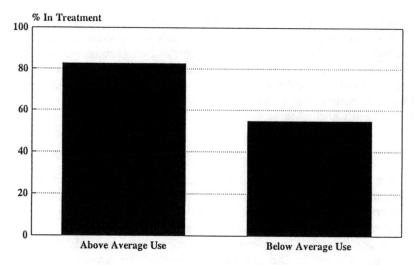

78 cocaine addicted pregnant patients.

FIGURE **13.2.** More network use, more treatment compliance.

system did not lead to any significant differences between the control and the experimental groups. But the use of the system did.

Subjects who used the systems more than 3 times a week were 1.5 times more likely to show up for formal drug treatment (see Fig. 13.2). There seemed to be a threshold after which the use of the systems had a more positive impact on treatment compliance. However, despite our success in bringing patients to drug treatment, participation in formal drug treatment was not effective in reducing drug or alcohol use in this population.

Computers Helped Answer Health Questions from Drug-Using Parents

To focus attention on specific telecommunication systems, the second study[22] analyzed data from the study reported above to examine the use of one of the systems: Community Health Rap (CHR). We evaluated the utilization of the CHR by 82 pregnant, Medicaid-dependent, drug-using or recovering women for whom a 6-month post delivery follow-up interview had been completed.

Forty-five percent of experimental subjects utilized CHR. Among those who used the system, 38 percent asked questions, and 89 percent listened to health messages. Use of the system varied considerably. The median number of health messages listened to per experimental subject per month was 1.7, the mean was 7.1, and the standard deviation was 10.9. According to this data, almost half of subjects used the system.

The impact of CHR on health status was examined by comparing randomly chosen patients who had access to CHR to a randomly chosen comparison group with no access. Analysis of covariance was used to control for baseline differences between the two groups. No statistically significant difference was found between the control and the experimental group in terms of health status or drug use. Therefore, we concluded that this component of the telecommunication systems did not lead to a change in the clent's health status.

Electronics Support Groups Reduced Cost of Care

In the third study,[23] we examined the use of Talknet (electronic and asynchronous discussion groups). A portion of the 179 drug-using pregnant patients in the first study were approached roughly 2 years after their first enrollment to participate in a new study and 53 volunteered to do so. Clients in the control group were asked to participate in biweekly face-to-face meetings. Clients in the experimental group participated in the voice bulletin board. The content of communications among the experimental group was recorded and utterances were classified as to the type of communication. Clients were paid to complete baseline and exit questionnaires; 94 percent completed the exit questionnaires. Subjects reported their level of drug use, health status, and utilization of health services. They also reported on their symptoms, attitudes toward use of physician services, loneliness, willingness to disclose information in groups, and sense of solidarity with their group.

On the average, experimental clients used the bulletin board 2.18 times per week; 96 percent of the clients used the bulletin board. We used analysis of covariance to statistically control for differences between control and the experimental group at base line. Results reported in Fig. 13.3 showed that clients were more likely to participate in the voice bulletin board than in the face-to-face meeting (alpha < 0.005).

The mean number of people who participated biweekly in the voice bulletin board was 8.09 times higher than the number in the face-to-face group. The majority (54.6 percent) of the comments left in the bulletin board were for emotional support for each other. There was as much expression of emotional suport in the early parts of the meetings as in the later parts. No "flaming" or overt disagreements occurred. The more clients participated in the voice bulletin board, the more they felt a sense of solidarity with each other (alpha < 0.001).

Members of the experimental group reported significantly lower rates of use of health services than members of the control group (alpha < 0.06). Lower utilization of services did not lead to poorer health status or more drug use (see Fig. 13.4).

These data suggest that voice bulletin boards may be an effective method of providing support to drug-using or recovering addicts and that electronic

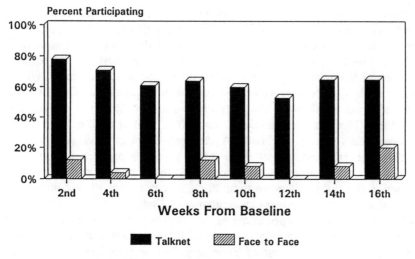

FIGURE **13.3.** Participation in self-help groups.

support groups reduce the use of health services without any apparent impact on the health status of patients.

Computer Reminders Increased Ontime Immunization by 23 Percent

The fourth study,[24] examined the impact of computer reminders on on-time immunization rates. We included in the experimental group 119 consecutive

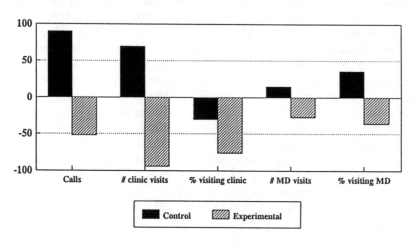

FIGURE **13.4.** Impact on use of services. All findings significant at 0.05 level. Analysis of covariance controlled for initial base line values.

infants who were less than 6 months of age, were being seen at the outpatient clinic for a first visit, and were patients of three attending physicians and three nurse practitioners. These infants were compared to 77 infants from the same clinic who were under 6 months of age and seen for the first visit during the same time period by the same providers. Unlike earlier studies, patients were not selected based on drug use. Patients were selected from mothers in the outpatient clinic of Rainbow Babies and Children's Hospital of Cleveland, an urban pediatric clinic that serves predominantly minority clients. A research assistant reviewed patients' medical records and collected birthday, mother's age, race, source of payments, and the immunization record. Immunization was considered to be late if the child was more than 30 days past any of the recommended immunizations of the American Academy of Pediatrics.

The show rate for appointments for the experimental group was 82 percent, while the comparison patients of these providers, during the same time period, had a show rate of 69 percent. The on-time immunization rate for experimental subjects was 68 percent, while the comparison group had a rate of 45.5 percent (differences were significant at alpha levels lower than 0.001). These data suggest that computerized reminders led to an increase in on-time immunization.

Summary of Findings

The findings described here were surprising to us: when we first started we did not expect that these systems would be used, much less have an impact. But they were used, and used by uneducated, poor, drug-using patients – a population that is extremely hard to reach. Because our computer would call patients, the use of voice mail was not surprising. What was more surprising was the use of the Talknet system, where patients called in on their own initiative. The heavy use of this system suggests that electronic support groups are addressing an unmet patient need.

Another surprise was how the use of some of the systems affected care outcomes. Participants in the combined Care Mail, Announcement, Follow-up, and Community Health Rap group were more likely to show up for formal drug treatment. Participants in Talknet had the same health status as the control group but much lower utilization of services. Participants in the reminder system had more on-time immunization rates. Despite these positive results, the question of the impact of telecommunication systems on care of patients seems naive to us. The real question is, why there should be an impact. For example, why should participation in electronic support groups lead to lower use of some health care services? What is the mechanism that leads to these results? Several theoretical models have been proposed to explain how social support affects care but these theories need to be reexamined in the context of electronic communications. Without a theory we have two phenomena that co-occur without any explanation of why they should.

Our data indicated that systems differ in impact. Experimental studies need to be devised to explore which component of a system makes a difference and for whom. Anecdotal data indicate that the use of the system depended on a variable that we did not measure: the content of messages being sent to the patient. Future researchers need to control more carefully for differences in the content. In short, the telecommunication systems described here are the medium, not the message. What makes a difference for people is the message, and studies need to examine the messages being sent.

These studies found associations between use of the system and outcomes of care, but readers should not interpret these findings as causal relationships. Further, because subjects decided to use the system on their own accord, self-selection may explain some of the relationships observed in the studies reported here. The generalizability of the findings needs to be established more clearly.

Implications for Organization of Practices

We had to evaluate the new technology in an environment where less than 1 percent of the patient load was accessible via the new system. A more appropriate test would require having the entire patient load on the system, so that the use of the electronic network would be the norm and not the exception. Then, patients and clinicians would be in the habit of going through the computer services for their care, and doing anything else would be unusual. We do not have experience with such complete adoption of the new technology (a project to enroll every new mother in Cleveland is underway), but in the remainder of this chapter we speculate about the future so that we, as a society, can think about where these technologies are taking us.

More Remote Management of Patients

One obvious impact of the new technology is that clinicians, especially physicians, will be more involved in remote management of patients in the community. Remote management of patients is not new. Clinicians have used telephones to manage patients, but mostly they have done so for prescription refill, prevention assessment, and triage. In the telecommunication practice model, remote management means a great deal more, including allowing the computer to collect a history, signs, and symptoms, allowing visiting nurses in the community to report on their physical examination of the patient, directing patients to appropriate laboratories for needed tests and allowing laboratories to report the results to the physician, advising patients over the telephone, prescribing medicine over the telephone, and allowing computers to automatically follow-up with the patient.

Life for physicians will be different than before. Traditionally, physicians have attended to the care of patients who visited them. Under this practice model clinicians will direct a host of services in the community including mobile test units, home test kits, pharmacy services, triage decisions, and visiting nurses. Many clinicians will contact the patient and some even may meet with the patient, but the role of the patient's physician will be to orchestrate these services and analyze the data from these services, *not* to actually deliver the services. In the end, the primary care physician may spend most of his or her time in a communication center, not with patients. Are physicians ready for this? No. Is this change necessary?

There are too many benefits to remote management for us to ignore it. First, it promises to reduce the costs of care by reducing capital costs (fewer visits mean smaller clinics) and improving the efficiency of services through better triage decisions (the computer will help the patient see the physician after and not before a laboratory test is done, thus avoiding unnecessary visits). Second, remote management will reduce the spread of infection. When patients do not wait together in a common area, the chances of iatrogenic infections are reduced. Third, with remote management, patients can remain at home, where they are most comfortable. And finally, if remote management is more protocol based (especially the collection of medical history, signs, and symptoms), then it will be more standardized and possibly the quality of care will be better. If remote management is more convenient for the patient, costs less, and is of better quality, then it is likely to be a viable mode of practice. Obviously the benefits of remote management must be investigated further, but data from studies that have looked at some of the components of remote management suggest that there may be great benefits attached to it. For example, when physicians were asked to call patients instead of scheduling a follow-up visit, the cost of care of patients dropped by roughly one quarter, while their health status did not change.[25] In the existing atmosphere, a one-quarter drop in health care costs cannot be ignored.

The part that some physicians find hardest to accept, besides the role of the computer, is that in the new system of care they will be held accountable for the health of patients who may or may not visit them. Many physicians are now comfortable with being held accountable for the cost of care of patients in capitated plans. But these patients still visit them and ask their advice, and decisions about care are still made during the visit. In the new system, physicians will need to think about health issues of patients who are not in their office and who when contacted may not be pleased about the physician's meddling in their life. Physicians must be prepared to contact, advise, and care for noncompliant patients, because now they will know who is not taking their medications.

Remote management of patients increases the physical distance between the patient and physician yet makes the physician more accessible. Over time it will make the relationship between the physician and the patient a more lasting one.

Administrators Will Be Lonely

If patients are managed remotely, then clinicians do not need to come to the office; so why have an office at all! There will be a few small offices spread over the community to deal with rare occasions in which a clinic visit is necessary, but no real central clinics. Who will stay in the central office? Perhaps administrators and computer programmers. Administrators' main task will be to allocate funds, personnel time, and support systems to care for patients in the community. For example, if the clinician is expected to contact a patient for follow-up, then the time to make telephone calls must be scheduled on the clinician's workload, no matter where the physician is.

The Gatekeper Will Change

It used to be that you received health education through the physician's office. With the new technology, health educators have direct access to the patient and they are the first gateway to clinical care: they will refer patients to primary care physicians. This change in who makes referral decisions will also change the nature of practices. Today, there is a frenzied rush to sign up primary physicians to capitated or preferred provider plans that restrict their ability to refer patients. If health educators have direct links to patients, and make triage decisions (perhaps under supervision of a physician), then it is likely that future health care contracts will focus on the activities of these individuals.

The gatekeeper will also change in a different way. Currently, the chronically ill must visit a primary care provider before visiting a specialist. In the telecommunication practice model, because care can be delivered remotely, it will be possible to put patients in diverse geographical settings in the same capitated plans. Thus, capitated plans will emerge that specialize in one type of illness. For example, all patients with HIV who live in Ohio may belong to the same capitated plan. The presence of telecommunications makes it possible to deliver care to large enough groups of chronically ill patients that they can be organized into an HMO of their own. The gatekeeper for services will then be a specialist, not a family physician or internist. An infection specialist may decide that the patient's complaint can be addressed by a family physician. The referral will be from the specialist to the family physician, reversing the current pattern. As a consequence of this arrangement, patients will be under the care of a specialist who is most knowledgeable about their illness, and thus they will receive better-quality care.

Medical Records Must Change

As more care is managed remotely in the community, care will become more fragmented. Fragmented care requires greater attention to the coordination of care through medical records. One reason that patient care is not well coordinated is that the patient's medical record is often unavailable. There are many reasons for this. The medical record may be in use by another provider, may be in transit from or to the record room, or may be kept at another institution. Some investigators have suggested that computerized medical records can solve the problems with the unavailability of paper medical records. Unfortunately, data entry into computer records cannot occur immediately and often lags behind by several weeks, making such records less useful.

A voice medical record is an alternative that avoids the pitfalls of both paper and computerized medical records. Providers dictate their notes about the patient into the telephone receiver. These dictations are recorded by the system and are available on a last-in-first-out basis to other providers. When more than three notes are entered, a health professional listens to the notes and gives an updated summary note about the patient. Notes are transcribed and sent back for inclusion in the patient's paper record, so that providers do not need to update records twice. Transcriptions can be searched by keywords to find specific notes. Providers from other institutions can obtain access to the information through a simple phone call, reducing the waiting time for the transfer of records. The advantages are many: voice entry is easier than writing; transcribed notes are easier to read than handwritten notes; information on the patient is immediately available without access to a paper record; information entry into the computer is not delayed; transcription can be searched by keywords; and information can be easily transferred to people outside the institution.

More important than the technological change in medical records is the change in ownership. Medical records will belong to patients, kept by their insurance company, and will cut across various health delivery organizations. Only then can the record be complete, reflecting the care received through various sources. When medical records are owned by patients, it stands to reason that they will be allowed to review the record and address its errors. Patients will control who puts information in their record, what information is made public, and to whom. Thus, the entire relationship between the medical record and institutional care will change.

Patients Will Change

Patients' expectations of what illnesses require health services and what should be accomplished in a visit are likely to also change. Compare the status of the health care system to banking before automatic teller machines. Today, we expect to have access to money any time of day or night. We transfer funds by telephone and think little of it. We did not need to do this before. When the technology made the service possible, consumers became aware of it and adjusted their expectations. Likewise, as the new telecomunication aids are implemented, consumers are likely to demand more services and services that we have not thought through yet.

One consequence of electronic support groups is that health care consumers will be more organized as a group. Today, only a small portion of patients participate in support groups. Our data showed that 96 percent of patients may participate in electronic support groups. Thus, almost everyone who has a chronic illness may belong to a support group. As a consequence, they will be more informed and motivated individually. And patients, collectively, will also be more articulate. Patient advocacy groups, such as Act Up for AIDS/HIV illness, will be more common. These groups will insist on participating in funding decisions about research, encouraging quality care and making information about quality public, sharing medical decisions with their physicians, and a host of other patient rights.

Patients will also change because they will know more. One can imagine a day when, as a consequence of intensive education, some patients with chronic illness will know more about their illness than a primary care provider who sees patients with a variety of problems. What will be the role of the clinician in such a situation? It is quite possible that chronically ill patients will visit their primary care provider with a copy of an article recently published and ask for modification of their care plans. Anecdotal reports from a Wisconsin team who provided services to patients with breast cancer through CRT indicated that clinicians knew who belonged to the experimental group because this group was more prepared for the visit. In the new era, the patient will come to the visit with lists of questions and concerns, fully aware of potential alternative methods. In the end, the physician may be acting as a librarian—helping the patient sift through massive amounts of information.

Conclusions

We are all familiar with computers assisting a clinician or an administrator. But what can computers do for a patient? A great deal, but only if patients have computers at home. However, recent advances in computer technology have solved the problem of patient access to computer services. This chapter describes a number of telecommunication systems that could help in remote management of patients. The data show that these systems can improve the care of the patient. We have not done a definitive study of the potential impact of these telecommunication systems. A lot remains unanswered. One of the most important weaknesses of our studies is that we did not control for the content of the messages sent. That is, our studies were like studying the impact of television programs without regard to what was being broadcast.

Clinics can use telecommunication systems throughout their services. Some may consider the telecommunication practice model described above as science fiction. Others may object to what it means for our society and the relationship among patients and clinicians. But no matter what the conclusion, this is the time to work on these issues; otherwise, the technology will force them on us and we will be unaware of what we have sown until it is too late.

Acknowledgment. Work on this research was supported by National Institute of Drug Abuse Grant #5-R18-DA06913-02 for Extended Case Management of Cocaine Abusing Pregnant Patients, the Cuyahoga Metropolitan Housing Authority Contract for Electronic Community Outreach, and the Robert Wood Johnson Foundation for the All Kids Count grant. The views expressed herein do not necessarily relfect those of the funding agencies. Projects reported in this chapter were directed by Doctors Farrokh Alemi, Sonia Alemagno, and Richard C. Stephens. The project's computer programming directors were John Butts and Ali Ghadiri. Programmers included Hilarity Okoye Roe Schnarrenberger, Hetal Thakkar, Frank Guo, Jyh-Yung Lin, Chandana Hathi, Murgesan Govindasamy, Pallav Bhatt, Jeffrey Ilersich, Paresh Chauhan, and Ann Bush. The evaluation team included Theresa Roebuck, Patrick Duhon, Shirley Llorens, Maghboeba Mosavel, Hayne Dyches, Dr. Michael Sabiers, Dr. Mary Jackson, Kellie Moehring, Michele Bailey, Marilyn Orr, Wendy Schmidt, Tonya Johnson, Angela Harvey, Angela White, Shauna Mack, Cassandra Griffin, Vanessa Ray, and Karen Pickard. The administrative staff included Erika Korodi, Angela Benning, Denise Ivan, Achuta Ramarao, and Prashant Deshpande. Manuals were prepared with the help of the Cleveland State University Department of Marketing and Advertising. The project benefited from collaboration with University Hospitals of Cleveland's Women Health Center, University Hospital's Rainbow Babies and Children's Hospital and Clinic, MetroHealth's Clement Center, and Saint Vincent Charity Hospital's Rosary Hall. In particular, we wish to express our gratitude to Belinda Cavor, Ken Gill, Leslie Williams, Connie Moehring, Leatrice Ash, Nettie Toth, and Drs. Ted Parren, Bob Kliegman, Jeff Goldhagen, Kevin Muise, and Rachael Garber. Finally, and most importantly, we wish to express our appreciation to the patients and the approximately 300 providers who received and sent care-related messages through our telecommunication system.

References

1. Anbar M. (ed.). *Computers in Medicine.* Maryland: Computer Science Press; 1987.
2. Alemi F, Stephens R, Butts J. Llorens S. Computer initiated calls: Reactions of

employees of one firm. Working Paper, Cleveland State University Health Administration Program, Cleveland, OH 1996.

3. Havice MJ. Measuring non-response and refusals to an electronic telephone survey. *Journalism Quarterly,* 1990;67(3):521–530.

4. Nicholls WL II. CATI research and development at the Census Bureau. *Soc Meth Res.* 1983;12:191–197.

5. Fink JC. CATI's first decade: The Chilton experience. *Soci Meth Res.* 1983;12:153–168.

6. Shangraw RF. Telephone surveying with computer: Administrative, methodological and research issues. *Eval Program Planning.* 1986;9:107–111.

7. Evan WM, Miller JR. Differential effects on response bias of computer versus conventional administration of a social science questionnaire: An exploratory methodological experiment. *Behav Sci.* 1969;14:216–227.

8. Johnson DF, Mihal, WL. Performance of blacks and whites in computerize versus manual testing environments. *Am Psycho.* 1973;28:694–699.

9. Kiesler S, Sproull LS] Response effects in the electronic survey. *Public Opin Quarterly.* 1986;50:402–413.

10. Lucas RW, Mulins PJ, Luna CBX, McInroy DC. Psychiatrists and a computer as interrogators of patients with alcohol related illness: A comparison. *Brit J Psychiatry.* 1977;131:160–167.

11. Greist JH, Klein MH, Erdman HP, Bires JK, Bass SM, Machtinger PE. Comparison of computer and interviewer administered versions of the diagnostic interview schedule. *Hosp Community Psychiatry.* 1987;38(12):1304–1311.

12. Lucas RW, Mullins PJ, Luna CBX, McInroy, DC. Psychiatrists and a computer as interrogators of patients with alcohol related illnesses: A comparison. *Br J Psychiatry.* 1977;131:160–167.

13. Angle HV, Ellinwood EH, Carroll J. Computer interview problem assessment of psychiatric patients. In: Orthner FH. (ed.). *Proceedings of the Second Annual Symposium on Computer Applications in Medical Care.* Washington DC: Institute of Electrical and Electronics Engineers; 1978:137–148.

14. Sawyer MG, Sarris A, Baghurst P. The use of computer interview to administer the Child Behavior Checklist in a child psychiatry service. *J Am Acad Child Adolesc Psychiatry.* 1991;30(4):674–681; Sawyer M, Sarris A, Quigley R, Baghurst P, Kalucy R. The attitude of parents to the use of computer assisted interviewing in a child psychiatry service. *Br J Psychiatry.* 1990;157:675–678.

15. Bungey JB, Pols RG, Mortimer KP, Frank OR, Skinner HA. Screening alcohol and drug use in a general practice unit: comparison of computerized and traditional methods. *Commun Health Studies.* 1989;13(4):471–483.

16. Carr AC, Ghosh A, Ancill RJ. Can a computer take a psychiatric history? *Psychological Med.* 1983;13:151–158.

17. Erdman H, Cline MH, Greist JH. Direct patient computer interviewing. *J Consult Clin Psychol.* 1985;53(6):76–77.

18. Alemi F, Higley P. Reactions to talking computers assessing health risks. *Med Care.* 1995;33(1):227–233.

19. *Computer to Help Mom-to-be Shun Drugs.* Plain Dealer, October 16, 1990:1.

20. Alemi F, Stephens RC, Javalghi RG, Dyches H, Butts J, Ghadiri A. Managed self care: A telecommunication practice model. *Medical Care Supplement on Telecommunication Practice Model.* In print.

21. Al Hays RD, Ware JE. MOS Short Form General Health Survey. *Med Care.*

1988;26(7):724-732.

22. Alemi F, Stephens RC, Muise K, Dyches H, Mosavel M, Butts J. Educating patients at home: Community health rap. *Medical Care Supplement on Telecommunication Practice Model.* In print.

23. Alemi F, Stephens RC, Mosavel M, Ghadiri A, Krishnaswamy J, Thakkar H. Electronic Self Help and Support Groups: A Voice Bulletin Board. *Medical Care Supplement on Telecommunication Practice Model.* In print.

24. Alemi F, Alemagno SA, Goldhagen J, Ashe L, Finkelstein B, Lavin A, Butts J, Butler K, Ghadiri A, Heineke N. Computer reminders improve on-time immunization rates. *Medical Care Supplement on Telecommunication Practice Model.* In print.

25. Wasson J, Gaudette C, Whaley F, Sauvigne A, Baribeau P, Welch G. Telephone care as a substitute for routine clinic follow-up. *JAMA* 1992;267:1788-1793.

Section IV

Logistical Issues and Information Networks

The final section of this book presents four perspectives on key concepts that underpin the successful implementation of CHINs: the relationship between CHINs and telemedicine, the nature of clinical practice delivered to patients via an electronic environment, management of privacy, confidentiality and security considerations, and the business−industry−CHIN interplay. These four topics represent an extension of this volume's key premise of the essential role of CHINs in the organization, delivery, and financing of health care. They provide operational considerations common across the examples of CHINs delineated through Sections II and III.

Shirley Moore draws on her experiences as the clinical nurse moderator for a special computer network service, the ComputerLink. Moore identifies key clinician responsibilities necessary to effectively use computer networks to provide clinical care to patients. Issues such as interface design and user training are treated from a clinical, rather than a technical dimension. Enumerating such challenges as relationship development and establishment of group norms, Moore provides a blueprint for clinical practices that wish to make use of CHINs in the delivery of care. Importantly, she presents scenarios where CHINs will, and will not, serve as vehicles for reaching patients where they live and work.

Dena Puskin posits that telemedicine initiatives and CHINs each provide unique services while sharing a technical overlap. Telemedicine is the use of modern telecommunication and information technology for the provision of clinical care to individuals and the transmission of information about that care. It is distinguished from CHINs by the emphasis on clinical over financial benefits. Puskin calls for the design of CHINs to arise from the information needs and practice styles of clinical care providers, not from the technical capabilities of computers and networks. She envisions a televillage within which telehealth services (health promotion, community wellness programs, etc.), as well as telemedicine practices, enrich the lives and well-being of citizens everywhere, including remote rural areas.

Issues of privacy, confidentiality, and security, well recognized in enterprise-specific information systems, are compounded by the interorganizational linkages characteristic of CHINs. Randolph C. Barrows and Paul D. Clayton provide an excellent enumeration of challenges and solutions. CHIN developers must foster public trust by setting policies that maintain confidentiality of the individual, insure appropriate access to data by authorized users, and preserve the integrity of health data.

Neilson S. Buchanan responds to calls presented throughout this volume that a business case must be made for CHINs. Employers are buyers of health services and, he argues, will find health services supported by CHINs as the best value for money. CHINs can support the clinician by providing access to information about patients, access to the professional literature and knowledge basis, access to consulting clinicians, and access to the clinician's own experiences. However, CHINs themselves represent important business entities. At present they exist on an emergent trajectory, early in their maturational stage.

These four perspectives (clinical, health service, security, and business) address unique dimensions of CHINs, formalizing lessons extracted from the organizational and clinical examples presented in Sections II and III. They complement the technical, organizational, community, and personal aspects of CHINs advanced in Section I.

14

Telemedicine: Building Rural Systems for Today and Tomorrow

Dena S. Puskin, Carole L. Mintzer, and Cathy J. Wasem

A Vision:

A rural community where residents do not have to travel long distances to receive specialty care from urban centers of excellence; where all providers have access from computers in their offices to their patients' records, including x-rays, lab tests, and video recordings of specialty consults; where rural residents have access to up-to-date health information and patients have access to their own medical records from home computers; where homebound rural patients can visit with their doctor or nurse by turning on the TV; where rural school nurses consult with adolescent health experts about students' medical conditions over the TV; and where health professions students at the local rural hospital and clinic are supervised daily over the TV by their teachers at a distant medical center.

This vision is still only a dream for most rural communities, many of which struggle with isolation, poverty, and a chronic shortage of health care providers. Yet the telemedicine technologies to implement it are here today.

Telemedicine is the use of telecommunications and information technologies to provide clinical care to individuals at a distance and to transmit the information needed to provide that care. The key to this definition is information. This information may be in various forms — audio, video, or text — but all typically contribute to a telemedicine consult. Generally, however, references to telemedicine have come to mean services in which some video link is provided, such as transmission of x-rays or video consults.

Telemedicine holds great promise for improving the services and quality of life in rural communities. Experience to date, however, suggests that with low population density, many rural communities lack sufficient demand for services to support the sophisticated telecommunications infrastructure required to sustain advanced telemedicine systems.

The prospects for sustainable rural telemedicine systems improve when we can use the technology to address a community's broader health information needs through multi-use systems.[1] However, experience also suggests that there are many logistical challenges to building these systems.[1]

This chapter outlines what we have learned from past and current telemedicine projects about building sustainable, integrated, multi-use systems.

Background

Telecommunications technology has been used to exchange medical information between sites via video since the 1960s. One of the earliest applications was at the University of Nebraska where psychiatric consultations were conducted on two-way closed-circuit TV using microwave technology. Somewhat later, a video link was established between the Massachusetts General Hospital and a clinic at Logan Airport. The National Aeronautics and Space Administration (NASA) and the National Library of Medicine (NLM) also pioneered telemedicine in the 1960s by jointly supporting satellite-transmitted services to Alaska and to the Appalachian and Rocky Mountain regions. Then, in the 1970s, NASA sponsored the STARPAHC (Space Technology Applied to Rural Papago Advanced Health Care) project, which was implemented with the Indian Health Service and the Department of Health, Education, and Welfare on the Papago Indian Reservation in Arizona.

These early projects began with much promise and then faded away, largely due to the high costs and limitations of the technologies used. Recent advances in telecommunications and information technology, however, have overcome or minimized many of the technical problems encountered in earlier telemedicine projects, and have actually lowered the cost of the technology.

Thus, after almost two decades of obscurity, telemedicine is experiencing a revival. The resurrection is being energized by the twin and sometimes contradictory imperatives to increase access to health services for underserved populations and reduce or stabilize the costs of health care in this nation.

Telemedicine is currently operating on a much larger scale and with a much wider scope than in the past. Large-scale demonstrations are being supported by the federal government, and most states have at least one telemedicine system in either the operational or planning stage. For example, the Eastern Montana Telemedicine Network is a joint federally/privately funded project that uses interactive video to connect Deaconess-Billings Clinic with five remote rural communities, one of which is nearly 300 miles from Billings. In a recent 12-month period, over 200 consults, mostly for mental health services, were provided to patients in those communities. In addition, the system is used for continuing education and is rented out to businesses, which use it to conduct meetings to which their executives and employees otherwise would have to travel.

Telemedicine systems also are becoming more versatile. The Mid-Nebraska Telemedicine Network, connecting Good Samaritan Hospital in

Kearney with five rural communities, uses software that allows the referring practitioners to choose between store-and-forward technology[2] or interactive video for obtaining consults. The software integrates medical record information with the images transmitted for a consultation so the specialist has access to complete patient information in one place. The practitioners also can type in their referral questions, or send a voice recording of their questions to accompany the patient information. Practitioners can use the system at the level of technology that makes the most sense for addressing the patient's problem.

Telemedicine's promise lies in its ability to provide a wide range of health and health education services without the simultaneous presence of provider and patient (or teacher and student) in the same place.[3] Today's telemedicine systems are being supported in the hope that they will address some of the most pervasive problems in the U.S. health care system; that is, geographic maldistribution of health resources, including persistent shortages of health care personnel in rural areas, uneven quality of health services, and high costs.

Despite the recent surge of activity in telemedicine, current projects are still in their infancy. As one author recently remarked: "Telemedicine is on its way (although it has not yet arrived)."[4] Moreover, while telemedicine has been practiced for over 30 years in one way or another, there is very little empirical information about the requirements for sustaining such systems in rural areas.

We have learned, however, that for many, if not most rural communities, telemedicine systems cannot exist in a vacuum. Except for the simplest applications using the telephone or fax machine, the systems require greater revenues than can usually be generated in a small population by clinical care alone.

For example, assume that a clinic wants to conduct specialty consultations requiring a telephone (T1) line that costs $2000 per month to rent. If the clinic only generates 10 consults a month, the cost of the line, alone, would be $200/consult, not a sustainable cost. However, if the clinic shares the use of the line with the nearby hospital and perhaps allows the local business community to rent the line for special purposes, the costs become more sustainable.

Thus, in rural areas, hospitals, schools, government, and other community service providers might well aggregate demand and share a network to spread the costs of developing and maintaining it. In its 1991 study on rural telecommunications, the Office of Technology Assessment suggested that this aggregation could be done through the formation of multi-use systems referred to as "Rural Area Networks," or RANs.[5] RANs were envisioned as shared usage networks, configured to include a wide range of users in rural communities. These networks would allow rural communities to meet their own needs while achieving economies of scale and scope.

A similar concept—the televillage—also addresses the need for aggregation of demand.[6] However, whereas the focus of the RAN was on the network itself, the focus of a televillage is on the participants and the strategic process for creating a "virtual village of services."

The Televillage and Telehealth – The Promise of the Televillage

It is useful to consider the development and deployment of telemedicine systems in rural areas within the context of the larger transformations taking place in society as new information and communication technologies change how we live, learn, and conduct business. Moreover, it is important to recognize the interdependence of these technologies, health care facilities, and the "health" of rural communities. That is, the future of health facilities in rural areas is tied to the economic future of the communities they serve; conversely the future economic "well-being" of the community is tied to the viability of its health facilities.

Rural communities now have opportunities to decrease their isolation, increase their connectedness, and improve their health and the overall health of their region, all through the innovative use of new information and telecommunication technologies.[7] One means of harnessing this potential at the community level, and, in the process, fashioning sustainable telemedicine systems, is by creating a *televillage*.

A televillage can be conceptualized as a "virtual" community of people, firms, government agencies, schools, libraries, health care providers, and others who share telecommunication networks and related services and who use the technologies to link to each other and the broader global information economy. A televillage is characterized by dynamic, new patterns of human interaction, communication, and development. In essence, it is a development strategy – not a thing. Each televillage will be unique because it will be structured to meet the unique needs of its area.[8]

The concept of a televillage has been applied for over a decade in numerous countries, including several Scandinavian countries, Poland, Australia, and, more recently, the United States. Originally conceived as a center at which new computer and telecommunication technologies would be available to community members for business, health care, education, and so forth, it has more recently assumed a broader scope that includes the integration of community services to form a virtual village.[9]

The process of creating a televillage can be effective in addressing a troubling phenomenon seen in many rural communities today – a lack of coordinated planning among all the potential users of a telecommunications network.

Telecommunication technologies are increasingly deployed along sectoral lines in education, business, health, or law, without regard for the need to develop a shared infrastructure—such as roads and water or sewer lines, that are laid for the entire community.[10] Deployment of individual telemedicine systems may be viable in urban or larger rural communities with adequate resources, but it is not a viable strategy in small, resource-poor ones.

Moreover, development solely within the health sector may not be able to address the health resource problems telemedicine seeks to solve. For example, a plan to enhance recruitment and retention of clinicians through the lure of a telemedicine system may fail if schools remain substandard because of lack of access to advanced courses (e.g., advanced science courses) and other services available through telecommunications technology and if employment opportunities for clinicians' spouses are limited.

Unfortunately, a narrow focus has been more the pattern than the exception for telemedicine systems in the United States. Many of these systems currently serve only users within the health care system and they have focused on a limited set of medical users and uses. For telemedicine systems to be sustainable where they are most needed in smaller, more isolated rural communities, they must engage other partners both within and outside of health.

As difficult as it is to conceptualize the adoption and adaptation of these new technologies in one's own sector, it is even more difficult to imagine how they will be deployed in other sectors. Yet this understanding is critical to creating the partnerships necessary for a successful televillage. Examples of potential partners within health care are provided in Box A. Examples of how telecommunications technologies are used in other sectors are provided in Box B.

Telehealth and Telemedicine

The terms telemedicine and telehealth are often used interchangeably. However, telemedicine is a narrower, more specific field of activity while telehealth is broader. Telemedicine involves the use of telecommunication and information technologies to provide clinical care to individuals at a distance and to transmit the information needed to provide that care. To date, most telemedicine systems have focused on two-way interactive consultation capabilities; few have built in the component of computerized patient records.

Telehealth includes clinical care but also encompasses the related areas of health professions education, consumer health education, public health, research, and administration. Telecommunications applications in this larger arena include distance learning for degree and continuing education, both didactic lectures and clinical precepting; consumer health services, such as electronic support groups and consumer health information bulletin boards; administrative uses, including electronic billing and administrative teleconferencing; and telemedicine.

(For a schematic representation of the concepts of televillage, telehealth, and telemedicine, see Fig. 14.1 and Table 14.1 and for examples of applications of telehealth and telemedicine within the televillage, see Table 14.2)

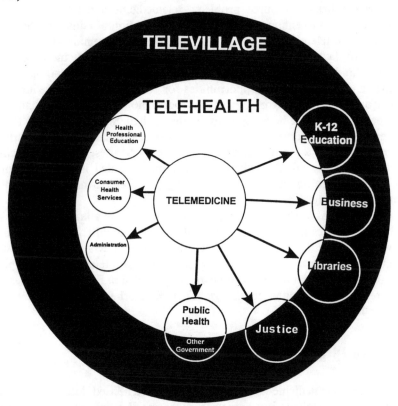

FIGURE 14.1. Interrelationships: Telemedicine, telehealth and televillage. Televillage—a virtual community of people, firms, government agencies, schools, libraries, health care providers, and others who share telecommunications networks and related services and who use the technologies to link to each other and the braoder global information economy. Telehealth—the use of modern information and telecommunication technologies to provide health care services and access to health information for health professionals and consumers; to train and educate health professionals; to increase awareness and educate the public about health-related issues; and to facilitate research about health care issues aross a distance. Telemedicine—the use of telecommunication and information technologies to provide clinical care to individuals at a distance and transmit the information needed to provide that care.

TABLE **14.1.** Potential health partners in the televillage.

dental hygienists	nutritionists and dieticians
dentists	occupational therapists
discharge planners	optometrists
emergency medical technicians	pharmacists
health educators	podiatrists
medical technologists	physical therapists
mental health workers	physical therapy assistants
psychologists	physician assistants
clinical social workers	speech therapists
psychiatric nurse clinicians	social workers
psychiatrists	substance abuse counselors
nurses (e.g.)	veterinarians
home health nurses	
nurse practitioners	
clinical nurse specialists	
diabetic nurse educators	
enterstomal nurse clinicians	
public health nurses	

Telemedicine and CHINs

Clearly, community health information networks (CHINs) represent one application within telehealth, but the relationship of CHINs to telemedicine is less well defined. Both transfer or exchange health care information. CHINs, however, exchange financial and nonimage clinical information, while telemedicine systems to date have focused almost exclusively on the video exchange of clinical information. CHINs and telemedicine overlap to the extent that a telemedicine system provides for the electronic exchange of patient records, and CHINs provide for the exchange of clinical information that includes images.

It is important to recognize that the development of both telemedicine and CHINs is evolutionary, and the two will probably merge in the future. Even today, some CHINs include telemedicine activities, while some telemedicine systems are aligned with CHINs. For example, the Southern Idaho Medical Information Network (SIMIN) is a CHIN in rural Idaho and Nevada that incorporates telemedicine applications into its network, while the telemedicine system being developed at Mary Imogene Bassett Hospital in New York will interface with the hospital's institutional CHIN.

A Prescription for Building Sustainable Systems

Whether building a televillage, a telemedicine system, or something in between, the logistical challenges are daunting. Although there is little concrete data about successful and unsuccessful strategies for building

TABLE 14.2. Televillage.

Examples of current and potential uses of telecommunication and information technologies in a rural community

General Applications:

Education—Math and language instructors are shared among rural schools, and rural schools downlink nationally broadcast classes.

Business—Companies use video-conferencing to hold meetings and minimize travel (e.g., in eastern Montana the telemedicine network has been used by rural bankers of several towns to hold meetings).

Libraries—Small rural libraries use the technologies to conduct business, such as processing interlibrary loans, and to provide community members access to a broad range of information via the Internet.

Justice—Arraignments are held using video conferencing, mitigating the need to transport prisoners.

Government—State governments, early creators and users of telecommunication and data networks conduct state business over the network.

TeleHealth Applications Within Nonhealth Sectors of the Community:

Education—High School students receive health seminars taught by health department personnel and university instructors over a video-conferencing system, and vocational education students are precepted at the hospital by instructors at the high school over the system.

Business—Employee health seminars are offered using video conferencing with a local community college.

Libraries—A library, through Internet connections, provides enhanced community access to AIDS information resources and environmental health.

Justice—Substance abuse and HIV prevention seminars are provided to prisoners using video conferencing.

Other Government—Critical pubic health information (e.g., on immunizations) is broadcast from the CDC to local health officials and clinicians; downlinks at hospitals and county extension offices are used to receive the program.

Telehealth Applications Within the Health Care Sector:

Health Professions Education—Using a range of telecommunication and information technologies (e.g., computer conferencing, two-way interactive video conferencing, and one way audio conferencing) health professions degree programs and continuing education are offered to individuals in rural communities. Computer conferencing and two-way interactive video sessions are used to provide precepting to health science students in rural facilities.

Consumer Health Services—An "electronic support group" is created for caretakers of individuals with Alzheimer disease by linking them, via computers, to an electronic bulletin board on the community's free-net. In addition to accessing support group members, caretakers are able to access a nurse clinical and numerous resource databases on Alzheimer's.

TABLE 14.2. *Continued*

Administration—Meetings of the hospital administrators of a rural hospital network are held using video conferencing. Physicians from several towns in a rural county hold their monthly county medical board meeting over the system. Computers, connecting several rural spoke clinics and hospitals to a hub hospital, are used for billing purposes and quality improvement activities.

Telemedicine Applications

Education—The school nurse is linked to a physician's office and a mental health clinic for consultations.

Business—A plant's occupational health and safety clinic is linked to a multispecialty clinical practice and a mental health clinic for consultations.

Libraries—Health science libraries provide, via a link to the National Library of Medicine, clinician access to medical databases on skin lesions for comparison of patients' rashes.

Justice—State prisons are linked to academic health centers for consultations with specialists, eliminating transport of inmates and travel by specialists.

Other Government—Public health nurses, using laptop computers with cameras and modems, access State immunization records to check on children's immunization status when conducting an immunization clinic and confer with nurse specialists at the referral center on wound and stomal care during a home visit.

telemedicine systems, there is enough anecdotal evidence to suggest the difficulties and how they can be mitigated. In this section, we consider some of these logistical considerations in building sustainable telemedicine systems, and how those lessons might apply to televillages.

Building a Common Vision

The first challenge is to build a common vision among all the participants that is based on the needs of the community. What will the telemedicine system look like? What will it be used for? Who is going to use it? What kinds of technologies will be employed? Several interrelated steps must be taken to arrive at a common vision. Although they can only be discussed one at a time, this is a multifaceted and simultaneous set of processes.

Building a common vision requires bringing together all the potential users of the system for numerous planning sessions. In telemedicine, this includes administrators, physicians, and other health care professionals, patients, and technical experts. It might also include business leaders, teachers, and others if the system will be available for use by those outside the medical community. Coordinating schedules for this new activity, making sure everyone speaks the same telemedicine language, and reaching consensus on the vision will take considerable time and effort. But this is essential to developing a system that will be used and sustained.

Unfortunately, the world of telemedicine is full of systems that do not start with a common vision among all the participants because they are developed without the input of all the potential users. For example, administrators and technical gurus may plan a telemedicine system without the input of the health care professionals who will actually use it. Although they may ask one or two physicians for their input along the way, they do not consistently involve them from the beginning. The risk is that the telemedicine system will not fit well into established referral patterns, it will not be located where the health care professionals practice, and the technology chosen will not fit their needs. Then the unfortunate result is that the telemedicine system is not used enough to justify its costs, and it takes considerable effort after the fact to persuade professionals to use the system.

Building a common vision for a televillage requires people to work together who have never worked together before—people who come from entirely different professions and who speak different professional languages. Within the health care field alone, it can be difficult to get physicians, administrators, nurses, patients, and allied health professionals to find a common vision for a telemedicine system. And presumably they have a common mission! Imagine bringing together health care professionals with teachers, librarians, police, lawyers, and business leaders to build a common vision for a community-wide telecommunications system that meets all their needs. Coordinating schedules and making the time for this new activity will be easy compared to the challenge of developing a common language and achieving commitment by all the players, including the skeptics.

The Need for Leadership

A key factor in creating a team from disparate partners is finding a strong leader. Every successful telemedicine project has someone at the helm with vision and authority, who can inspire people to work together and gain the commitment of the various partners to achieve their common goal. This person also must have the wisdom to resolve differences without losing team members. A strong leader will be essential not only to developing a common vision of the televillage but also to realizing the dream.

Telemedicine systems also require champions among users who have credibility with their peers and speak the same language they do. Convincing physicians and other health professionals to use the new technology is one of the biggest challenges to implementing a telemedicine system. They may, however, overcome their reluctance if one of their colleagues uses the new technology first and demonstrates how well it works. In implementing a televillage, it probably will be necessary to have a champion in each sector to pave the way for others to use the system.

Matching Needs to Technology

The common vision should be realistic and based on the needs of the community. The planning process should include a thorough examination of the community and its needs.[11] Telecommunications technology can do many amazing and wonderful things, and people are often seduced by the possibilities. It is tempting to develop applications around the capabilities of the technology. To build a sustainable telemedicine system, however, the challenge is to focus on the applications the community needs and is likely to use. Then look for the technologies that will help achieve those goals.

Determining which technologies and applications will best serve the community's needs requires learning about and understanding the capabilities of the new technologies. Physicians often say that they are unable to identify their needs for information technologies because they do not know what the technologies can do. They cannot imagine how they would use the equipment because they have never seen it in use or talked to anyone who used it. In matching needs to technology, it is essential to talk not only to vendors of equipment and software, but also to people who currently use the technology. Find out what it can do, what it cannot do, how easy it is to learn to use, and how easy it is to use on a routine basis. If technology education is integrate into the needs assessment process, the telecommunications system is more likely to have the support of users and meet the needs of the community.

Although the jury is still out on which technologies will work best for telemedicine, there are many examples of projects that developed around the technology rather than around the information needs and practice styles of health care professionals. For example, interactive video looks like a terrific medium for providing specialty consults to rural residents, but it typically requires the patient and two practitioners to be present for the consult at the same time — a scheduling nightmare. When information needs are considered, it may be that for most patient care applications, store-and-forward technology is sufficient — and it fits better with physician practice patterns. Perhaps the best solution will be provided by new software that allows practitioners to choose between using store-and-forward or interactive video.

A televillage should be built first and foremost around the needs of the community. Each sector should first examine its own needs along with the technological possibilities. Then the televillage members should consider the extent to which the needs of different sectors are compatible. Opportunities to share equipment or telecommunications lines should be explored. Needs should be differentiated from wants, and both should be prioritized as part of realistic discussions about resources and funding.

Need for an Inventory

Before the common vision can be implemented, there must be a careful inventory of available telecommunications capabilities and equipment, including computers. The inventory may be revealing in both what is available and what is not. For example, some small rural hospitals may discover that the only computers they have are for billing purposes. For them to join a telemedicine system will be a considerable, and perhaps welcome, leap in technological capabilities.

The inventory also should consider how much of the existing equipment can be used for the telemedicine system or televillage before deciding what new equipment to buy. Some existing equipment may be underutilized and could become part of the telecommunications system. It also is necessary to determine whether the needed telecommunications capacity (e.g., bandwidth) is available to each site. If not, preparations must be made to assure that each site has sufficient bandwidth.

Coordinate with External Partners

By definition, telecommunications projects involve outside partners. Telemedicine systems and televillages should build on existing relationships, rather than trying to forge completely new partnerships that bypass existing alliances. Telemedicine systems that bypass existing referral patterns are less likely to be used by health care professionals because it means giving up trusted colleagues and referring patients to practitioners they do not know.

The technology to be used must be coordinated with all the members of the system. The equipment and software at each site must be able to talk to all the other sites. To date, most telemedicine systems have been developed from the ground up, with all sites purchasing their equipment simultaneously. In the future, we are likely to see more sites added on to existing systems. These sites will have to purchase equipment that is compatible with the equipment of the network they are joining.

In developing a televillage, each sector will have to coordinate activities and equipment needs with their external partners. This can have major implications for the ability to share equipment or telecommunications lines. For example, if two sectors of the televillage need to conduct business with external partners at the same time, they may not be able to share the telecommunications lines if they cannot split the line. Or, if one sector's external partner uses still-image telephones, and another sector's partner uses interactive video, they will not be able to share equipment even if internal analysis of their equipment needs suggests that they do so.

Protocols for Sharing Lines, Equipment, and Expertise

Telemedicine systems often are used for multiple purposes allow maximum utilization of the system. The same system that is used for patient care also can be used for continuing education and administrative meetings. However, shared uses pose some logistical challenges. One challenge is scheduling. Protocols need to be established that allow regularly scheduled meetings to be interrupted when medical emergencies require immediate consultation. Another challenge is locating the equipment in a room that can accommodate multiple uses. A patient examination room may not be appropriate for educational seminars attended by several people, and conversely, a conference room may not be suitable for a patient consultation. Some telemedicine projects try to overcome this problem by using portable equipment, but the equipment is heavy and fragile and may not withstand frequent moves.

The different sectors of a televillage also may want to consider sharing telecommunications lines, equipment, and expertise. Sharing some aspects of the system may reduce costs and encourage greater coordination and cooperation among the different sectors. The logistical considerations are similar to those found with telemedicine.

If telecommunications lines are to be shared, but not equipment, it will be necessary to establish protocols for scheduling time on the system. If a high school class has connected for a special session on the space program, what happens if the hospital has a medical emergency requiring immediate access to the system? How much time will each sector have for regularly scheduled programming? Must access time to the system be fixed—e.g. the justice system has it every Monday morning from nine to noon? Or will there flexibility so the school can take advantage of a special program at 10:00 a.m. on Monday? How long in advance must scheduling requests be made? Scheduling should be centralized with clear rules that are developed and understood by all sectors.

If utilization of the system by several sectors is low, it may make sense to share equipment as well as telecommunications lines. In this case, it is essential to locate the equipment in a place that accommodates all the different users. For example, a telemedicine system located in a nursing home may offer limited access to other users if there is no waiting room. Evening use of the system could be disturbing to residents, making it unavailable to the school system for adult education. A system located in an elementary school may not be appropriate for use by the justice system when school is in session. Patient privacy must be assured if the system is located in a public building.

Telecommunications systems require considerable technical expertise. Sharing technical personnel among the different sectors is an excellent way to assure efficiencies in and coordination of the system. However, shared technical staff must have clear priorities and protocols for serving the different members of the system. Which parts of the system get installed first? If two different sectors have technical difficulties at the same time, what is the protocol for determining who gets assistance first? Many disagreements can be avoided by establishing protocols in advance of problems.

Funding—Affordability, Cross-Subsidization

After building a common vision based on needs, inventorying existing lines and equipment, and deciding what can and will be shared, it is time to decide what equipment and software to purchase. Although this decision will be based on the above factors, the costs of purchasing, maintaining, and using equipment also must be considered. Telecommunications equipment costs are coming down, but the costs of using the equipment (e.g., transmission costs, maintenance, staffing, etc.) remain high, and must be considered if the system is to be sustainable.

Three important questions must be answered when considering funding for the project: What are the sources of funding? How much funding is available? Will there be cross-subsidization among the partners (i.e., will some partners pay more than their share of the network costs while others pay less)? The answers to these questions may dictate much of the development of the system.

If the sources of funding are internal (i.e., not from grants) then the system can be developed without any of the constraints that a grant program might impose. Grant dollars typically come with strings attached about what the system should be used for and how the money can be spent. While grants may allow the partners to develop a system that they could not otherwise afford, grants also may tempt the partners to purchase a system they cannot sustain after the grant ends. Regardless of the source of funding for the initial start-up of the system, long-term sustainability must be considered from the outset.

Although grant dollars may help develop a system, few grants will sustain it in the long run. Therefore, all options for long-term funding of the system should be explored, including charging users, negotiating reduced rates for telephone usage, soliciting donations, and cross-subsidization.

Telemedicine systems typically look for reimbursement of clinical services as a means both of increasing utilization and financing the system. However, the reluctance of fee-for-service insurers to pay for teleconsults means that reimbursement may not be a viable source of income. In addition, fee-for-service payments to health care practitioners may not necessarily be accessible to the health care facility that incurs the expense of the telemedicine system. Alternatively, managed care plans may find telemedicine extremely valuable for assuring access to care, especially as they expand to rural markets. Consequently, it may make sense to court managed care plans and seek their financial support for the system.

The issue of cross-subsidization poses interesting challenges and must be explicitly addressed to avoid conflicts. Telemedicine systems may be used for multiple applications within and outside the health care system. Whether by design or circumstance, different users cross-subsidize the costs of the system. For example, a telemedicine system is purchased and operated with funds designated for providing clinical care to patients. But this system also is used to provide continuing education to health care professionals. If the health care professionals are not charged for the continuing education class, then the costs of transmitting the class are subsidized by the clinical care dollars. If businesses use the system for meetings among distant affiliates and are charged more than the costs of operating the system for their meetings, then they are cross-subsidizing the costs of providing clinical care over the system.

Such cross-subsidization is acceptable if it is understood and agreed that it is necessary for sustaining a telemedicine system that serves the greater good of the community. In a televillage, similar cross-subsidization may take place among different sectors, with the wealthier sectors supporting the telecommunications needs of the poorer sectors. They will agree to do this if the system is based upon the needs of the community and they perceive that the system as a whole benefits them as well as the community. Clear, unambiguous contracts among the sectors will avoid the conflicts that will arise if some sectors believe they are paying more than their fair share for no justifiable reason.

Conclusion

Through the wonders of modern telecommunications technology, communities have immediate access to a world of services. As a part of this world, telemedicine holds much promise for improving access to health services in rural, underserved communities. At the same time, many of our rural communities are still traveling the "dirt road" of information technology. For these communities to enter the information superhighway, multi-use systems will be required that create an effective economic demand for the sophisticated telecommunications infrastructure necessary to support them. However, as noted earlier, the building of these multi-use systems creates significant challenges, not the least of which is getting disparate segments of the community to work together.

We have outlined the model of the televillage as one approach to creating such multi-use systems. This model may not be appropriate for all rural communities, but many of the principles outlined in building the village should be useful for any community contemplating development of multi-use systems. We must remember that although building the televillage or its equivalent for many rural communities is fraught with difficulties, not building it could very well result in death or permanent "third world" status for these communities.

References

1. Puskin DS. Opportunities and challenges to telemedicine in rural America. *J. Med Syst.* 1995;19(1):59.
2. Store-and-forward technology allows a practitioner to send patient data and images for review by a distant practitioner at a later time. The two practitioners do not interact simultaneously over the telemedicine system.
3. Anonymous. Telemedicine: Fad or future? (editorial). *Lancet* 1995;345:73–74.

4. Franken EA et al. Telemedicine and teleradiology: A tale of two cultures. *Telemed J.* 1995;1(1):7.
5. U.S. Congress, Office of Technology Assessment. *Rural America at the Crossroads: Networking for the Future.* OTA-TCT-471. Washington, DC: U.S. Government Printing Office; April 1991.
6. Kimel KW. *The Rural Televillage: Creating a New Strategy for Rural Development.* A Conference White Paper Presented at the Creating the Televillage Conference. Tampa, Fl: 1994.
7. Cisler S. *The Library and Wired Communities in Rural Areas.* Unpublished manuscript, 1994.
8. Kimel, *loc.cit.*
9. Two televillages currently being developed in Kentucky, however, do include the development of centers, one of which is located in a community hospital.
10. Witherspoon JP et al. *Rural TeleHealth: Telemedicine, Distance Education and Informatics for Rural Health Care.* Purchase Order No. 92–1208 (P). Rockville, MD: Office of Rural Health Policy.
11. One example of a planning process is provided in volume III of *Telemedicine — Assessing the Kansas Environment: Community Planning Guide*; November 1993. Prepared for the Kansas Telemedicine Policy Group, sponsored by the Kansas Department of Health and Environment and the Kansas Hospital Association.

15

Computer Networks as Environments for Care: Dynamics of the Clinical Encounter

SHIRLEY M. MOORE

Clinicians have used computers primarily for business functions, record keeping,[1] computer-assisted instruction,[2,3] decision assistance[4,5] and more recently, patient assessment and evaluation.[6,7] Of late, however, computers have been envisioned as a way to directly deliver interventions. Thus, clinicians are challenged to consider the types of clinical situations and interventions most suitable for computer use, the best way to deliver interventions using computers, and the most effective way to use computers as interventions. This challenge is not simply a matter of adapting to a new medium; rather, clinicians must learn to use computers as new environments for therapeutic clinical encounters. This chapter describes the dynamics of clinical therapeutic encounters using a computer network to deliver client interventions over nearly 3 years. Illustrations are from a project designed to provide homecare support to two groups of clients, persons living with AIDS (PLWAs) and caregivers of persons with Alzheimer's disease (AD), using a computer network, ComputerLink.

ComputerLink[8] consisted of separate electronic networks for PLWAs and AD caregivers; computer terminals placed in clients' homes allowed them 24-hour access to a variety of features, including a communications module, an information module, and a decision assistance module. The communications module included a Forum, where clients and the moderator publicly posted and read messages; a question and answer section (Q&A) in which clients could anonymously post questions to a registered nurse moderator; and a private mail system. The Electronic Encyclopedia provided several hundred indexed screens of information about the disease course, diagnosis and treatment, symptom management, care issues, and community resources. The decision support module guided clients through decisions using an analysis process that incorporated their own words and preferences, thus assisting them to make choices consistent with their values.

Nurse moderators interacted with clients on ComputerLink via typed messages. Because messages were posted and read at times convenient to users, most communication was asynchronous. The nurse moderators read all public messages daily, reviewed any personal mail, and typed responses to individuals or the group. Nurse moderators employed both individual and group interventions of support, information-giving, encouraging expression of feelings and ideas, acceptance, reassurance, clarification, and interpretation. They used the advice of expert panels for assistance in responding to the wide range of clinical questions arising on the network.

Clinical Interventions

Several types of clinical interventions can be delivered over computer networks. Interventions can be group- or individual-focused and as in ComputerLink projects, they may include information, social support, emotional support, resource support, and decision support. The use of the clinical process (assessment, diagnosis, intervention, and evaluation) via a computer network requires the traditional professional knowledge and skills of clinicians, as well as new knowledge and skills. Clinical interventions over computer networks require the clinician to have an understanding of how the technology involved affects client participation, communication, relationship development, and group norms, both social and computer behavior.

This chapter focuses on the group interactions of clinical encounters through computer communication. Specifically, the chapter describes interactions on the Forum, the public communication area of ComputerLink. The Forum was an unrestricted bulletin board on which users could read, post, and respond to concerns and interests. Messages consisted of requests for information, comments describing frustrations and daily hassles, suggestions for coping and management of problems, and simple acknowledgements. A series of messages on a common topic often comprised "conversations" on the Forum by participating members and the clinician moderator.

Ensuring Client Participation

One of the most important challenges for clinicians in computer clinical encounters is assisting clients to master the computer technology. Client comfort and skill in using computer technology are necessary for clinician-client network interactions, and the clinician must take an active role in designing aids to facilitate this mastery. One way to assist clients using the technology is to provide a user guidebook or manual. In the ComputerLink projects such a user manual was used in the initial training and clients were instructed to keep it by the computer for future problem solving. A telephone help number was included in the manual so that clients could call for assistance in using the computer if necessary.

Several techniques were used to simplify the complexity of computer use.

For example, "hot keys" were used to gain access to the system. On ComputerLink, hot keys were created that consisted of user access numbers, ID and passwords programmed on the function keys. A client needed only to push F1, F2, and F3 in sequence to gain entry into the main menu of the system, requiring only minimal typing and effort. Clients' use of different program features was facilitated by "seeding the system" with messages prepared in advance of installation to be used during the home training session. These seed messages instructed clients to respond and interact with specific aspects of the network, thus providing them immediate opportunities to experience different components of the system. To reinforce learning from the initial training session, subjects also were sent messages in the first 24 hours following installation of the computer that required them to use specific program features, such as the decision support module, the electronic encyclopedia, and the Q&A section.

Assisting clients to master appropriate command sequences to use the network requires coaching them through the desired experiences. ComputerLink was menu driven, with language specific to users. Clients were taught how to use "help functions" on the computer and were given assurance that nothing drastic would happen if they exited the system and started over. Further, participants observed all steps in the installation of the computer in their homes. The computers were purposely assembled in their presence so that they could observe and be instructed about the location of the power cord and keyboard attachments to the computer and see how the modem was hooked to the telephone and computer. Clients were encouraged to participate in assembling and setting up the computers in their homes, and simple computer maintenance and technical problem-solving issues were discussed. ComputerLink clients often commented that "this really isn't such a complicated machine after all."

Communication

Clinical interventions often take place in the context of exchanging information, giving emotional support, and providing counseling and individual or group psychotherapy. New communication challenges exist when computers are used for clinical encounters. They include the asynchronous nature of computer communication, multiple simultaneous conversations, diffuse time referents, and the absence of face-to-face visual cues.

The asynchronous nature of computer network communication is one of the most unique aspects of the medium. This asynchrony requires the clinician moderator and client participants to include *context* in posted messages, because messages remain over time and are available to be read and interpreted in both the near and distant future. Context can be built into messages by including references to preceding messages and by rephrasing questions or comments from other messages on the network that are pertinent to the discussion at hand. Another way to build context into messages is to use a title for a message that is consistent with the discussion. In the ComputerLink projects, each conversation strand had a unique title, allowing one to search and read all the titles making up a particular discussion. Here is the series of messages under one title:

From: MO
Subject: Driving HELP

My husband and I are having a big problem. We had to take the KEYS to the car away from dad. The doctor really did this but he does not remember, all he knows is that we have the keys. He will not even talk to my husband (his son) and we have to go over this again and again. We even had his attorney talk to him about why he can no longer drive. I have just about had it with him. At one point I just wanted to give him the keys and just say go. But I know in my heart that we can not do this. But it does not make it any easier. I HATE BEING THE BAD GUY.

From: S
Subject: Re: Driving HELP

TO MO

THIS IS S

I ALSO HAD TO TAKE THE KEYS FROM MY HUSBAND. WE HAD LOST OUR INSURANCE COVERAGE BECAUSE HE HAD SEVERAL ACCIDENTS IN THE PREVIOUS YEAR. HE WAS PERSUADED TO REQUEST CANCEL-LATION OF HIS DRIVING LICENSE AND I WAS ABLE TO OBTAIN INSURANCE IN MY NAME FOR MY CAR. I WENT ONE STEP FURTHER. I ASKED OUR OLDEST SON TO TAKE THE CAR SO THAT MY HUSBAND WOULD NOT SE IT AND WANT TO DRIVE. HE KNOWS NOW THAT WE ARE IN MY CAR WHEN I TAKE HIM TO THE PLACES THAT HE GOES.

THIS MIGHT NOT FIT YOUR SITUATION. BUT I BELIEVE THAT AS TIME PASSES YOUR HUSBAND WILL FORGET ABOUT DRIVING. DON'T GIVE UP!

From: KK
Subject: Re: Driving HELP

I don't know if this would be of help to you, but at our support group several months ago the same topic was discussed.

It didn't apply to me, because in our case once the Dr. told Mom she could no longer drive, surprisingly stopped—even gave her car to my brother-in-law. But I learned from the group, those who had problems could discreetly request the state to re-test an individual. They are then sent a letter, which informs them of the re-test and a date. If they don't come to the test someone is sent to the home, officially, to take away the keys and license. They never know who made the request.

Many times this makes for an easier transition for both the patient and the family. Hope in some way it might be helpful for you.

The ComputerLink system of titling messages also assisted the clinician and clients to manage the multiple simultaneous conversations that constitute computer network interactions.

Diffuse time referents are present in computer communication in that space and time take on different dimensions than in concurrent discussions. Because of the asynchronous interactions of most computer communication, feedback on questions and comments occurs over a longer time frame than in synchronous communication modes. The inclusion of a date and time on all posted messages provides orienting information for users.

The diffuse time referents are a special challenge to clinicians applying therapeutic group concepts on computer networks. Group therapy, for example, requires the clinician to grapple with the decision about how fast to respond to a silence in the group. Silences are used to give group members opportunities to formulate responses and to consider their contributions as members of the group. Leaders "wait out" a silence to allow group members the opportunity to participate more fully and to encourage participation by all members, rather than a discussion between the leader and selected members. In concurrent, face-to-face group interactions, leaders often "wait out" silences for a minute or two. However, in the asynchronous communication of computer networks, clinicians must learn what is an appropriate "waiting out" time for a group silence. On the AD caregivers ComputerLink group network, it was found that at approximately 24 to 36 hours a group member would break the silence with a comment. Thus, clinicians using computer networks must learn what constitutes reasonable response times in computer-mediated communication.

The absence of face-to-face visual cues requires the clinician to rely on a new set of cues, many of which differ from those of clinical encounters involving face-to-face or voice communication. Important communication cues are found in the content of the written messages themselves as well as in the clients' uses of message spacing, word selection, grammar, punctuation (such as exclamation points and dashes), and the frequency and length of messages.

Relationship Development

Developing and maintaining relationships is a goal in any therapeutic clinical encounter. There are challenges to relationship development in computer clinical situations. On the ComputerLink Forum, which used group interactions, a critical mass of users (6–8) was necessary to ensure enough interaction so that individuals' comments would receive attention by other group members. Therefore, when starting new groups the clinician should ensure that a large enough cohort of people simultaneously join the network.

In any therapeutic relationship, rapport and trust must be developed between the clinician and the client. When using computers, "introductions" must be designed by the clinician who serves as moderator. The introduction of new members is particularly important for group interventions. On ComputerLink this was facilitated by having an introduction system in place whereby a common set of information was requested of all new members to be shared on the network as they entered the network group. For example,

> From: TS
> Subject: Greeting from New Member
>
> hi my name is Tami
> my husband is in early stages of the disease and I live IN CLEVELAND HEIGHTS
> look forward to communicating with you.

Clinicians should also share information about themselves on the network including background and training and current role on the network.

Acknowledgment and encouragement of group members are also important in relationship development. On ComputerLink a relaxed tone was set by the moderators, who posted messages that encouraged (through modeling and responding) conversational language. For example, members were instructed not to worry about complete sentences when constructing messages, and the nurse moderators used "feeling-toned" words early in the computer discussions to demonstrate their use in computer communication.

Clinicians who are leading group interventions must encourage members to take responsibility for the group. The nurse moderators on Computer-Link used posted messages that encouraged individuals to feel a part of the group, for example, by starting messages on the Forum with "Dear Group" or by referring to a specific person on the network who might have had an experience similar to one currently described by another member. "Quiet" people (those who seldom posted messages) were gently encouraged to participate more by occasionally acknowledging that there were many people out there who were participating by reading but not posting messages and that their comments were welcome. As with any support group, balancing factual information with emotional support was a challenge for the clinicians on ComputerLink. Analysis of the use of the ComputerLink functions indicated that clients considered the support received from the computer group members one of the most important benefits of being part of the network.[8]

On ComputerLink several types of psychosocial support, including instrumental support, emotional support, and spiritual support, were provided to clients.[9,10] Contrary to what might be expected on a computer, people interacted on an emotional level, sharing intimate feelings and problems. Clients' emotional support to each other included expressions of sympathy, understanding, and a sense of community—for example, "I know what you are going through," "We are all in this together," and "I am sorry you have had such a rough time lately."

The clinician moderators paid attention to the feelings of members by noting clues to emotions communicated in the posted messages. The moderators provided validation and feedback to those people who took risks in the group by disclosing information that might be considered difficult to share publicly. Yalom's[11] group therapeutic factors of instillation of hope, universality, information, altruism, corrective recapitulation of the primary family group, development of socializing techniques, imitative behavior, interpersonal learning, group cohesiveness, catharsis, and existential issues were employed using the computer groups. The use of these therapeutic factors in the ComputerLink projects has been described in detail elsewhere.[12]

Group Norms

Social Norms

Facilitating group norms is important in group interventions. In computer network groups this involves both social norms and computer behavior norms. Social group norms are based on group purpose (therapeutic group, support group) and group membership (elders, teens, chronic or acute illness, etc.). The group leadership style of the clinician moderator has an important influence on group norms. For example, a group in which the clinician uses a model of the clinician-as-expert will have different group dynamics from a group in which the clinician routinely draws upon the expertise of the members. In the ComputerLink projects, both the AD caregivers and the PLWA group members often provided more support and information in a given discussion than the clinician moderators.

Another group norm involves management of issues of confidentiality. As in all groups, confidentiality issues for computer network groups must be discussed with the members. On the ComputerLink projects, confidentiality issues involved printing out messages and the use of the network by persons who were not members of the ComputerLink group. Because the computers were in subjects' homes, other members of the household obviously had access to the computer. ComputerLink participants were encouraged not to share their passwords, and periodic reminders were given by the moderators about the importance of the confidentiality of discussions on the network.

As is common to any group, members of the ComputerLink groups needed to learn that it was safe to bring up sensitive topics, such as those having social stigma or that might be viewed as taboo. Among the AD caregiver group, sensitive topics included wanting a divorce from a spouse with AD, wanting one's own life free of the responsibilities of caregiving, and euthanasia. In the PLWA group sensitive topics included suicide, sexual behavior, and alternative treatments. The risk of bringing up such topics in a computer network group may be perceived by clients as greater than the risk in face-to-face groups because computer network messages often remain on the network for some time after posting. The clinician moderator can encourage this risk taking by posting messages that model acceptance of the feeling or topic and inviting group members to comment on them.

An unexpected issue that ComputerLink project clinicians encountered was handling a client posting that contained dangerous or inaccurate advice. Client messages such as "I'd suggest you slip some extra pills tonight" or "Take some arsenic and end it all" were not removed by the clinicians despite technical ability to do so. Instead, moderators responded to dangerous or inaccurate messages with a posting that clearly indicated they did not support the content of the message, and when possible they gave a "professional opinion" about the issue.

The ComputerLink project involved a target group of clients that clinicians came to know well. However, in computer network situations in which there is no target client group (organized around a specific issue or for a specific timeframe) or opportunity to know clients well, the clinician-moderator's central role may be to assist communication among members. Clinicians may also rely more on direct information giving and referral to community resources as methods of client interaction.

Computer Behavior Norms

Computer behavior norms that the clinician-moderator can influence include the use of conversational language in posted messages, the acceptance of typographical errors, the frequency of member participation, and "acceptable" topics. On ComputerLink, interesting computer behavior norms developed concerning the frequency of posted messages near the planned termination of the groups. In both networks, clients engaged in weaning behaviors near the predetermined project end. That is, clients posted messages indicating that they had plans to decrease their use of the system slowly over time so that they would not be too dependent on the network when it ended. Analysis of client use of the system near the end of the project indicated that clients did in fact decrease their participation as the end of the projects neared.

Computer Features and Clinical Intervention Approaches

Maintenance of a therapeutic milieu on a computer network is facilitated by the use of a philosophy of care to guide clinician decisions. For example, in the ComputerLink projects, self-care[13] was emphasized. The goal of encouraging clients in self-care guided the nurse moderators' decisions about how much information to directly give clients and how much information they should be encouraged to seek on their own through the use of resources on the network. Consistent with the philosophy of self-care, clients on ComputerLink were linked with other individuals on the network and referred to other sections of the network, such as the Electronic Encyclopedia and the Decision Support Module. Also, the techniques used by clinician moderators to support relationship development and group social norm development emphasized the expertise of the group as well as the clinician's professional expertise.

Computer Features and Clinical Encounters

Several features of computer interactions affect the boundaries and contexts of clinical encounters. One important feature of computer communication is the necessity of translating information into text. Computer communication is restricted to a set of cues present in the pattern and context of posted messages. Cues frequently used by clinicians, such as facial expressions, rate of speech, and body position, are not accessible. Instead, clinicians are dependent on client-reported cues, symptoms, and descriptions. Individuals who only read messages and seldom or never post messages are participating in the network in ways that provide few cues for the clinician. Dependence on the keyboard to transmit ideas may also impede the communication of large amounts of information at any one time.

At the same time, because there is no face-to-face contact in computer communication, some physical signs of power that affect relationships (e.g., white lab coats, skin color, physical size) are removed from the interaction. Thus, computer interactions may promote more equal status in the clinician-client relationship than often exists in face-to-face encounters.

The temporal nature of computer communication (delayed time vs. real time) offers less opportunity for on-the-spot validation and feedback. However, in computer communication, the clinician is provided unlimited time for reflection, composing, editing, sending, and retrieving messages. And unlike spoken words that are lost after they are said, computer messages remain and they can be repeatedly read or interpreted by network users. An additional feature of computer clinical environments is the potential to systematically analyze recorded clinical interactions. Thus, clinicians can engage in continuous improvement of their interventions if desired.

Interventions Not Supported

One of the drawbacks of computer communication is inability to handle emergencies. The clinician moderator should be open to cues in messages that indicate health emergency situations. In the ComputerLink project, emergencies included a suicide threat, possible elder abuse, and manic behavior. In such situations there is need for a more immediate form of communication than the computer network provides. In the emergency situations that arose with ComputerLink, telephone calls were made either to the clients themselves or other resources for assistance with the problem. Also, a standard message should be placed on the network that clients see on entering the system, which instructs them not to use the network for emergency situations.

Summary

Advances in technology suggest that clinical interventions in the future will occur in many environments, including locations remote from acute care centers such as homes, long-term care settings, and community health clinics. Computers can enhance clinicians' abilities to intervene with clients because they afford opportunities to provide interventions in a timely manner, overcoming geographical and social barriers.

The unique features of computer networks offer both advantages and challenges. Advantages for the delivery of clinical interventions include the ability to (1) access clients in an efficient, yet supportive manner; (2) respond to multiple levels of need in multiple clients; (3) attend to emotional as well as concrete needs; and (4) provide the opportunity to systematically analyze interventions over time. Client benefits include the opportunity to (1) use the service at a time, frequency and duration of their choice; (2) be supported in self-care efforts, rather than in a more dependent role; and (3) engage in a normalization of their experience. Challenges of computer networks for the delivery of clinical interventions include (1) the lack of physical presence of members; (2) diffuse time referents; (3) asynchronous communication; and (4) and necessity for clients to learn to use the technology. Computers provide a unique context for interpersonal communication.[14] The dynamics of clinical encounters on computer networks require a new set of knowledge and skills on the part of the clinician to optimize this technology.

Acknowledgments. Funded by Grants #AG8614 and NR 2001 from the National Institute of Health.

References

1. Behrend S W. Documentation in the ambulatory setting. *Semin Oncol–Nursing.* 1994;10:264–280.
2. Skinner CS. The potential of computers in patient education. *Patient Ed Counsel.* 1993;22:27–34.
3. Malik RL, Horwitz DL, Smyth-Staruch K. Energy metabolism in diabetes:

Computer-assisted instruction for persons with diabetes. *Diabetes Educator*. 1987;13:203–205.

4. Brown-Ewing LJ, Finkelstein SM, Budd JR, Kujawa SJ, Wielinski CL, Warwick WJ, et al. Implementation of a home-based program for early detection of clinical deterioration in systic fibrosis. *Med Instrumentat*. 1988;22:240–246.

5. Paperny, DM, Aono JY, Lehman RM, Hamar SL, Risser J. Computer-assisted detection and intervention in adoescent high-risk health behaviors. *J Pediatr*. 1990;116:456–462.

6. McNamara DM. Health-oriented telecommunication: A community resource. *Nursing Manage*. 1994;25(12):40–41.

7. Gustafson DH, Bosworth K, Chewning BJ, Hawkins R. Computer-based health promotion: Combining technological advance and problem solving technique to effect successful halth behavior changes. *Ann Rev Public Health*. 1987;8:387–415.

8. Brennan PF, Moore SM, Smyth KA. The effects of a special computer network on AD caregivers. *Nursing Res*. 1995;44:166–172.

9. Brennan PF, Moore SM, Smyth KA. Alzheimer's disease caregivers' uses of a computer network. *Western J Nursing Res*. 1992;14:662–673.

10. Gallienne RL, Moore SM, Brennan PF. Alzheimer's caregivers: Psychosocial support via computer networks. *J Geront Nursing*. 1993;19:15–22.

11. Yalom ID. *The Theory and Practice of Group Psychotherapy*. 2nd ed. New York: Basic Books; 1985.

12. Ripich S, Moore SM, Brennan PF. A new nursing Medium: Computer networks for group intervention. *J Psychosocial Nursing*. 1992;30:15–20.

13. Orem DE. *Nursing: Concepts of Practice*. 3rd ed. New York: McGraw-Hill; 1990.

14. Hesse BW, Werner CM, Altman I. Temporal aspects of computer-mediated communication. *Comput Human Behav*. 1988;4:147–163.

16

Privacy, Confidentiality, and CHINs

Randolph C. Barrows, Jr. and Paul D. Clayton

The clear emerging benefits of electronic medical records (EMRs) and Community Health Information Networks (CHINs) are discussed elsewhere in this volume: they include sharing patient data between remote generalists and specialists, sending prescriptions to pharmacies, providing access to vital health information in an emergency, ensuring that standards of care are being met, and so forth. Because the purpose of CHINs is to increase the accessibility and sharing of health records (among authorized individuals), public concern about the unauthorized disclosure of health information is understandable. Privacy of the information collected during health care processes is necessary because of significant economic, psychological, and social harm that can come to individuals when personal health information is disclosed.[1-3] With remote access to distributed health data in a CHIN environment, or the pooling of health data from multiple CHIN participants in a central repository, the potential for loss of information privacy is greater than in isolated institutional EMR systems or paper medical records. However, with appropriate safeguards, computer-based medical records may actually offer more security than traditional paper record systems.

In this chapter we examine the extent to which fears of the loss of privacy are justified, and discuss measures to protect the security of health data. We also consider the tradeoffs between accessibility and security of electronic medical records compared to paper records. In our discussion, we use "security" to refer to issues of confidentiality, integrity, and availability of health data.

We believe that currently available security mechanisms are sufficient to enable CHINs to exist while using inexpensive public and commercial communication systems and media. Security technologies have proven effective in the banking and military sectors, but experience is lacking to demonstrate that similar technologies are satisfactory for healthcare. As yet no model security implementations exist in any clinical computing environment,[2] although awareness of risks and possible technical solutions is increasing.

Goals of Informational Security in Health Care

While there is currently a lack of cohesive security policy across institutions, counties, and states, governmental and nongovernmental committees are grappling with difficult policy details that have far-reaching consequences. Although it may be challenging to establish and implement security policies, the goals of information security in health care can be simply stated[1,4,5]:

1. To ensure the confidentiality of health care data and the privacy of patients (prevention of unauthorized disclosure of information);
2. To ensure the integrity of health care data (prevention of unauthorized modification of information); and
3. To ensure the availability of health data for authorized persons (prevention of unauthorized or unintended withholding of information or resources).

The goal of information privacy raises issues of access control (user authentication and authorization) and the use of cryptographic protocols for data transmission and storage. The goal of data integrity introduces the need for electronic user and data authentication.[6,7] The goal of data availability raises issues of access control and system reliability and backups. The policy and technical aspects of these and related issues are discussed below.

Security Policy

As many have pointed out,[1,2,8-10] the main problem with information security in health care is not technology, but a lack of cohesive security policy. It is policy that must shape technology, not vice versa. CHINs are "cutting edge," so implementors must set interinstitutional policy where none has previously existed, and they must find applicable technologies to implement their policy.

Security policy defines what is to be protected, to what reasonable degree protections will be afforded, and who is privileged to access protected items. A policy is influenced by:

1. the functional requirements of an information system (what users need to accomplish from the system);
2. the security requirements for the system (items that need to be protected); and
3. a threat model (the expected motives and resources of potential perpetrators).

It is the role of policy to balance the functional and security requirements of a system, which are typically at odds. Security requirements can often be tempered by the practical concerns of a threat model, because costs and user inconveniences rise sharply with stricter security.

As an example of a threat concern, consider that the most routine kinds of security transgressions are "inside attacks," that is, from persons who are legitimate system users with privileges, but who abuse their privileges in search of gossip material or for other personal or financial reasons. The monetary value of health data obtainable on most individuals, however, is relatively low (unlike some financial data or military secrets), so it is reasonably safe to assume that an attacker will not spend inordinate resources (money and time) in attempting to acquire such data by computer break-in or cryptanalytic attack. Specifically desired information, as always, might be available with less trouble and expense via "social engineering" techniques (bribery, extortion, personal misrepresentation of identity, etc.). Health data on celebrities and VIPs may be of greater monetary value in certain markets, but currently available (although not necessarily implemented) security mechanisms, such as system management, access control, and encryption techniques, are sufficient to detect and thwart the covert activities of hospital employees, newspaper reporters, relatives, and other unsophisticated attackers.

Other potential threats come from information-hungry employers, insurance companies, and managed care organizations. These organizations have greater economic resources, along with the motivation of significant profit from what they can know about individuals. Unethical operations in such industries could allocate a high-end computer to the task of breaking a cryptographic key used in the transmission of health data over inexpensive public channels. The 1995 cost of a machine capable of breaking a DES (Data Encryption Standard of the U.S. Government) key within 1 year (with an 8 percent chance per month) is only $64,000.[11] Profit-motivated health care-related organizations and unethical "private investigators" might be willing to make this investment and, for example, gather HIV data that could be used covertly to deny medical insurance coverage.

These threats are to data confidentiality, but threat models should also consider attacks on the integrity and availability of health data. Such threats might come from malevolent "hackers," natural disasters, or mechanical failures, and they could potentially cost the data guardians of CHIN implementations more than any breach in confidentiality.

The Data Security Policy and Standards developed for the Mayo Clinic/Foundation provide one model of a clear institutional security policy statement.[12] Columbia-Presbyterian Medical Center (CPMC), in approaching a statement of policy, hired external consultants to facilitate security policy development for its Integrated Advanced Information Management System (IAIMS) project.[13] After 24 meetings with 80 people from numerous departments in two institutions, 14 (overlapping) topic areas for policy development were identified:

1. *User authentication*—issues related to the identification of users to the system, and how the system might know that users are who they claim to be.
2. *Physical security of data center sites*—issues related to physical access to computer hardware, theft prevention, backup and disaster recovery, and the security at sensitive terminal locations such as console or control and publicly accessible terminals.
3. *Access control to system resources*—issues of the physical devices and logical mechanisms, such as computer programs, that control access to system resources.
4. *Data ownership*—issues of who will own which data, delegation of authority over data, and delineation of the duties and responsibilities of data ownership.
5. *Data protection policies*—issues of minimally acceptable and consistent protections to be afforded by systems crossing organizational and functional boundaries, anticipated implementation barriers to those protections, and the punitive measures for organizational members abusing system privileges.
6. *Building security into systems*—issues of how to ensure that security requirements are addressed in central and local participating systems, how to divide security responsibilities between central and local systems, and how to ensure that security requirements are satisfied when systems are modified or expanded.
7. *Security for hard copy materials*—issues of how to prevent security breaches from paper copies of sensitive electronic documents and data.
8. *Systems integrity*—issues related to the accuracy and reliability of system data, and the integrity and reliability of physical computer and network systems.
9. *User profiles*—issues related to defining user types and roles that serve to distinguish the functional needs and security levels of users.
10. *Legal and liability issues*—issues related to the uses and misuses of the system that involve potential liabilities or legal concerns for participating organizations, including protections under existing computer crime laws, liabilities when a record is compromised, and requirements for user penalties under union contracts.
11. *Problem identification and resolution*—issues of system audits and auditability, intrusion detection and notification of intrusions, and detection and notification mechanisms for other types of security problems.
12. *Network security*—issues related to the security management of computer networks and the movement of data over such networks, including the security of bridges and routing equipment, the passing of

authorization tokens, data encryption, electronic signatures, and non-repudiation of messages.

13. *Informed consent*—issues related to the use of medical information collected about patients and obtaining consent from patients for desired and potential uses of medical data.

14. *Education of users*—issues related to the education of users regarding their responsibilities as system users and the risks created by their actions, including activities on the system and degrees of nonvigilance.

From these 14 areas, a list of 65 policy items needing definition were identified. These items were then ranked, resulting in a list of 17 urgent actions. Of particular note, the number one action item was to establish a mechanism for making institutional policy!

Privacy and Confidentiality in Health Care

The health care provider-patient relationship is characterized by intimacy and trust, and confidentiality is embedded, at least implicitly, in patient-provider interactions. The notion of confidentiality in health care has a strong professional tradition that has suffered progressive erosion due to third-party reimbursement schemes, managed care and other healthcare organizational structures, and the perceptions and culture of professionals in modern health care systems.[14] One third of medical professionals have indicated that information is given to unauthorized people "somewhat often."[3]

Unfortunately, information privacy currently has an incomplete and inconsistent legal basis.[15] Federal law prohibiting information disclosure only pertains to Federal agencies, not to the private sector or state and local governments. Most states have laws that at least minimally address the privacy of medical records, but they do not consistently recognize computerized records as legitimate documents. Thus, in most states laws are inadequate to guide CHIN developers with respect to obligations to protect the privacy of computerized medical information within state or across state borders.

One reason that it is difficult to set policy is that the legal concept of privacy is relative and shifts from time to time to reflect the public versus private interests of society.[16] Consider, for example, airline passenger and baggage inspection policies now compared to 30 years ago, and laws that require the reporting of infectious, especially sexually transmitted, diseases. In addition, privacy is partly in the eye of the beholder, and an intrusion of privacy perceived by one person may be considered a convenience by others (targeted marketing, mail-order catalogs, solicitations by insurers and preventive health service providers, etc.).

In a 1993 survey, 80 percent of persons said they believed consumers had lost control over information about themselves.[3] CHIN developers should strive to maintain the confidentiality of personal health information to foster public trust in information systems that hold promise for improving health care quality and decreasing the costs of care. For their own benefit and the benefit of society, patients should not feel reluctant to share medically relevant information with health care practitioners.

It should be recognized, however, that the goal of strict information privacy conflicts with the goals of optimal patient care, medical research, public health, and social policy, all of which may require access to patients' confidential medical records without their knowledge or explicit consent. In addition, healthcare providers have a working need for high data availability and are intolerant of cumbersome security procedures. For instance, when access hurdles are too steep, logon sessions and passwords may be shared among providers. Because the use of information technology in healthcare is still relatively new and not yet ubiquitous, there is generally too little awareness of the risks created by such actions.

Technically, the confidentiality of medical records on computers can be maintained by access control mechanisms, and by audit trail logs, which can be inspected proactively or in response to suspicious events. Other mechanisms for assuring confidentiality include the education of CHIN organization members regarding security concerns, professional responsibilities, and personal accountability; time-outs on system terminals; hard-copy control; clear policies; and consistent disciplinary actions. Human factors, however, such as errors, negligence, and unethical activities, can result in breaches of confidentiality despite optimal security implementations.

Accordingly, it is the view of the American Civil Liberties Union (ACLU) that a privacy policy for health information should be based on the following principles[17]:

1. Strict limits on access and disclosure must apply to all personally identifiable health data, regardless of the form in which the information is maintained.
2. All personally identifiable health records must be under an individual's control. No personal information may be disclosed without an individual's uncoerced, informed consent.
3. Health record information systems must be required to build in security measures to protect personal information against both unauthorized access and misuse by authorized users.
4. Employers must be denied access to personally identifiable health information on their employees and prospective employees.
5. Patients must be given notice of all uses of their health information.
6. Individuals must have a right of access to their own medical and financial records, including rights to copy and correct any and all information contained in those records.

7. Both a private right of action and a governmental enforcement mechanism must be established to prevent and/or remedy wrongful disclosures or other misuse of information.
8. Establishment of a federal oversight system is necessary to ensure compliance with privacy laws and regulations.

Data Ownership and Legal Accountability

Data ownership is a legally complex issue. Ownership of a medical record is at best a limited right that is primarily custodial in nature, and information contained in the record is often characterized as the patient's property.[18] It does not appear that there will be any immediate and clear legal assignment of electronic health data ownership from which may follow assignment of responsibility. As an issue of concern to CHIN participants, it is reasonable to state that all parties who are entrusted with health data, both movers and users, should be considered as stewards of that data, and they may be held liable for irresponsible acts and breaches of confidentiality. Thus, a heightened sense of personal responsibility for health data among CHIN participants is warranted.

According to Dierdra Mulligan, an expert in privacy policy at the Center for Democracy and Technology (a nonprofit public interest organization based in Washington, DC) and a consultant to the John A. Hartford Foundation for their Community Health Management Information System (CHMIS) projects, data ownership is actually a "red-herring" issue for CHIN/CHMIS implementors, who would be better served by not focusing on this unresolvable issue (though it is difficult to entirely avoid) and by focusing instead on the problem of access control.[19]

Informed Consent to Disclosure

Informed consent to disclosure of information typically requires that the patient:

1. be told what information is to be disclosed;
2. understand what is being disclosed;
3. be competent to provide consent; and
4. consent willingly, free from coercion.

There are many potential difficulties with implementing this doctrine, and "informed consent," as it pertains to typical uses of health care data, is arguably neither. Infirm or confused patients cannot meaningfully sign an informed release, and no informed release specifically covers all potential or desired uses of medical data that may be collected on an individual. Also, patients are coerced into giving up personal rights to confidentiality when they apply for insurance or sign a hospital waiver that allows medical information to be shared. (In recognition of such concerns, a general release of medical information in New York State no longer applies to HIV data.) Finally, patients are typically asked to authorize disclosure of medical information, yet only about half of the states guarantee patients' rights to see their own medical record. Traditionally patients have difficulty gaining access to their own records, but without knowledge of what is contained in the record, consent for disclosure cannot be fully informed. The position of the American Health Information Management Association (AHIMA) reflects a balance of opinion, and states that a computer-based patient record requires that patients have greater access to their own medical record.[20]

With these problems, alternatives to the use of an informed consent policy might be considered by CHIN participants. One competing notion suggests that individuals gain medical benefits in exchange for reasonable uses of their medical information for prescribed purposes. Once reasonable uses are defined, the CHIN must protect data and enforce only defined uses. Informed consent would be required for special uses of the data. Because CHINs potentially limit an individual's ability to control the use, disclosure, and security of personal and sensitive information, policy that errs on the side of caution is warranted.

Use of Medical Data

The primary uses of medical records are to provide health care, pay for it, and assure its proper delivery. Secondary uses of medical data include uses by various business and governmental organizations such as life and auto insurers, employers, licensing agencies, public health agencies, the media, medical researchers, educational institutions, rehabilitation and social welfare programs, and uses for legal purposes. Responsibility for the protection of patient privacy and the confidentiality of computerized medical information must extend to these secondary users. CHIN policy should dictate how patient data may be used and to whom information will be released.

When electronic records are used for research, valid epidemiological studies may be conducted using aggregates of nonidentifiable patient data. In other cases, encrypted patient identifiers might provide acceptable research results and still adequately protect patient privacy.

User Authentication and Access Control

Originators of the few landmark computer-based patient record systems have grappled with the conflicting goals of security and functionality in health care systems.[21] Generally, systems use some form of password security for user authentication, and user-specific or role-specific menus may be used to further limit access. However, standard password access controls do not prevent insider threats, and they are not helpful when authentication has been compromised.

In addition, tight access control at the level of type of user, computer application, or patient fails in critical ways in the healthcare environment.[4,6] Sensitive data (e.g., mental health data or HIV status) are often among the most important items necessary to take care of a patient. This information may need to be made available and shared among numerous care providers and ancillary health personnel. Generally, numerous persons at multiple levels in multiple roles (medical students, residents, nurses, therapists, dietitians, social workers, administrators, consultant physicians, covering physicians, as well as a private or personal "attending" physician) are routinely involved in a patient's care, and it is difficult to predict which person in which role will validly need access to a person's health record at some particular time. Provisions for emergencies, when none of the patient's usual care team is around, must also be made. Similar concerns apply to CHINs. Thus, in an EMR (Electronic Medical Record) setting it is often not practical to prohibit access by most medical users to most data on most patients. For this reason, clinical system pioneers have generally allowed all clinical personnel access to the computerized medical record of all patients in a hospital, and usually the records of patients not in the hospital as well (i.e. discharged patients and/or their ambulatory care records).

Improved multilevel and role-based access models for health care that better accommodate user needs are under development.[22–25] A "need to show" model (vs. the military "need to know" multilevel security model) and its supportive technical platform have been proposed to extend the notion of personal professional accountability for health data to interaction with information systems.[26] Such accountability may help discourage information sharing across unauthorized informal human networks,[27] a problem that is difficult to address by technology.

It is a matter of institutional and CHIN policy to decide how much effort should go toward authenticating a person. User identifiers with password authentication are commonly employed; other technical solutions such as biometric authentication by morphometric hand measurements or voiceprints, system-synchronized random number generating cards, and passphrase-encrypting smartcards are more expensive but can be more effective alternatives when appropriate.

The CPMC Clinical Information System (CIS) implements an access control matrix with user roles along one axis (attending physicians, residents, medical students, hospital nurses, clinic nurses, various types of technicians, etc.) and data types (laboratory data, radiology reports, discharge summaries, demographic information, etc.) along the other. We defined 68 user types and 6 classes of data. Departmental leaders determine access privileges for each user type, subject to the approval of the hospital medical board. Users receive a menu of options specific for their defined access privileges. Login screens remind users that information is limited to legitimate medical purposes and misuse can lead to dismissal as well as civil and criminal penalties. Access to data on VIPs and hospital employees invokes an additional screen message warning that all user activities are recorded.

Cryptography

Cryptographic techniques applicable to the goals of privacy, integrity, and access control have not yet been widely deployed in the health care environment, and experience is needed before confidence can be gained that they can provide security solutions compatible with the diversity of health care needs.[28]

As a trivial example of an encryption cipher, the famous Caesar Cipher uses a "shift by three" rule, so that every 'A' in a message is replaced by a 'D', every 'B' by an 'E', and so forth. The algorithm is said to have been used by Julius Caesar to encode communications with his generals via human messengers whom he did not trust. Many more complicated and secure mathematical algorithms for encryption exist. Private-key, or "secret key," encryption depends upon a number or string of characters, shared only between the communicating parties, that is used by an encryption algorithm to encode and decode the message. The exact encryption algorithm need not be a secret. The best known such encryption algorithm is DES. One of the main problems with private-key encryption protocols is that communicating parties must somehow manage to securely share and use the secret key.

Public-key encryption can avoid some of the pitfalls of a secret key by making use of a mathematical technique that creates an "asymmetrical cryptosystem" that is, the keys to encode and decode a message are different but intimately linked so that they are, in effect, functional inverses of each other and can only be used together. In public-key cryptography, one key is published and the other remains private to a user. To send a secret message, the recipient's public key is obtained by the sender and is used to scramble the message, which only the recipient can decode with the private key. In addition, the creator of a message or document can "sign" it by encoding a piece or algorithmic digest of the document with his or her secret key, and anyone can then verify the "signature" by decoding it with the signer's published key.

The New York State CHMIS Confidentiality and Data Security Policy says "All data collected into or handled through the repository and defined as 'deniable' (identifiable) . . . shall be encrypted, both when being transmitted through the network or if written to a local system. Software and/or hardware shall be supplied with secure algorithms which will encrypt/

decrypt all such sensitive data".[29] For practical purposes, due to the imbedding of sensitive data in text documents, it is reasonable to recommend that all health data in a CHIN environment be encrypted when transmitted over public or insecure channels and when residing on storage devices in local machines.

The Massachusetts Institute of Technology's Kerberos is a secret-key cryptographic protocol for the provision of authentication and authorization services in a distributed environment. Its use has been outlined for the health care setting but not implemented.[6] Public key cryptographic protocols have been proposed to address the need for a universal (across institutions and states) patient identifier.[30] Software toolkits for the secure transmission and archiving of files by medical applications are beginning to appear.[7] In the near future, vendor products will supply encryption technology embedded within computer systems for health care. Until then, CHIN developers must create their own implementations of well known and secure cryptographic algorithms and protocols.[11]

Data Integrity

Electronic patient data can be assumed valid based on software testing and verification, access control mechanisms, and error-checking protocols used in data transport, or (in addition) it can be authenticated with digital signatures, as discussed above. Most lapses in data integrity will continue to be due to human error and malfunctions or bugs in medical computer systems.

Firewalls

Firewalls are computers that are positioned between a site's internal network and an unsecured public network such as the Internet; they may be particularly useful at CHIN sites. Firewall computers are configured to monitor and regulate the messages passing into and out of a site's private network and thus can prevent unauthorized users from entering local computer systems from the outside, or can prevent particular programs and services from operating through the firewall. Such functionality can help protect private information from leaving a CHIN site, or can impose an extra layer of password security on authorized users.

Reliability, Redundancy, and System Backups

As discussed above, threat models should consider "attacks," whether natural or manmade, accidental or intentional, on the integrity and availability of health data. Hardware or software failures, including "denial of service" attacks, can cause downtime or loss of vital health care data for CHIN participants. The reliability of CHIN systems and data should be considered a security concern and covered in security policy and system management activities, usually via mechanisms that support data redundancy and system backups.

Audit Trails

Primarily due to limitations on the applicability of access control methods in health care, the audit trail is a critical tool for managing data security issues. In any large computing environment there is significant risk for misuse of the system by authorized users. For this reason, the audit trail has become an important reactive security mechanism, used commonly to detect security violations post hoc and support disciplinary actions.

For example, at CPMC the CIS records the identity of any individual who looks at patient data and the type of data accessed. In one instance, a resident physician in obstetrics harassed a nurse about being pregnant before the nurse had announced her pregnancy to any individual. The nurse complained, and review of audit trail data showed the resident physician had looked at the nurse's test results and, without a valid "need to know," this led to an official reprimand. In another instance, a resident physician contracted a serious illness that required a hospital stay. He requested a list of all those who accessed his data to see if colleagues had violated his privacy and was relieved to see that only those who provided his care were on the list. Such reassurance could not be obtained from the paper medical record.

One problem with audit trail data is that typically the data are far too voluminous for human processing. A level C2 (a Department of Defense computer security classification requiring auditing and the unavailability of encrypted passwords) audit mechanism for a multi-user system can fill 1 gigabyte of disk space within an hour.[31] One published prototype system generated 7 megabytes (MB) per day per average user, and up to 136 MB for a busy user.[32] The CIS audit trail logs as implemented at CPMC fill about 100 MB of disk space per month. Typically 95 percent of audit data is of no security significance,[33] and use of the data accumulated in security audit files is at best minimal. Extraneous data in the files obviously makes it harder to detect suspicious behavior, especially behavior that can be detected only by examining complex relationships between data features, something particularly difficult to discover.

Automated reduction and analysis tools for audit trail data could help immensely, but their availability is still limited. Discussing data reduction methods for intrusion detection, Frank[34] gives an example of selection methods to identify a subset of data features that best classify some audit data. Systems that implement some kind of automated analysis of audit trail data are relatively recent. Early approaches to audit trail analysis only categorized threats as due to internal versus external penetrators, but the goal is to identify threats by any users or processes that attempt an illegal action within their authorized boundaries (abuse of system privileges), not within their authorized boundaries (exceeding system privileges), as well as any action by unauthorized system users, such as intruders who masquerade as authorized users or otherwise evade system authentication and security controls.[35] Recent models for intrusion detection have used statistical user profiling or expert system techniques that examine the deviation of actual user behaviors from anticipated or usual behaviors on the system.[36]

Intrusion detection methodologies differ based on the type of intrusion: anomaly versus misuse.[30] Misuse detection refers to well-defined patterns of intrusion, exploiting weaknesses in software that can be detected directly. Because it looks for known vulnerabilities, misuse detection is of little use in detecting new or unknown intrusive behaviors. Anomaly detection depends on unusual behavior or use of system resources, and seeks to detect the complement of normal behavior. Generally, intrusive activity is expected to be some subset of anomalous activity, but intrusive behavior does not always coincide with anomalous behavior, and might be the sum of individual nonanomalous activities.

Nine intrusion detection tools are reviewed by Marshall.[33] Most of these systems do both anomaly and misuse detection. Statistical techniques lend themselves to anomaly detection but are inadequate to detect all types of intrusions and do not prevent users from gradually training their usage profiles so activity previously considered anomalous might be regarded as normal. Expert systems and model-based techniques lend themselves to misuse detection, but specifying the orderings on facts, for the pattern matching of events, is inefficient.[31] Thus, in the best systems, anomaly and misuse detection methods complement each other.

Each system is, out of necessity, somewhat ad hoc and custom designed. Few systems are general or flexible enough to be easily portable or adaptable. More generic systems, capable of reuse and retargetting, are likely to be inefficient or of limited power. Also, the cost of building an intrusion detection system is high and requires specialized knowledge input from system and security experts who can make an appropriate choice of statistical metrics and specify expert rules. Moreover, testing and validation of intrusion detection systems is difficult because potential attack scenarios can be difficult to simulate, and the lack of a common audit trail format precludes easy comparisons between the performance of existing systems against common attack scenarios.

Consequently, no commercially available audit analysis tool kit exists, and there is as yet no known application of software tools for audit analysis in the health care sector. The idea, however, was discussed by Shea[6] and is apparently being implemented in the European community.[35]

A Comparison of Paper and Electronic Record Environments

Many security issues apply to paper-based as well as electronic records. The most obvious new risk factor afforded by electronic records is also the benefit that pushes us toward that format: more convenient access to, and distribution of, health information. A related and potentially troubling capability is the ability to query for a population of patients who have a common feature (such as the same surgeon or a particular test result). Any risks of an electronic breach of security must be weighed against analogous risks in paper record systems, and against the recognized disadvantages of paper records. Electronic records are arguably more secure if proper policies and currently available technologies are in place.

For example, with paper medical records it is not possible to keep an accurate audit trail of who has seen the record and what portions of the record were accessed. It is also difficult to restrict certain classes of users only to particular types of information. Paper records are easily altered by removal or substitution of documents, but an electronic document signed with an encrypted digital signature is much more difficult to alter. The paper record can only be in one place at a time, whereas the same information in electronic format can be available to multiple users simultaneously. It is also possible to present the content of the computer-based medical record in a clearly organized and legible fashion so that caregivers are more likely to respond to important information. In a paper-based environment, it is not possible to generate real time rule-based suggestions and warnings when standards of healthcare are missed. Also, costs may soon favor the use of electronic medical record systems. For example, at CPMC the cost to find and pull a paper record from the file room for doctors, for just a single patient visit, has been estimated to be between $5 and $10. In contrast, we estimate that the total cost for the creation and lifetime maintenance of an electronic record for our patients is between $25 and $50.

Thus, substantial advantages to the electronic record exist, and it seems prudent to move ahead with electronic record implementations, including the policies required to guide the use of available security technologies.

Conclusion

In summary, while security concerns surrounding health data in CHIN environments are justified, problems are surmountable with currently available technologies. In the banking industry, electronic security mechanisms have enabled increased personal conveniences that include access to bank accounts from a choice of locations and at all times of day. Although neither automatic tellers nor electronic medical records are free from abuse, protocols for electronic systems probably provide better security than those that exist in analogous manual systems. In any security system, the weak links are most likely to be human.

A major challenge will be enticing developers, who are eager for working medical computer applications, to make the financial and time investments in designing and building adequate security features into their systems. Institutional and CHIN policies will be a key stimulus in this regard. Chief financial officers will probably come to regard security investments as insurance policies: although we must pay for the policies, we are pleased when there is no need to file a claim. In our opinion, a more formidable barrier than security requirements to sharing records in a CHIN environment is the current lack of convenient and acceptable ways to acquire data from patients and providers in an electronic format. Security issues should not deter progress toward solving this more substantial problem.

References

1. Gostin LO, Turek-Brezina J, Powers M, Kozloff R, Faden R, Steinauer DD. Privacy and security of personal information in a new health care system. *JAMA.* 1993;270(20):2487–2493.
2. Shea S. Security versus access: Trade-offs are only part of the story. *J Am Med Inform Assoc.* 1994;1(4):314–315.
3. Davis R. Online medical records raise privacy fears. *USA Today,* Section A:1, March 22, 1995.
4. Bakker AR. Security in medical information systems. In: van Bemmel JH, McCray AT (eds). *Yearbook of Medical Informatics.* Shattauer, Stuttgart-New York; 1993:52–60.
5. Bengtsson S. Clinical requirements for the security of the electronic patient record. *Int J Biomed Comput.* 1994;35(Suppl 1):29–31.
6. Shea S, Sengupta S, Crosswell A, Clayton PD. Network information security in a Phase III Integrated Academic Information Management System (IAIMS). In: Frisse ME (ed.). *Proceedings of the 16th Symposium for Computer Applications in Medical Care;* November 8–11, 1992. New York: McGraw-Hill; Health Sciences Division: 283–286.
7. Bleumer G. Security for decentralized health information systems. *Int J Biomed Comput.* 1994;35(Suppl 1):140–145.
8. Curran WJ, Stearns B, Kaplan H. Privacy, confidentiality and other legal considerations in the establishment of a centralized health-data system. *N Engl J Med.* 1968;281(5):241–248.
9. Brannigan V, Beier B. Standards for privacy in medical information systems: A technico-legal revolution. In: Miller RA (ed.). *Proceedings of the 14th Symposium for Computer Applications in Medical Care* (Nov. 4–7, 1990). Washington, DC: IEEE Computer Society Press. 1990;266–270.
10. Latham L. Network security, part 2: Policy should come first. Inside Gartner Group This Week; April 26, 1995.
11. Shneir B. *Applied Cryptography.* New York: John Wiley & Sons, 1994.

12. Information Security Subcommittee, Mayo Clinic/Foundation. Data Security Policies and Standards; September, 1994 (provided by Dr. Christopher D. Chute, Section of Medical Information Resources, Mayo Clinic/Foundation, Rochester, MN).

13. Clayton PD, Sideli RV, Sengupta S. Open architecture and integrated information at Columbia-Presbyterian Medical Center. *MD Comput.* 1992;9(5):297-303.

14. France FH, Gaunt PN. The need for security—a clinical view. *Int J Biomed Comput.* 1994; 35(Suppl 1):189-194.

15. US Government, Office of Technology Assessment. *Medical Privacy Report, 1993.* Chapter 1: Introduction, Summary and Options.

16. Robinson DM. Health information privacy: Without confidentiality. *Int J Biomed Comput.* 1994; 35(Suppl 1):97-104.

17. American Civil Liberties Union. *Toward a New Health Care System: The Civil Liberties Issues.* An ACLU Public Policy Report (a5BN 0-914031-24-4); February, 1994.

18. US Government, Office of Technology Assessment. *Medical Privacy Report,* 1993. Chapter 3: Computerized Health Care Information.

19. Personal communication at the NYS CHMIS Executive Policy Meeting, Albany, NY; April 2, 1995.

20. Position Statement of the American Health Information Management Association, Chicago, IL; March 1992: 1.

21. Murphy G. System and data protection. In: Ball MJ, Collen MF (eds.). *Aspects of the Computer-based Patient Record.* New York: Springer-Verlag; 1992:201-213.

22. Orr GA, Brantley BA. Development of a model of information security requirements for enterprise-wide medical information systems. In: Frisse ME (ed.). *Proceedings of the 16th Symposium for Computer Applications in Medical Care,* November 8-11, 1992. New York: McGraw-Hill, Health Sciences Division; 287-291.

23. Henkind SJ, Orlowski JM, Skarulis PC. Application of a multilevel access model in the development of a security infrastructure for a clinical information system. In: Safran C (ed.). *Proceedings of the 17th Symposium on Computer Applications in Medical Care,* October 30-November 3, 1993. New York: McGraw-Hill, Inc., Health Sciences Division; 64-68.

24. Dargahi R, Classen DW, Bobroff RB, et al. The development of a data security model for the collaborative social and medical services system. In: Ozbolt JG (ed.). *Proceedings of the 18th Symposium on Computer Applications in Medical Care;* November 5-9, 1994. Hanley & Belfus, Inc; 349-353.

25. Brannigan VM. A framework for "need to know" authorizations in medical computer systems: Responding to the constitutional requirements. In: Ozbolt JG (ed.). *Proceedings of the 18th Symposium on Computer Applications in Medical Care;* November 5-9, 1994. Hanley & Belfus, Inc; 392-396.

26. Kowalski S. An accountability server for health care information systems. *Int J Biomed Comput.* 1994;35(Suppl 1):130-138.

27. Lincoln TL. Privacy: A real-world problem with fuzzy boundaries. *Meth Inform Med.* 1993;32:104-107.

28. Barber B, Bakker A, Bengtsson S. Conclusions and recommendations. *Int J Biomed Comput.* 1994;35(Suppl 1):221-229.

29. New York State CHMIS Executive Policy Committee. *NYS CHMIS Confidentiality and Data Security Policy*. Draft; December 21, 1994.
30. Szolovits P, Kohane I. Against simple universal health-care identifiers. *J Am Med Informatics Assoc*. 1994;1(4):316–319.
31. Kumar S, Spafford EH. *An Application of Pattern Matching in Intrusion Detection*. Technical Report CSD-TR-94-013. COAST Project, Department of Computer Sciences, Purdue University, West Lafayette, In, June 17, 1994.
32. Picciotto J. The design of an effective auditing subsystem. *Proceedings of the 1987 IEEE Symposium on Security and Privacy*.
33. Marshall VH. *Intrusion Detection in Computers*. A summary of the Trusted Information Systems (TIS) Report on Intrusion Detection Systems (TIS Report #348). Booz, Allen & Hamilton Inc; January 29, 1991.
34. Frank J. Artificial intelligence and intrusion detection: Current and future directions. Division of Computer Science, UCD, Davis, CA: June 9, 1994.
35. Hayam A. Security audit center — a suggested model for effective audit strategies in health care informatics. *Int J Biomed Comput*. 1994;35(Suppl 1):116–127.
36. Lunt LT. A survey of intrusion detection techniques. *Comput Security*. 1993; 12(4):405–418.

17

Business, Industry, and CHINs

Neilson S. Buchanan, Alan Peres, and John Fleming

What is the value of a Community Health Information Network (CHIN) to an employer? The easy answer, of course, is that CHIN costs relative to benefits equal value. However, during the next 3–5 years, agreement on *true* costs and *real* benefits will be difficult. On the positive side, it is clear that citizens, employers, payors, and providers in a few communities across the United States (all early adopters) are evaluating the value of a CHIN in their community. In typical American fashion, these early CHINs are evolving in numerous shapes, sizes, and visions for the future. Each CHIN is providing rich experience to the stakeholders who experiment with CHIN concepts.

Eventually experimentation turns into proven business value and that value will be transferred to those other communities who appropriately sit on the sidelines and wait for definite answers about the value of CHINs. In the meantime, the most honest answer about the value of a CHIN to employers is simply that the "jury is still out," but as the juries return, there are likely to be generally positive answers varying widely in clarity and intensity.

Clearly, employees and, therefore, employers can benefit from improved information systems supporting clinicians. However, there is a gap between this perception and the actions taken by stakeholders who can cause such systems to evolve. The objective of this chapter is to establish a framework for anticipating the needs of employers and the ability of CHINs to meet those needs. Figure 17.1 depicts a model that shows CHINs providing a relatively small amount of perceived value to employers in 1995 but a great deal more over the next 10 years. The issue is not what level of value fledgling CHINs are providing in 1995; the real issues are to what degree the perceived value of CHINs will increase in the minds of employers and whether CHINs will move from a relatively unknown concept today to a highly valued management tool of tomorrow.

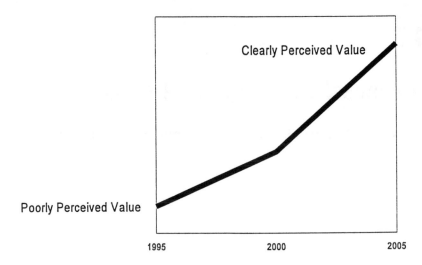

FIGURE 17.1. Perceived value model.

What Do Employers Really Want, Information Technology or Perfect Knowledge?

Information technologies (ITs) can assist a buyer to monitor a supplier's adherence to the buyer's specifications. In the case of health care services, employers (buyers) adopt a variety of specifications expressed in the form of clinical processes and outcomes such as length of stay, immunization rate, or absence of complications. Early in the next century, ITs will become a critical factor in the success of any healthcare provider seeking a preferred supplier status with an employer or health plan. Collecting data and reporting performance to specifications is virtually impossible without ITs. Employers understand the value of ITs and will evaluate suppliers of healthcare services on the basis of their IT utilization. This does not, however, mean that employers desire to understand the details of the data or know how providers and health plans actually collect/use the data. More importantly, it has become obvious to managed care physician executives that IT can directly support frontline clinicians who are caring for patients on an everyday basis. Thus, use of ITs simply for data capture and reporting is an inadequate goal for a health care provider, health plan, or employer.

The employer's concept of a CHIN may eventually coincide with the thinking of managed care executives. Simply stated, an employer wants a health service supplier with the greatest expertise to provide acceptable quality/service at the lowest cost. It can be argued that ideal service (perfect quality, perfect costs, perfect consumer satisfaction) can be delivered if the supplier has perfect knowledge and know-how. Mark Wheeler, MD, recently described "perfect knowledge" for the clinician (the most critical production worker) as the confluence of the following four areas of knowledge:

1. Medical and procedural facts (textbooks, articles, PDR, etc.);
2. Access to other clinicians;
3. Complete, accurate patient information; and
4. Experience and skills stored in a clinician's head.

The concept of perfect knowledge is naive, if not dangerous; for the purposes of this chapter, we will assume that perfect knowledge means "almost perfect knowledge," to allow for the fact that clinicians must strive to be perfect, but invariably fall short to some degree.

It stands to reason that employers would want to place their business with health plans whose clinicians and executives have "perfect knowledge." CHINs contribute significantly to the four areas of knowledge cited by Wheeler; however, CHINs are merely supporting mechanisms to clinicians with perfect knowledge. Furthermore, clinicians with perfect knowledge are merely supporting mechanisms for the clinical outcomes desired by employers on behalf of their employees.

Complicating Circumstances

A definitive answer about the value of a CHIN to employers is difficult because both employers and CHINs are complex, vague entities. Consider the following complexities that CHINs encounter:

- employers of various sizes, expectations, and so forth;
- impact of managed incentives;
- rapidly changing technology;
- consolidation among traditionally disparate healthcare providers;
- inherent business risks in a restructuring marketplace;
- individual and family emotional attachments to health care services; and
- legal issues, such as confidentiality.

The term "employer" is very broad. In this chapter, we use the term *employer* to mean the broad spectrum of employers (big or small, local or national, providing health benefits or not). The term *leadership employers* describes those employers, generally large employers but occasionally smaller employers, who provide leadership and resources to CHINs. Employers who express themselves through a coalition or trade association can also be considered leadership employers. This differentiation among employers is important when generalizations are made about employer attitudes and behavior.

There is (and will be) little agreement among employers about what a CHIN is or could be. Leadership employers hold quite varied opinions about what a CHIN is and who should finance and control it. Further, the vast majority of employers have not given CHINs any serious consideration, and many employers do not have executives with the skills and time to devote to developing of a major new business such as a CHIN.

From the individual employer's perspective, the value of a CHIN is unclear. Some of the potential value may not accrue directly to the employer, but to employees, their families, and the general community, in such a manner that an employer perceives an indirect benefit difficult to evaluate.

The issue of fairness and parity arises with employers who devote early capital and sweat equity to the development of a CHIN. If the CHIN successfully evolves in a community, it is possible (in the absence of compulsory participation) for many employers to receive benefits without contributing of capital and operating expenses. This tends to discourage potential leadership employers who might otherwise be willing to support the CHIN with start-up capital and operating revenues. If long-term CHIN benefits are transferred broadly to leadership employers' competitors, these initial investments are difficult to justify.

Technology seems bewildering as ever-improving equipment hits the market and competing information superhighways emerge to serve various sectors of the economy. Ironically, however, technological architecture and capabilities, although complex and ever-changing, are simple in comparison to economic, organizational, and legal issues. Divergence of opinion about organizational issues such as policy setting/ownership/capitalization tends to paralyze decision-making in those CHINs who depend upon a wide variety of stakeholders in the community.

Economic issues are becoming more intense. Managed care is reducing the quantity of health care services and lowering prices; in today's environment of consolidating health care providers and health plans, business plans for CHINs are risky. Competition among providers and health plans tends to reduce collaboration; however, the bigger issue for the community is that competition may reduce the benefits envisioned for a community-driven CHIN.

Employee relations and community politics also complicate employers' support of CHINs. Confidentiality and other ethical and legal issues add to the complexity. It is unclear that the American public has confidence in large private or public databases containing sensitive personal information.

CHINs, providers, health plans, technology vendors, and employers have to deal with differences in incentives and expectations. Ideally, all stakeholders may advocate a robust database with real-time price and quality information; however, it is hard to imagine how five competing clinical laboratories will have unbridled enthusiasm for a CHIN when their services and prices will be presented on a CHIN-enabled "spot market" to health plans and physicians who select lab services on the basis of quality and the lowest acceptable price.

In summary, the complexities of a CHIN are recognized by all early developers, but it is important for these pioneers not to become paralyzed by the acknowledged obstacles and unanswered questions. A more constructive form of analysis is needed to anticipate the needs and actions of employers.

Early-Stage, Complex Systems Development

The lack of current literature about employers and CHINs suggests that CHINs have entered a period known as early-stage, complex systems development (ECSD). ECSD has the following seven characteristics:

1. There is reasonable agreement among diverse leaders that "something new" is needed. In other words, the current business paradigm is not working satisfactorily and needs improvement. In the case of CHINs, leaders of health care organizations, employers, the general community, and technology companies seem to be reaching agreement that "something new" is needed.
2. There is little acceptance at the basic organizational level that the business paradigm needs improvement. Thus, there is a divergence of opinions between stakeholders at the "top" and "bottom."
3. There is at least one driving force or facilitating mechanism that unifies leaders and creates a "can do" spirit among the diverse stakeholders. In the case of a CHIN, the "information super-highway" *technology and hype* may be that driving force. Adoption of Health Plan Employer Data and Information Set (HEDIS) cost, quality, and satisfaction standards by regional employer coalitions may be another facilitating mechanism.
4. There is no obvious, preexisting champion. Risks, benefits, and need for change exist across a wide constituency.
5. It is possible for any stakeholder to obscure and/or exercise "near-veto" power on major policy issues.
6. Leaders in the early stages of change usually are preoccupied with "organizational form and control" rather than "value-added functions."
7. There are significant social, economic, organizational, and legal barriers to the rapid development and deployment of solutions. These barriers tend to be greater than technological barriers; in fact, reasonably viable technological solutions are fairly obvious to the leaders of ECSD.

Importance of Process in the ECSD Paradigm

CHINs may not be definitive organizations in 1996; CHINs may be imperfect amalgams of disparate information systems and fragmented decision-makers. CHINs today may be simply a response to new demands, including but not limited to the following:

- gaps between costs of healthcare services and value perceived by employers;
- new consumer (enrollees and patients) demands;
- increasing willingness of clinicians to challenge the status quo, especially fee-for-service principles;
- changing employer expectations;
- a vacuum of government policy; and
- movement from "illness" health care delivery to population-based health care delivery.

Many health care experts today concede that the fee-for-service, cottage industry of stand-alone hospitals and independent physicians is changing to some new form of health care. This change is simplistically labeled "managed care," "integrated delivery systems," "population-based health care," and so forth. CHINs today may not be organizations or even a set of specific functions but the initial expression of demand for new processes in the financing and delivery of managed care.

Perhaps a CHIN is not a noun; perhaps it is a verb. Creating Health Information NOW (CHIN) might be the definition of a CHIN in the long run. Many leading businesses today maintain that they are market-driven, information-dependent, and must regularly reinvent themselves. If health care enterprises, providers, and health plans are to follow in these footsteps, then CHINs, defined as a "verb," may have a real future.

Because the conditions of ECSD seem to be applicable both to CHINs and health care in general, it is counterproductive to prescribe a single answer to the question of value. This chapter provides a *flexible framework* for defining what CHINs could be and how employers will perceive value. There is no simple definition of a CHIN; and there is no simple definition of an employer. Therefore, the question of the value of CHIN to an employer requires multiple answers.

Overall Lack of Urgency

At this early developmental stage there is ample evidence that CHINs are being defined by a wide variety of employer actions (and nonactions). A literature search and telephone calls to CHIN experts have confirmed that leadership employers and employers in general have been relatively inactive in overall CHIN development in the United States. However, some exceptions exist — for example, in regions such as Memphis, Wisconsin, and western Michigan.

Health Care as an Outsourced Service

The practice of outsourcing has become much more sophisticated during the past 10 years, particularly in the manufacturing sector and more recently in the service industry. Outsourcing allows a business to concentrate on its core competencies by shedding noncore functions and deliberately avoiding any new function which does not qualify as a current or future core competency. There are 10 basic principles of outsourcing:

- strong buyer/supplier agreement on product/service specifications;
- buyer emphasis on a supplier's outcomes rather than processes;
- supplier's ability to more effectively produce the product/service (i.e., the supplier has superior *knowledge, know-how)*;
- buyer's desire for long-term accountability from a few prequalified suppliers;
- periodic informal renegotiation or formal rebidding of price;
- mutual, open commitment to continuous improvement and quality;
- active, arms-length, yet collaborative planning and problem-solving;
- buyer receptivity to suppliers' suggestions for product/service design and redesign;
- electronic exchange of information between buyer and supplier; and
- rapid, "fast-cycle" buyer/supplier response to market forces.

Very few employers in the United States have found that direct provision of health services is compatible with their core business. Because health care services (i.e., services delivered via various health plans) are likely to remain outsourced services, the emergence of CHINs raises a question about the extent to which leadership employers will significantly involve themselves in the capture, transmission, storage, and manipulation of health care data. It is highly unlikely that employers, as defined earlier in this chapter, will ever involve themselves with CHIN issues.

If direct health care services for employees, retirees, and their families remain an *outsourced* service, then employers are likely to prefer that health information network(s) and health plans evolve as an outsourced service. If this trend prevails, then CHINs will evolve primarily at the alpha end of the continuum of employer expectations described below.

It may also be argued, of course, that CHINs will evolve at the other end of the continuum. Some business and health policy leaders think that employers should become more active participants in the creation and operation of CHINs. For example, employers in western Michigan have examined their needs and taken an activist role in the formation of a CHIN. Their health plans (generally self-insured, Third Party Administrator [TPA] arrangements) by default or by design have not assumed roles as data integrators. Initially these employers established basic CHIN specifications on their own and later they began to collaborate with local hospitals and physicians. A vendor has been selected as a strategic partner in the ownership and control of the local CHIN, which transcends the TPAs. The approach is based on the argument that outsourcing is impractical and inappropriate. And indeed, the following points are persuasive.

- There are few reliable standards (specifications) for health care services. Buyers should have a role in creating and articulating these specifications.
- Human resource professionals generally have little understanding of health care outcomes or processes; therefore, collaboration with providers can be productive.
- The degree of provider integration is generally low throughout the United States, and it is difficult to hold large numbers of fragmented health care providers accountable.
- Employers are reluctant to selectively contract with preferred providers.
- It is difficult to change health care providers and health plans. Employers cannot make quick changes in health plans without incurring employee dissatisfaction; consequently, strong control mechanisms are more effective than switching suppliers.
- Individual health care providers effectively obscure price/quality.
- Most health care providers, especially individual physicians, who are the most critical suppliers, are not committed to mutual, open quality assurance.
- Hospitals do not have access to meaningful cost and quality information, particularly in the outpatient-driven managed care paradigm.
- Health plans are not oriented to the capture and use of information to support clinicians' decision-making.
- There are legal and social barriers to the rapid exchange of information.
- Demand for health care services is largely driven by enrollees (employee and family members), not employers.
- Suppliers, not buyers, have a clear-cut lead in the design and redesign of specifications for health care services.
- True market forces have been historically slow and are perhaps non-existent.

The proponents of Omega-CHINs argue that only the following two outsourcing principles apply to health care services:

- supplier's ability to produce the service more effectively than buyers; and
- buyer's desire for long-term relationships with suppliers.

Dichotomy Between Principles and Practice

Many businesses have successfully outsourced vital services outside their core competencies; for example, security, janitorial services, employee cafeteria, and so forth. The principles of outsourcing, practiced most visibly in modern manufacturing, are often applied to vendors of these support services and even to certain types of manufacturing. However, very few employers have applied the principles of outsourcing to health care providers or health plans. It may be useful to examine the reasons for this.

It has been accepted practice in the business community to *not* directly challenge the delivery of health care. Executives usually can find larger and less controversial internal costs to manage. Human resource executives are usually not challenged or rewarded by top management for initiating change and managing health care costs in the same manner as product, engineering, or manufacturing managers manage costs. Health care services are not directly "bought" because consumption occurs between providers and employees/family members. Finally, it is very difficult to establish price, service level, and quality specifications for health care services when services are obtained through a complex distribution network controlled by health providers and health plans. Thus it is easy to see why employers find it more difficult to focus on health care costs than on other costs. (For a more in-depth review of this situation, see Paul Starr's *Social Transformation of American Medicine*.)

Emergence of Outsourcing Principles in Health Care

Health care may never fit into the purist outsourcing paradigm perfected by manufacturers, but it is obvious that leadership employers have begun to apply outsourcing principles to health care. For example, acceptable standards (HEDIS) are capturing the attention of large employers and employer coalitions. Organizations such as the National Committee for Quality Assurance, the National Business Coalition Forum on Health, CalPERS, the Pacific Business Group on Health, and other leading employer coalitions may be examples of the ESCD facilitating mechanisms noted earlier. All of these organizations are transferring knowledge to health benefit managers and CFOs to use in managing employee health benefit programs.

It is reasonable to expect that for the foreseeable future, a relatively small number of savvy human resource executives will increasingly demand, on behalf of their employees, maximum value from health care suppliers (health plans and/or providers from whom they receive "outsourced" services). The bottom line for outsourcing is that employers will seek (1) the lowest level of involvement with the details of healthcare production; (2) the greatest amount of expertise to be held by a few, preferred, prequalified health care providers and/or managed care organizations; and (3) effective financial incentives, clinical outcome standards, and new informal methods of accountability (e.g., HEDIS; contract specifications; close, face-to-face trusting relationships) to assure that price and quality are actively managed. Because most employers within the United States are constantly reexamining their core competencies and making outsourcing decisions, it is reasonable to expect that in time most employers will apply outsourcing principles to suppliers of health care services. This prediction is based on the assumption that there will be minimal state or federal regulatory pressure to compel employers and health care providers to participate in a "mandated" CHIN of some type.

A Continuum of Employer Expectations

By placing demonstrated employer actions (as opposed to verbal promises and public statements) onto a continuum (from Alpha to Omega), it is possible to provide a framework for analysis of CHINs, however defined, in any community of the United States. This continuum is not designed to dictate "either/or" choices; it simply illustrates the many opportunities that a CHIN may have in a given community. Because employers, individually and collectively, are only part of the decision-making process, there will be a wide variety of CHINs, at least in the early stages, before some models prove themselves to be more functional than others:

The CHIN Continuum

<Alpha CHINs   Omega CHINs>

Alpha CHINs—The Health Care Enterprise Model

(CHIN is a verb!)

Alpha CHINs—The Health Care Enterprise Model

The alpha end of the continuum assumes that a CHIN is the composite of the health information systems inherent in the production of health care. Clinical information systems supporting clinical workers are rapidly evolving as a result of competition, health care enterprises reaching critical economic mass, and sheer passage of time. Thus if the current changes in U.S. health care result in a few large, fully integrated, accountable health care enterprises such as Kaiser in California or Henry Ford Health System in Michigan, these health care enterprises may be compelled through competitive and regulatory pressures to develop strong internal information systems that support their most important workers.

Information systems are not in widespread use in health enterprises today, but it is reasonable to expect that the majority of large health care enterprises early in the 21st century will depend heavily on internal information technology (IT) for optimal delivery of cost and quality. These health care enterprises will probably be highly integrated with hospital and physician services; many will also be integrated with managed care financing services such as HMOs and PPOs. The marketplace, especially employers and employees, will hold these enterprises increasingly accountable for quality, cost, and enrollee/patient satisfaction. More importantly, the leading health care enterprises will distinguish themselves from competitors by population-based health care and improved clinical outcomes achieved by clinicians with proper real-time IT support.

It is reasonable to assume that these relatively large, accountable health care enterprises will maintain a basic proprietary interest in their own information systems, driven by self-interest, priorities, capital, internal development skills, and strategic alliances with key vendors. Although IT usually does not produce a sustaining competitive advantage, there is significant, short-term competitive advantage to controlling IT system development within the health care enterprise. Long-term advantage depends on the enterprise's ability to access IT services and innovations at lower costs than competitors.

Basically, the Alpha CHIN is the intrinsic information system of a large, highly integrated health care enterprise within a given geographic region. The Alpha CHIN model also assumes that the obstacles to joint development of IT systems by competing health care systems are great, but development costs can be carried internally by each health care enterprise or through strategic relationships with prime technical and service vendors. Thus, in the future the information systems within large health care enterprises could essentially be more than 90 percent of an Alpha-CHIN.

This discussion has not addressed the very real entrepreneurial and public health pressures for certain data to be shared among competing enterprises. In fact, several large health care enterprises in the United States are already merging selected quality and cost data for epidemiological and outcome studies that require very large numbers of patients, encounters, and so forth. As a practical matter, of course, no health care enterprise can have sole access to the universe of vital data. Parallel systems will occur at various levels. For example, pharmacy/laboratory benefit management (PLBM) companies may create clinical and commercial value from their clinical pharmaceutical, clinical laboratory, and financial databases. Various levels of abstracted PLBM data could eventually be transferred to health care enterprises and/or to a higher level "Super-CHIN," which takes responsibility for assembling the complete universe of data needed in the region.

With its ability to compile reliable databases and support large, retrospective studies, this "Super-CHIN," sometimes referred to as a "Double-CHIN," has value for employers, employees, patients, and health care enterprises. The greatest value, however, accrues to the health care enterprise that uses outcome studies, and so forth, to improve delivery of patient care. Data can also help a health care enterprise to differentiate itself from competitors. Employers will clearly benefit as health care enterprises engage in constructive, meaningful competition based on valid clinical quality and cost performance indicators. Further, employers will have more confidence in the validity of marketing claims when the data are subject to the validation and audit capabilities of the Super-CHIN.

The Super-CHIN's success will depend on health care enterprises to make outcome information available to clinicians on a real-time basis as they practice medicine, nursing, and so forth. This feedback loop is often omitted from CHIN design; but without meaningful feedback to clinicians, much of the value to employers is lost.

The following are common assumptions about employer financing for a Super-CHIN.

- A few employers will donate sweat equity, initial capital, and operating expenses with no expectations of cash return on investment.
- A few employers will invest capital with expectations of true return on investment.
- The founding/sustaining organizations (including a few leadership employers in conjunction with providers, payors, etc.) will provide capital and operating costs through a permanent "dues" structure.
- The Super-CHIN will charge a basic tariff (e.g., a charge to each health care enterprise, provider, etc. based on volume and quality of data submitted).
- There will be a charge to health care providers, health plans, clinical researchers, the public, therapeutic companies, policy makers, and others for accessing the database and its analytical capabilities. Most long-term operating revenue will be generated from charges to health plans and providers, who will pass on the costs to employers in their normal charge structures. If the Super-CHIN is cost-effective, then the net cost incurred by employers should drop as the CHIN helps health plans and providers lower their costs and improve quality.
- There will be a reliable government subsidy of some type.
- Because the alpha-CHIN is an inherent operating cost of a health care enterprise, all employers indirectly finance a portion of the Alpha-CHIN. Employer-driven competition among health care enterprises for quality, price, and satisfaction (e.g., CalPERS in California) implies that employers accept alpha-CHINs as a valued service whose cost is passed on through the premiums charged for health care services.

In summary, nearly all (more than 90 percent) of the "ALPHA" model is composed of the clinical and administrative information systems used by health care enterprises during the normal course of operations. It is reasonable to assume that there is a great need for information beyond the health care enterprise itself and that the remaining 10 percent of the Alpha-CHIN will involve information collection, processing, and analysis at a level *other* than the health care enterprise itself.

Omega CHINs — The Community Utility Model

This model assumes that health care delivery in the United States will continue to be fragmented and that no health care enterprise can capture a reasonably complete database in the course of its operations. The Omega-CHIN presupposes that a wide variety of small, fragmented, decentralized health care providers (voluntarily or through regulation) will submit transaction-based and abstracted clinical data to a regional CHIN, which will turn the data into useful information.

The Omega-CHIN provides a clear, tangible focal point for the definition, collection, and analysis of health care data. In contrast to Alpha-CHINs, in which employers place primary data responsibility on health care enterprises, Omega-CHIN creates the expectation that providers, health plans, and others will submit prescribed data to a central clearinghouse. The Omega-CHIN is inherently larger than the Super-CHIN described above and employers will be more involved in the active use of data than with the Alpha-CHIN. Employers endorsing the Alpha-CHIN will place primary reliance on those health care enterprises that are accountable for the collection and internal use of data. The Super-CHIN is an organization that tends to operate on an "exception" basis; that is, it does only those functions that cannot be accomplished by enterprise information systems. In contrast, the Omega-CHIN is responsible for all elements of the information network.

To recover its costs, Omega-CHINs must create significant economic value from the basic transmission of health care transactions and from the database created. Proponents generally make one or more of the following assumptions in their business plans:

- A few employers will donate sweat equity, initial capital, and operating expenses with no expectation of cash return on investment.
- A few employers will invest capital with expectations of true return on investment.
- The founding/sustaining organizations (including a few leadership employers in conjunction with providers, payors, etc.) will provide capital and operating costs through a permanent "dues" structure.
- The CHIN will charge a basic tariff to large numbers of providers for individual transactions (e.g., charges for eligibility checks, bills submitted to health plans, various types of financial and clinical inquiries, creation of an electronic medical record, etc.)
- Various forms of managed care, especially capitated health care enterprises, will require special incentives to submit data because they may not need the financial transactions (such as billings) inherent in the fee-for-service system.
- There will be a charge to health care providers, health plans, clinical researchers, policy makers, and others for accessing the database.
- There will be a government subsidy of some type.

Employers and Operational Issues

The following issues are frequently cited as the most difficult issues in the creation and operation of any CHIN: capital costs; operating costs; governance and control; IT technical issues, such as connectivity, scalability, input methodologies, storage, and access speed; confidentiality; access rights to data; research skills and methods; data ownership; adherence to technical and linguistic standards; equity among like stakeholders with varied levels of interest; individual and community acceptance of large personal databases; provider willingness to reveal competitive advantages; and appropriate application of emerging technologies.

This list offers one way to determine the value that employers perceive from "their" CHIN. The more the value employers perceive from their CHIN, the more employers will be involved with the difficult operational issues cited above.

Employer action (investment of time, money, and leadership) is an objective measure of employer perception of the value of a CHIN. To the knowledge of the authors, there is no comprehensive survey process to establish baseline data on employer activities in the formation of CHINs. Periodic surveys of employer activities in CHINs could create an objective baseline for the value of CHINs to employers in the United States.

Employers and Policy Issues

Leadership employer involvement in CHIN policy matters can be expected to indicate when and where employers anticipate deriving value from a CHIN. The issues listed below are frequently cited as the most difficult policy issues in the creation and operation of any CHIN:

- Population-based health care versus illness-oriented health care.
- Accountability standards for outcomes and services. Health care enterprises and larger health care providers can be held openly and increasingly accountable (via HEDIS and various accrediting organizations) for clinical processes/outcomes and selected treatment patterns for defined populations (e.g., well babies, diabetics, mammography for women aged 45–54, immunization rates, etc.).
- Real-time clinical information systems: most data required for practice improvement should be gathered as a byproduct of routine care rather than through retrospective analysis of healthcare financial transactions.
- "CHIN function" before "CHIN form;" that is, clinical, administrative, and technical leaders within the CHIN movement must subordinate their fascination with governance/control/technology and concentrate on how clinicians can achieve clinical practice improvements.

Evaluation Models

It would be easy to conclude that there is no quick, easy way for an employer to appraise the potential value of a CHIN; however, there are several "back-of-the-envelope" options. The following models are informally used today by leadership employers:

Evaluation Model 1

What, How, Who, When Analysis

The question, WHAT is a CHIN? becomes more complex when it is combined with the decision-making process (HOW will employers evaluate a CHIN?). In our pluralistic, capitalistic economy, it is clear that in the first generation of CHINs, value will largely be "in the eye of the beholder."

An employer's search for definitive value becomes exponentially more complex when it is necessary to include all the formal and informal decision-makers (i.e., WHO will make value decisions?). It will be easy to identify a small number of employer leaders within the business community who want to influence the strategies and tactics of a regional CHIN, but there are thousands of employers in the United States and many decision-makers within the employer community. By design and by default, small business owners, human relations vice presidents, compensation/benefit managers, and union officials will be defining what a CHIN is by influencing employer decisions such as requirement of a health plan to submit claims; requirement of a provider to submit claims; requirement of a provider to report various processes/outcomes; requirement of a health plan to report various process/outcomes; and requirement of both a health plan and provider to engage in certain internal quality assurance/utilization review (QA/UR) processes.

Given the complexity of health care and the elusiveness of clear-cut cost/benefit figures, it is likely that a definitive endpoint (i.e., WHEN will the value of a CHIN be established clearly?) will not occur in the short remainder of this century.

First Consulting Group presents its concept of the value of benefits/ services in Table 17.1. An employer is not limited to the categorization of benefits/services suggested by First Consulting. The major question is whether or not a CHIN's cost effectiveness is transferred to the employer. For example, a vendor of medical supplies can lower its ordering and billing costs by using the CHIN electronic data transmission; however, those savings are not necessarily transferred to an employer. In contrast, an employer will directly benefit if communicable disease reportings reduce the incidence of employee exposure to tuberculosis.

Evaluation Option 2

Gross Economic Modeling

If the cost of employer-provided health benefits is $4000 per employee, and a CHIN has 100 percent probability of creating 15 percent net savings

TABLE 17.1. Value of CHINs to participants.

Participants	Immediate benefits/services	Future benefits/services
Employers and purchasers	+Cost reductions +Electronics enrollment +Demographic updates	+Comparative outcomes +Cost/benefit studies +Expense modeling
Patients	+Administrative simplification +Improved quality and service	+Health education +Effectiveness reports +Home care improvements
Public health interests	+Communicable disease reports +School immunization verification +Electronic indigent referrals	+Data collection and analysis
Medical supply and ancillary service vendors	+Increased electronic transmission +Lower cost of distribution	+Market analysis tools +Service applications

through reduced costs and improved quality, then value can be estimated at $600 per employee per year. This line of reasoning assumes that the continued presence of the CHIN is necessary to maintain this level of savings from year to year. If an employer has 1000 employees, then the CHIN represents a $600,000 increase in pretax income.

This provides a benchmark for an employer to evaluate the opportunity costs of the CHIN relative to other investment opportunities available to the business. The employer who feels that there is inherent value in a CHIN can make an investment and evaluate the return on the investment at any reasonable time in the future.

Option 3

Considerations of Community Well-Being

An employer may also be motivated by the potential of the CHIN to improve the well-being of employees and the general community. This line of reasoning assumes that an employer concludes there is inherent value in a robust information system directed to the well-being of the community. The employer then subjectively concludes that use of IT, creation of a database, and study of issues will produce direct and indirect benefits.

Evaluation Option 4

Epidemiological Considerations

An employer may be motivated by a desire to cure or reduce certain diseases or promote certain conditions of wellness. A CHIN could, for example, support complex cancer studies by evaluating various treatment processes and clinical outcomes. Long-term environmental causation studies could be much more feasible with a CHIN's database.

Summary

This chapter has not attempted to suggest that there is a single, definitive answer to the question about the value an employer will derive from a CHIN. Forecasts about CHINs beyond a 5-year period are prone to error; consequently, it would be misleading to conclude with long-range predictions. Short-range predictions are much more appropriate. The opinions of the authors about the probable actions that can be expected from employers are outlined below:

- A few self-directed leadership employers will continue to provide resources (leadership, direct and in-kind start-up costs) to the development of their regional CHINs.
- Leadership employers will increasingly require provider and/or health plan participation in a CHIN, especially when the CHIN clearly creates information that is understandable and valuable to the average employer (i.e., cost and quality accountability, such as HEDIS standards).
- Most leadership employers will continue their current wait-and-see policy toward CHINs.
- Employers will not support any binding regulation that requires all employers in a region to participate financially in a CHIN's operational costs.
- Employer trade associations will not adopt significantly supportive policies on CHINs. Employers who have a business stake in CHIN technologies may be an exception.
- Most employers will not be involved in or even aware of CHINs.

CHIN executive staff, health plans, and providers must assume the burden of convincing employers that CHINs have value.

Potential for Improvement

The significance of CHINs lies in their future, not in their present activities. The healthcare industry today is very much like the U.S. automobile industry a few years ago, during the period of initial foreign competition. Production costs of the old models (fee-for-service) are still high. Traditional services are experiencing price and service competition from brash new competitors with significantly improved models of service delivery and financing. Health care consumers, while occasionally cautious and contradictory, are steadily accepting and buying the new models of healthcare, especially managed care. Yet the medical establishment hangs on to the unfettered fee-for-service model with hopes that managed care is a fad, not a long-term trend.

In retrospect, it is clear that the U.S. automobile industry encountered competition, and competition made U.S. automobile executives and workers jointly accountable for their products. Consumers evaluated automobiles, developed preferences, and met their needs in a traditional capitalistic fashion. Change within the U.S. automobile industry required years; however, informed buyers and sellers eventually met each other in the marketplace.

Health care is a not a simple, understandable product like a self-financed automobile; healthcare is a complex, occasionally emotional service generally financed by a third party. Services are purchased indirectly at the time of selection of a health plan and directly at the time of consumption. Questions about the cost and value of health care services have steadily increased during the past 40 years, and now unanswered questions have reached a point where health care processes and outcomes must be made more understandable to the general public and the employers/government agencies who finance health care.

The gap between the costs and the perceived value of U.S. health represents an opportunity that CHINs must seize. The average citizen and the average employer, acting as individual buyers, simply cannot gather enough information to evaluate health plans, providers, and so forth. CHINs will vary in their organization and capabilities; nevertheless, all CHINs will consistently deliver information to the community that improves quality, lowers costs, and increases satisfaction with health care services. For example, if a CHIN sets an objective to improve breast cancer treatment, then it will pursue that objective until improvements can be demonstrated. A CHIN could collaboratively conduct the complex studies that evaluate treatment processes and outcomes, and the CHIN could eventually "specify" optimal treatment patterns and/or outcomes to providers. At the same time, a CHIN might be expected to adopt accountability standards for breast cancer outcomes and publicize the performance of health plans and providers in meeting those standards.

CHINs can find ways to present the true costs of individual health services as well as the packaged costs per course of illness, per outcome, or per member per month. Then employers and employees will be better able to understand the cost of health care. Finally, a CHIN can improve the information on basic consumer satisfaction with health services. For example, health plans may present their own surveys of customer satisfaction; however, that information probably does not permit a potential enrollee to evaluate satisfaction with competing health plans in a given region. A CHIN has the opportunity to directly or indirectly make that vital information available in the marketplace.

Community Benefit and the Common Good

Inevitably, the success of a CHIN is dependent on the vision, strength, and breadth of its leaders. Employers have a responsibility to join the community leadership network that designs the CHIN role and functions. The interests of employers go beyond optimal quality, cost, and satisfaction for employees, retirees, and their families. The common good and well-being of the whole community are also at stake. For example, the emergence of tuberculosis in the inner city may not be an immediate problem for a suburban employer. Yet with the aid of the CHIN, that employer can identify the community's problem and participate in finding a solution for the problem. It is unlikely that any one employer's health plan will be large enough to contribute to meaningful outcome and epidemiological studies. And thus, in the absence of a CHIN, it is unlikely that meaningful studies of health care will be conducted efficiently in the region. Ideally the employer can recognize the greater community good and contribute its database to the CHIN as an integral part of a community problem-solving process. CHINs that have a strong vision for improving the community's well-being may represent the most important improvement in public health that has occurred during the past 25 years.

Index